How Does *STOP THE INSANITY!* Work?

By explaining:

- Why 98 percent of all diets fail
- Why counting calories doesn't work
- Why you'll never get fit if it's left up to the fitness industry
- How you're set up to fail
- How trusted brands are lying to you

By showing:

- How to eat *more* and weigh *less*
- How easy it is to make the choices to change the way you look and feel forever.
- How to exercise at any weight, age, and fitness level
- How to lose body fat and increase your strength and cardio-endurance
- How to eat, how to breathe, and how to move
- How to stop treating the symptoms and solve the problem permanently

---

"*STOP THE INSANITY* is true Powter power. . . . The message is short. Food is fuel. Fat makes you fat. Eat more food, less fat. And move."

—Diane Eicher, *Denver Post*

"In *STOP THE INSANITY*, Powter not only tells readers how to embrace the healthy, well-conditioned fat-burning lifestyle, she also tells about her own journey."

—Deborah Beroset Diamond, *Cleveland Plain Dealer*

Stop the Insanity!

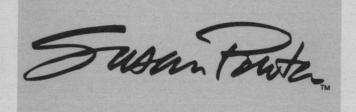

POCKET BOOKS

New York London Toronto Sydney Tokyo Singapore

Page 282 photo by Balfour Walker. Used by permission of the Susan Powter Corporation.
Page 328 photo by Scott Esteran.
Photos on pages 218–229 by Ted Munger.

Appendix material from *The T-Factor Fat Gram Counter,* revised and expanded, by Jamie Pope-Cordle, M.S., R.D., and Martin Katahn, Ph.D., by permission of W.W. Norton & Co., Inc. Copyright © 1991, 1989, by Katahn Associates, Inc.

POCKET BOOKS, a division of Simon & Schuster Inc.
1230 Avenue of the Americas, New York, NY 10020

ISBN: 0-671-52292-2

First Pocket Books printing February 1995

10 9 8 7 6 5 4 3 2 1

POCKET and colophon are registered trademarks of
Simon & Schuster Inc.

Cover photos © Sigrid Estrada

Printed in the U.S.A.

ACKNOWLEDGMENTS

I must start by acknowledging Rusty Robertson. If you ever want to "cut" the best deal of your life and have it done with honesty, integrity, and passion, don't do it without her. She is the best. She is half of me, and I couldn't have done a damn thing without her.

Sally Wilkins has organized everything I needed from the moment I met her. Without Sally I'd be in a padded room, spinning around in a circle, babbling about all there is to do. Thanks for keeping me sane, enlightened, and honest. Sally, I love you very much.

Ethel LaBranch has straightened me up and made me as pretty and fluffy as anyone could make me. When you see me all clean and pressed on tele, thank Ethel. The cards, gifts, and acknowledgments that get there on time with a nice note attached—I'm ashamed to admit it's not me, it's Ethel. When I write the checks from an account that I closed three months before, it's Ethel who saves me every time. When I am sixty-three years old, I want to be as beautiful, sexy, and cool as Ethel.

The staff at the studio: You guys work like hell to maintain the standards of this program. You've done such a great job. This studio is my blood, and when I'm out of town and I know our clients are being taken care of by you guys, I am at peace. That is very, very important to me. Thank you.

To the staff of RPR: You guys plugged me in, faxed me, and FedExed me every time I needed it. Thanks so much.

To Jan Miller, my literary agent, who went right along with the conversation about hats and going to the bathroom as if it were perfectly normal that day.

ACKNOWLEDGMENTS

Last, but certainly not least, Bob Asahina. Rusty and I walked into this man's office, blew him out of the water, talked about hats and going to the bathroom, and he got it. Instantly, he got it. That's my kind of man. Bob, Bob, he's my man, if he can't do it . . . nobody can, not edit like this man, not many people are that good at anything.

THIS BOOK IS DEDICATED TO . . .

The woman in New Jersey who is "like a mother." I know she's proud of me.

The raging redhead who believes and loves and never, never takes no for an answer.

The romantic soul of a friend who buys the case when she loves it.

The wonderfully funny woman who talked her way out of a ticket because she understood and believed so strongly.

The magical lady who collects praying mantises.

The drummer man who saw a person with very sad eyes and believed there was something underneath.

The man who suggested I read the Yellow Pages, and the woman who loves him.

The lady in Pelham who prophesied, "If you could ever get paid for talking, you'd make a nice living."

All the people who told me I'd never make it—dispositionally, that's just what I needed.

The lady who sees more clearly than most of us and is learning how to express it—what a joy she is.

The reason I live, Damien and Kiel.

People don't behave if they have nothing to lose.

I have so much to lose now in my life that finally I'll behave.

All of you have believed in me and loved me unconditionally.

Most people don't get this much love in a lifetime.

I am so very grateful. I love and thank you all.

CONTENTS

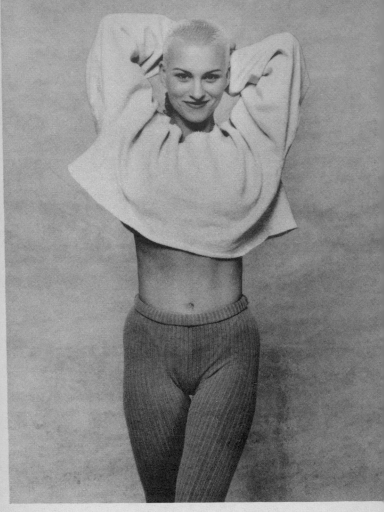

BONNIE SCHIFFMAN   From the video "Lean, Strong & Healthy with Susan Powter" (A *Vision Entertainment)

This is me now.

INTRODUCTION

*Men have moods,
women have periods.*

I'm not angry, damn it.

I'm passionate.

Passionate about getting this message to every woman on earth. Passionate about stopping the insanity.

The insanity of starvation, deprivation, and destroying our self-esteem for the sake of skinniness. The insanity that has affected, and all too often ruined, the lives of millions of women. Who wouldn't be passionate about stopping the insanity for Betty, who lost the enamel on her teeth and was hospitalized with a hiatal hernia from vomiting so much?

Then there's Julie, born with a medical problem. Several abdominal surgeries and thirty years later, she walked into my studio weighing 250 pounds. Her body fat was so high, it was off the chart.

This was where she was after having tried every diet under the sun and failing.

And what about Teresa? She lost 126 pounds on a doctor-sponsored liquid fast program. But she lost the weight so fast, her skin was hanging from her body. Her solution? Cosmetic surgery, leaving her with huge scars under both arms and inner thighs. When I met Teresa, she was desperately afraid. She was gaining the weight back—you know, the way 98 percent of us do on those liquid fast programs. Her doctor had forgotten to tell her that the odds were against her and that she could end up with huge stretch marks all over her body as the weight poured back on.

My passion (maybe there *is* a little anger) comes from having been through "it" myself. I was a 260-pound housewife, feeling desperately out of control, afraid, hurting physically and emotionally, trying every diet out there and, like Julie, failing. Failure—not being able to regain the control I needed so desperately, the breakup of my marriage, single parenthood, and all the emotions that went along with watching my life take a nosedive toward the gutter.

Somebody told me during the middle of my descent that all bad experiences bring new life and growth. Well, to say I wasn't open to this metaphysical wisdom would be an understatement. I have a really hard time following anything that intangible. "I know I'll grow from this, BUT RIGHT NOW I'M IN A HELL OF A LOT OF PAIN, SO BRING ON THE NUMBING, WHETHER IT'S FOOD OR DEMEROL . . . JUST BRING IT ON."

People come up to me everywhere I go—I am not exactly unrecognizable; it's not as if they look and say, "There's something about you that reminds me of that lady on the 'Home' show, give me a second, let me think" (with this hair either I am or I am not that woman)—and say, "Hey, you are that lady who talks to fat people." Not true—I speak to anybody who can't walk up a flight of stairs without sucking wind; it doesn't matter if you're as thin as a twig, you are unfit. Anybody who doesn't have the upper body, abdominal, or lower body strength to hold themselves up is unfit. Anybody with an unhealthy percentage of body fat—whether that's 10 percent over or 50 percent over —is unfit. Or anybody without decent flexibility. I don't speak to "fat" people. I speak to anyone who wants to look and feel better and improve the quality of their lives. Anybody.

I am not a physician, dietitian, nutritionist, or diet or fitness expert. I am a housewife who figured it out. Broke the system. Busted them.

The American Medical Association and the diet and fitness industries had fooled me for years, making me feel as if I needed a degree to figure it out—as if this whole thing were just too complicated for my simple little mind and I needed them to help me sort it out . . . making me believe I lacked the discipline, motivation, and control to stick to any diet for any length of time. Boys, boys, boys, you shouldn't have done that to me.

My life-style was killing me mentally and physically. I felt terrible. I had every ache and pain in the book. I weighed 260 pounds, I was suffering and being treated for depression, and I hated the way I looked and felt. I could no longer live feeling and looking the way I did. My motivation was desperation. Sitting around waiting for the heart attack, hypertension, osteoporosis, or whatever else would strike me down was one thing. Not being able to sit comfortably for more than a few minutes was the real problem. It was uncomfortable and it hurt. I could wait until it got worse or I could change my lifestyle. Scary thought when you are presented with the options given by the American Medical Association, the diet industry, and the fitness industry. Bland, boring, complicated foods; no more fun stuff. Low-calorie, got-to-get-that-weight-off shakes, pills, and powders. They are fun enough, but you are told to add those beat-the-hell-out-of-yourself exercise classes that leave you with lockjaw of the calf and feeling like a fat, uncoordinated slob.

Based on the options we are given, I can understand statements like these:

"Give up my sirloin? Life just ain't worth living if I gotta do that." (Notice the southern touch there.)

"I'm not spending the rest of my life eating this rabbit food."

INTRODUCTION

"What do you want me to do, turn into one of those health nuts?"

"I don't have time for this stuff."

When what you're offered in return is that instant, frozen, powdered blah stuff that's called diet or "good for you" food, it's no wonder you are frightened, cautious, and unwilling to change.

Each diet I tried led to failure, and each failure led to the next. When one diet didn't work, I'd go right on to another—liquid starvation, pills, shakes, diet bars, or whatever was being blasted at me as the answer. Why I thought one diet was any different from another is exactly why all of us who are trying to lose weight spend years going from one starvation plan to the next: desperation.

I would have done anything (and I mean anything) to look and feel better. To be skinny. If someone had told me that cutting off my right arm would have made me skinny forever, I would have severed the limb without anesthesia. If there was a diet on earth that worked, I would have found it, you would have found it—we've all done the same things. Eventually we would have bumped into the answer, the one that worked, the solution to the problem, and there wouldn't be a fat person on this planet. According to the Centers for Disease Control, over 34 million people in the United States are fat. You are not alone, this is a national epidemic. Collectively we spend $5 billion (I guess we've all got some cash to burn) trying—the operative word here is "trying"—over and over and over again to lose weight. But 98 percent of us gain back any weight we lose. The odds are not good, folks; this is not a good investment.

You give us your money and we'll give you some freeze-dried, instant, kaka-flavored substitute for food. You will be edgy, unhappy, and have no energy. It will work, you will lose some weight for a very short period of time, and like the other 98 percent of the people who have tried this program, you will gain the weight back and need us again in a few months.

You don't have to be a physician, dietitian, or nutritionist to figure it out. This is not a good deal.

But don't be discouraged—you've got the answer in your hands, so read on.

The aerobics industry humiliated me, the diet industry starved me, and the medical industry tranquilized me! I decided enough already—there has to be a better way!

Stop the Insanity! is about how I broke the system. How I figured it out and started talking. I have a story to tell. So do thousands of women like me. They are changing the way they look and feel. At times it's very funny and too often it's very sad. But as we share our stories, we come to understand that the effort required to do it right, to stop the insanity in our lives, will never be as great as the money, time, and self-esteem wasted on the endless diets, programs, pills, shakes, instant cures, and quick fixes.

Stopping the insanity in my life was more than a physical journey. It was an emotional journey.

I didn't always handle the process well. There was a lot of pain, anger, and frustration along the way.

I've written it all down, just the way it happened, and told you exactly how I handled it. Bear with me—if at times you think my anger is gonna jump off the page and move in with you, don't worry. A lot has been healed since then, and that's what this book is about.

STOP THE INSANITY IS THE ANSWER, the solution to the problem that faces millions of us: hating the way you look and feel; never-ending dieting, starvation, and deprivation, those self-esteem beatings that we live with every day of our lives. This is a book for women, about women getting well. It's about the thousands of women who have stopped the insanity in their lives, and it can be about you stopping it in your life. How to stop dieting and why you should never diet again. How to get lean, strong, and healthy. How to like the way you look and feel again, how to build a foundation of wellness that can change the way you look and feel forever. What could possibly be more important than that?

INTRODUCTION

I have been told over and over again: "Susan, nobody is going to listen to you. Number one, you are a woman. Number two, you are intelligent. Number three, you are opinionated. Number four, you are bucking the system. And number five—YOU ARE BALD." I was told that I would offend every woman in this country. I'm so glad I didn't listen.

During the past couple of years I've spoken all over the country to every group imaginable. These one-hour, four-hour, and half-day seminars have made it clear to me that we may have different life-styles, tastes, and opinions, but everybody wants to look and feel better. No one out there likes waking up every day feeling bad. Being so tired you can't get through the day. Squeezing into those large sizes and knowing that it's getting worse. Having every ache and pain in the book and trying every solution that's offered—and failing.

My seminars are not angry, male-bashing, bra-burning events.

That's not what I'm about.

These are very passionate, very precious hours spent sharing and solving the problems that have hurt so many of us. Solving the problems, not treating the symptoms.

I speak to women about women because I am a woman. Who better to understand what obese women are feeling than someone who has been there? I've worn the size 22, bought the baby powder by the case for the burning, chapped thighs and underarms, and felt the pain of not being able to ride the ride, run the race, play ball, swim (sheer embarrassment stopped me from that; Lord knows I could float better than the rest of the moms), and do all the things my children wanted their mom to do with them.

I can tell you that changing my life-style and improving my fitness level have given me more control and choices in my own life. I will share stories with you from some of the thousands of women who, like me, have been resurrected from the dead.

I will show you how to increase your cardio-endurance

without those hateful exercise experiences; how to increase your upper body, abdominal, and lower body strength, no matter how long it's been since you've seen or felt a muscle; how to decrease your body fat, even if it's a whole other person you need to get rid of; and how to get well. How to live, eating more food than you can imagine. How never to diet again—it's over, no more starvation, deprivation, and killing yourself.

I have a lot to say about the diet industry. I know why all the calorie counting, weighing and scaling, shakes and powders, don't work. After you read this book, you will, too. All of us who have dieted, or those of you who still are, know what it feels like to starve to death. Because that's what diets are. Starvation and deprivation. They are impossible to live on—nobody can succeed living with starvation.

As for the fitness industry, I have been to the "best" exercise studios in the country, and I'm amazed that there are not a hundred deaths a day in some of these classes. A monkey could get "certified" to teach what's being taught in these classes: no modification, unsafe movements, assembly-line fitness, kicking, jumping, and hopping till you drop.

That's not fitness. That's insanity.

Fitness is, or should be, for everyone. Any age, any fitness level, any physical consideration. You can get fit. You can get well. You can change your body by increasing your cardio-endurance, increasing muscular strength, decreasing body fat, increasing flexibility, and building a fitness level. This has nothing to do with willpower, behavior modification, control, or motivation. There is no magic or mystery involved, and it's got nothing to do with dieting.

Stop the Insanity! is a process that is easy to understand and apply to your life. You will learn how important it is to EAT. Without food you can't function. How important it is to BREATHE. Without oxygen you die. How easy and important it is to MOVE. No more fast music, crazy choreography, and jumping up and down like a lunatic, all in the name of fitness. Eating, breathing, and moving within your life-style, fitness level, and physical considerations are the answer.

Forget your health. Don't do it for that reason. That was never my motivation. I didn't lose 133 pounds to have a healthy heart. My motivation was to look better than my ex-husband's girlfriend, and my motivation now is to look and feel the way I want to look and feel. Getting healthy is a side effect of eating, breathing, and moving.

You may not be quite as superficial as I am, but don't be ashamed to admit it if you are. There are plenty of us out there.

Don't do this for your health; do it to love the way you look and feel. Do it for your thighs. Do it to feel sexy and pretty. Do it to spite all the people who think you can't. Do it for whatever reasons, just do it.

We are on an interesting journey together. This self-help, how-to, motivational book is not a step-by-step tip sheet to the answer.

It's a story, a prescription, and a bit of a personal diary. I want to engage your heart and your mind in the process. Along the way, you may find yourself angry, sad, hopeful, and sometimes afraid. My process, which is what you are about to read, gave voice to feelings that I hadn't found a way to express. That may happen to you, too.

I need your help. I'm relying on your patience—stay with me, hear me through, because as you read, you may just hear your own story mixed in with mine.

We will get to the answers, because that's what *Stop the Insanity!* is about—getting you the information you need to change your life. When we do, you'll have gotten there just like I got there. But I promise we'll make it less painful.

Knowledge is not power. Getting the right information and learning how to apply it to your life is power.

When we get to the prescriptions, they will be yours, because the only way to make the process yours is by understanding it . . . so read on.

Stop the Insanity! is not about perfection. Living in a perfect bubble of health and fitness is not for me, but I do make choices every day that make an enormous difference in my life. You may not be willing to change some things. It will be your choice. This is not an all-or-nothing deal. But there are some things we can no longer ignore.

We are not well. Most of us are the walking dead. We don't have enough oxygen in our bodies to get through the day. Our muscles have atrophied, our metabolic rates are in warp zone, we are lugging around tons of extra fat. We are physically ill. There's a lot on people's minds these days. The social and environmental issues that we spend millions of dollars trying to solve. We spend the cash, rally the rallies, talk and fight about it all—while individually we are dying. Dying of oxygen deprivation and lack of strength, and being crushed by fat.

Eighty-five percent of all disease can be directly attributed to life-style. Even if health is not your motivation or concern, this is important. Other than genetic inheritance, your life-style determines the length and quality of your life more than anything else. Well, let's not eliminate fate—when that eighteen-wheeler comes around the corner with your name on it, there are other things involved besides genetics and what you've been eating. But other than that, we do have a lot more control than most of us realize.

Your life-style is determined by what you are eating, whether you are moving, exercising. Exercise, movement—has it been ten years since you've done anything? When was the last time you moved within your fitness level and gave your muscles and cells the one thing they need to live—oxygen? Where's that coming from in your life? And how are you feeling?

You have lots of choices. I had lots of choices. You may not understand what they are or how to apply them to your life. I didn't understand my choices and had no clue how I was supposed to apply any of them to my life —but now I know. So will you. You will learn how to take the control back in your life, change the way you look and feel, and dramatically improve the quality of your life.

Or . . . you can give up:

INTRODUCTION

You can continue eating the way you're eating. Get fatter. Feel horrible. And live with all the symptoms of being unhealthy. Don't do that. You've had enough. It hurts. Please don't set yourself up for a heart attack, hypertension, cancer, diabetes, arteriosclerosis, or whatever may ruin your life. You are too valuable.

What I'm saying here is that we can no longer deny the connection—the connection between what you are living with daily, the way you look and feel, and what you are or are not putting in your mouth.

Let's look at some staggering facts. You should never make any decisions without the facts.

Do you know what the leading causes of death are? According to the National Center for Health Statistics, here they are:

Heart Disease	36.4%
Cancer	22.3%
Cardiovascular Disease	7.1%
Accidents	4.6%
Pulmonary Diseases	3.6%
Pneumonia, Flu	3.3%
Diabetes Mellitus	1.8%
Suicide	1.5%
Liver Disease and Cirrhosis	1.2%
Arteriosclerosis	1.1%
All other causes	3.4%

Heart disease, so the American Heart Association tells us, is the leader: 68,090,000 people in the United States have one or more forms of heart and blood vessel disease —often at the same time. Think about it. The number one killer, preventable and much easier to live without. Here are some numbers:

Hypertension	61,870,000
Coronary Heart Disease	6,080,000
Rheumatic Heart Disease	1,290,000
Stroke	2,930,000

INTRODUCTION

Heart attacks caused 511,050 deaths in 1988. This year, as I write this book, as many as 1,500,000 people will have a heart attack, and 500,000 will die from it. Strokes killed an estimated 150,300 people in 1988. Hypertension (high blood pressure) afflicts nearly one of every three adults in our country.

Mr. Surgeon General of the United States says that 1.5 million out of the 2.1 million deaths in 1987 were related to dietary factors; cholesterol and saturated fats were the big problems. And to think that 85 percent of all of it can be slowed down, prevented, or stopped by eating, breathing, and moving daily!

Changing your life-style—not dieting.

But this book is not about motivating you with disgusting medical facts, scaring you, making you feel guilty, or sending you to a 12 Step program. A born-again ex-fatty I'm not. Changing your body doesn't solve the problems we all face—the kids, the husband, the job. Life doesn't get magically better when you change your body, but it's all a whole lot easier to cope with when you're lean, strong, and healthy. Sophie Tucker said it best: "I've been rich and I've been poor, and rich is better." Excuse me, Sophie, but I've rewritten you: "I've been fit and I've been fat, and fit is better."

The insanity in my life has stopped. I have created my foundation of wellness and know what it takes to maintain it. The strength I have gained, the cardio-endurance, and the healthy percentage of body fat I have, the way I look and feel, are why I believe this is the most important information you can have. "Skinny" and "diet" are two words that no longer control me. They don't have to control you any longer.

Stopping the insanity means relearning what we've all been taught and learning how to eat, breathe, and move and get LEANER, STRONGER, AND HEALTHIER. Unless you're in an iron lung, you can get fit. If you can move anything, you can get fit. You can and will change the quality and direction of your life. Let's stop the insanity together.

This information will change the way you look and feel

forever. You can go from an unfit person to a fit person. It's changed my life, and it will change yours.

My life has changed. I have choices now that I never dreamed I'd have.

My kids asked me the other day to go bike riding with them. You should see me in a helmet—it's a sight.

Down the street we go, pedaling like mad. One of my sons, with the most beautiful face you've ever seen (it's okay to say your kid is prettier than mine, but please don't tell me about some distant cousin who is prettier), looks back and yells, "Hey, Mom, this is so much fun riding with you—I love you!"

Now add to the picture the crazy-looking mom in the helmet with tears streaming down her face.

There was a time when I couldn't bike ride with my sons.

I didn't have the choice.

I was too fat and unfit to think about getting a bike, forget about riding it.

Bike riding may be one thing, but flying from Los Angeles to Dallas sitting two seats away from Dolly Parton is another.

We met when she introduced herself at LAX.

"Hi, I'm Dolly Parton."

No joke—who else could you possibly be?

Five-inch stiletto heels at eleven in the morning.

The biggest hair I've ever seen.

Nails so long they could kill you.

And unbelievably beautiful.

Dolly Parton is my idol. My nails need just a bit more acrylic, and the high heels, I've got them down (see my "after" picture). I'll never be able to match the big hair, but let me strive. Strive to be Dolly.

During our flight a couple of people asked Dolly for her autograph. She was so polite, accommodating and sweet, but what was going on two seats behind her was blowing my mind. At least sixteen people came up to me asking questions, wanting an autograph, or just telling me that they were eating, breathing, and moving, and their lives were changing.

Wow. People changing their lives. Looking and feeling better. What a strange feeling. I'm not a movie star, I'm not in the entertainment business, and as hard as I try, I'll never be Dolly Parton.

During that flight I realized that this message must get out to as many people as possible. I was so grateful for the changes and choices in my life. The job that I love so much, the bike rides with the kids, the fabulous women I meet everywhere I go who are stopping the insanity in their lives, and to top it all off, to be sitting two seats behind Dolly Parton.

Yeah, I'm passionate about women getting well.

Passionate.

Not angry.

> Men are strong, women are bitches.
> Men are focused, women are obsessed.
> Blah, blah, blah. . . .

PART ONE

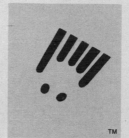

The Insanity

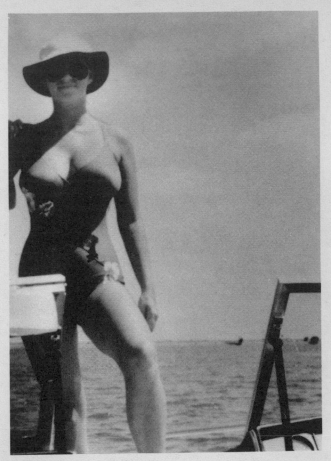

I was always a "big girl." Long before I breast-fed two babies I had boobs. Check it out. My body could easily fluctuate between 130 and 160. I always wore big, baggy sweaters and loose-fitting clothes and was never comfortable with my body. My stomach and my chest were the focus of my body self-hatred for years. Having a petite, little body (which to me meant feminine) was a dream of mine, so I started starving to get it.

Body Images

The body is a sacred garment. It's your first and last garment; it is what you enter life in and what you depart life with, and it should be treated with honor.
—MARTHA GRAHAM

"THERE IS NO DIFFERENCE BETWEEN AN EXTRA 10 POUNDS OF FAT ON SOMEONE'S BODY OR AN EXTRA 100 POUNDS." That's a big statement coming from an ex-260-pound woman who had to face changing a very fat, unfit body instead of just losing a couple of pounds.

Physically there's a big difference. Emotionally it seems to be exactly the same.

I was teaching a class a couple of years ago in my studio. There were a lot of different body types in the room, but none quite like the model-perfect, beautiful, tall, blue-eyed, unbelievably thin girl/woman who walked in, a little late, and started to take class with the rest of us normal-looking (standing next to her, hideously ugly) people.

I must admit my first thought was, What in the hell are you doing here? Everyone else was thinking the same thing, and we all thought it was big of us to let her take class. I couldn't wait to get through to find out why she was here looking the way she did.

Cindy was a model—no joke.

She had gained 10 pounds. Her extra 10 were interfering with her career. Thank God I was never a model. Can you imagine what an extra 133 pounds would have done to my career?

Cindy's work was not the only thing that her "weight gain" was affecting. Her husband had married model perfect and considered her extra 10 pounds unattractive.

There's not much I have less patience for than a man who demands model perfect or nothing. It doesn't fly with me—especially when he looked like Cindy's husband. Yes, his face was very, very pretty. And he had great hair—long and luxurious. But his body left a lot to be desired.

I think I may have offended him a bit when I asked him what he looked like naked—was he as perfect as he required his wife to be? Perhaps he had some extra weight to lose. I told him I was sure it wasn't in his brain, because that was obviously dangerously lean and malnourished. I don't normally attack my clients' husbands—but who could blame me this time?

For Cindy the process of becoming lean, strong, and healthy was the same as it was for me—a 260-pound, never-have-been and never-will-be model, mother of two. Cindy had very little cardio-endurance—she had to build that. Cindy had very little strength—she had to build that also. And Cindy had body fat to decrease, which meant cutting back on her fat intake.

Thinking about restricting anything was difficult for Cindy. She had never thought about food before in her life—you know, one of those people who can eat whatever, whenever they want, poor thing! So this was more difficult for her than it was for me. You see, all I did was think about food.

Exercise was also new to Cindy. Yes, she had been model perfect since the day she was born, with no effort at all. (Don't we just love women like that?) But exercising wasn't as easy for Cindy as it is for most people, because she was unbelievably uncoordinated. It was difficult for her to move her beautiful arms and her perfect long legs at the same time. I guess when you look like her, you don't ever have to learn how to move. I consider

4

myself almost saintly for not pointing out to the class her lack of coordination. I even modified the movements so that she could feel like part of the group. Call the Vatican and get me an application for sainthood!

Cindy had to learn how to eat, breathe, and move to change the way she looked and felt. That's exactly what I had to do; that's exactly what Cindy had to do; and that's exactly what you are going to have to do—no matter what your fitness level or your fitness goal is.

The only difference between Cindy, 10 pounds over, and me, 133 pounds over, is that my process took longer. I had more fat to burn, weaker muscles to strengthen— after all, it had been a long time since I'd done anything but pick up toys and wipe counters; at least she had to move during those strenuous modeling sessions—and cardio-endurance to build (and a lot of cosmetic surgery to go through if I ever wanted to look anything like her).

Emotionally, Cindy's extra 10 pounds were as difficult as my extra 133. That's hard for me to say. I think that those of us who have made a drastic physical change deserve more credit than somebody who loses 10 pounds.

But the truth is, there really is no difference. I have seen an extra 10, 20, or 30 pounds do as much damage to someone's self-esteem and body image as 60, 70, or more pounds. How much fat it takes to do the damage is not the issue.

Why are we all under so much pressure? Why do 10 pounds do the same damage as 133 pounds? Why do we all have such warped body images? Easy and obvious.

Every magazine you read, everything you watch and listen to on TV—everything you see and hear—tells you what you should look like. You know that.

You have a choice here. You can sit around and get angry about the responsibility of the media, the medical community, and the diet and fitness industries for your negative self-image, you can buy whatever it is they have to sell you and continue to live in the pain of trying to live up to standards that are impossible to attain, or you can choose not to believe it, turn it off, close the magazine—or better yet, not buy it, choose not to live by a standard that we all know is stupid and unattainable, and get well. Be as lean, as strong, and as healthy as you want to be. It's time to forget about the standard that Barbie set years ago, the one that none of us ever has been able to live up to. I've seen and heard so many stories from women trying to live up to that impossible image.

Let's start with these:

The Perfect Bosom. Women have ruined their immune systems trying to live up to that one.

Tiny Waist. I met a woman who had her two bottom ribs removed after the birth of her second child to reach that goal.

Hips and Buttocks Perfectly Proportioned to the Perfect Bosom. How much hatred have you directed at your butt and thighs over a lifetime? Every spring and summer there is more butt and thigh hatred in the world than could be imagined.

Big, Long, Perfect Hair. Well, Barbie, this is where you make me spin. I could starve, deprive, torture my body till the cows, pardon the expression, come home. Lipo it, cut it up, remove external and internal anything. But there's one thing I could never do—no, two things: have big hair or sleep with Ken.

Barbie, get a life. Babs, get a job, a personality, a new boyfriend, and do me a favor: STOP TELLING ME WHAT I'M SUPPOSED TO LOOK LIKE.

The "Insanity" doesn't need to be defined—you and I and millions of other women have spent a lifetime in it —but we must change it. Reprogram. Educate ourselves. Get well.

Love the way you look and feel. Be strong. Get out of it.

Let's do it right this time. Starting with body image.

Take off your clothes—yes, if you're reading this on an airplane, or at your desk, or waiting in a doctor's office for your appointment, go ahead and take off your clothes, remember you're proud not to look like Barbie. Or you can wait until you get home, but you've got to do this.

STAND UP NAKED AND BOND WITH YOUR BODY.

Look at your body without the sunglasses on. Get out of the denial for a moment—it's only you and me.

Butt naked, high noon, in a mirror.

Believe me, I understand how difficult this is, but you're not looking to criticize anymore. You're not looking to moan and groan about the starvation that lies ahead. You are looking at what your body is—all that dieting, money spent, months of effort and energy, have really paid off, haven't they?

You are looking at your body and deciding where you want it to be. Simple. Do you need to burn some fat? Forget that extra inch that we have all been told we shouldn't be able to grab, I'm talking losing fat here. How much do you want to lose to look and feel the way you want to look and feel? Look at your body and decide how much fat you need to burn. Do you want to see hipbones again? How about a collarbone? Where are your ribs— has it been years since you've seen a rib? Most of us have wads of fat that we need to lose.

Muscles? Where are they? Is it difficult to hold your body up? Do you have every ache and pain in the book, like I did? Are you tired and achy? If so, we've got to get you some strength and increase your cardio-endurance. Get you some energy, strength, and oxygen. If a flight of stairs is equal to the New York Marathon, then build the cardio we will.

Don't look at yourself, run to the fridge naked, and start shoving food in your mouth because you're so depressed by what you see. Because you've got the answer in your hands. It's okay, we are going to work together to Stop the Insanity that you and I have lived with for too long.

Your body should and can be as lean, as healthy, and as strong as YOU want it to be. YOU think about it, YOU design it, YOU work on it. With the right information it's easy and effective, and YOU make it happen.

Everyone has a different fitness level; everyone has a different fitness goal. The diet and fitness industries want us to believe we all should look like Heather Locklear, Cher, or Jackie Smith. Yeah, like there's a real chance of this happening.

My mother would have loved me to be Jackie Smith or any of the other "model" women.

Model perfect.

Model sexy.

Model vamp (it's Cher who fits into this category).

Model everything that we're all supposed to be.

Do we blame the industries for splashing these images at us? I mean, after all, perfect sells; sex sells. Or is it our fault for buying into it? I pick number two. Each time I tried to live up to the image of what I was supposed to act like, feel like, dress like, or be thin like, I failed.

Failed big. And each time I failed I ate. I know this sounds familiar to a lot of you.

Hey! Call me smart, but it only took me years and a million failures to learn that my body image was about MY body, MY goals, MY fitness level, and MY standard of looking and feeling better.

So what about Cindy? She increased her fitness level, as I did, lost the extra body fat, as I did, and reached her fitness goal looking better than I, or any other human being, could ever look.

God bless the Cindys of the world.

As long as I was sitting in front of a TV (not a mirror), I could fool myself into thinking I wasn't *that* out of shape.

—Comment from a client

The mirror image you're looking at, whether with sunglasses on or not, may be too much to bare (pardon the pun), but you are no longer going to be ruled by anyone else's standards. You want to change your body. But where do you go? Like millions of others, you go to the diet industry.

Dieting is an obsession in this country. I've had women come to me concerned about what their five-, six-, and seven-year-old daughters say about their own bodies.

(Funny, I never hear about their sons. I guess boys learn early that they don't have to be as attractive as girls to get a date.)

Like us, teenage girls are under enormous pressure to have the perfect body and will do anything to get one. Recent studies show that 63 percent of all high school girls are on diets—some go the extreme route of 500 to 600 calories a day. I've spoken at high schools and colleges all over the country and found that these young, precious girls are doing the same things that you and I do to get skinny—not eating, throwing up, living on fruit or salads—all in the name of getting a date to the prom and being skinny. Do you want that for your daughters? Let's stop the insanity where it is beginning, so that the children don't have to live through the same pain and mistakes we've all made.

Think about the insanity of starving a growing, hormonally whacked-out body. I don't know about you, but I know that I would not go back to being fifteen or sixteen for anything in the world, and I am sure my parents wouldn't like it, either. When one diet didn't work for me, I'd go to the next. I ate grapefruits for weeks (talk about gas), ate kelp (does anybody know what that stuff is?), swallowed lecithin capsules, and drank cider vinegar.

I've got a cider vinegar story. My little brother is eleven years younger than me. We dubbed him the "Catholic mistake" (I know, I know, he's scarred for life). He was born a perfect 10 pounds with beautiful curly hair, this perfect Catholic mistake, and was doted on by me from day one. I didn't need Barbies. I had him —the real thing.

Anything he did was brilliant. All the other kids were developing normally. But I thought this child was exceptional in every way and much prettier than the rest of them.

When he was two years old he toddled around for a couple of days saying something that sounded like "dirty socks." He would make this perfectly cute little face, squinching up his perfect little nose, and say, "P U— dirty socks!"

What a genius! Two years old and speaking so well. No need to bring up the fact that nobody understood what he was talking about—he could have been brilliant, or he may have been as nutty as a fruitcake.

After a couple of days the family realized that he was showing his brilliance only around me. I was the inspiration for this child's brilliance!

RIGHT?

Wrong.

I was on a lecithin, kelp, and cider vinegar diet. The cider vinegar was oozing from every pore in my body, and I smelled like—you guessed it—dirty socks.

My insanity, I'm sure like yours, started early. I was only thirteen when I was on the dirty sock diet.

I have the kind of body that has been enormously fat and very, very skinny. It required absolute starvation to keep it that way. Before I had kids I was a double-D bra size. (Nursing two babies changes that quickly!) I always had a stomach, and from the day I can remember I wore big baggy sweatshirts, slouched, and was very, very self-conscious about my large chest and big body image.

I never felt petite or cute. I was always the big girl. I was always 30 to 35 pounds overweight and never liked my body. But I have never been as desperate as when the scale tipped 260.

I was dieting at eight—fifty years later I was still dieting without success.

—Comment from a client

You may know all the diet information there is to know, have tried every diet on the market to create perfection, and think that you have heard it all—I thought I had. But believe me, there are a few things you have not heard:

We are the only nation on earth that not only volunteers to be starved, but WE PAY A WHOLE LOT OF MONEY FOR SOMEONE TO STARVE US (or *lots* of someones, because most of us have been on too many diets to count). If you really stopped and thought about the money you've spent to be starved, you'd get nauseated.

Think about this. Business 101.

You give "them" your hard-earned money.

Then they tell you what kind of starvation you'll be living on. Do you get the most extreme: 300, 400, 500, maybe even 600 calories a day? (A whole lot of people are living on those numbers.)

How about middle-of-the-road starvation? This is the 600 calories and up kind.

Or do you get the "healthful" starvation of 1,200 to 1,400 calories a day?

You'll spend hundreds of dollars on the yummy freeze-dried, instant, or frozen food that you'll need to live on forever to keep up this insanity. And while you're starving you may be coming in once a week to visit and get applauded—that's if you've lost a pound or two—or sit around and talk about all the reasons you are metabolically incapable of losing weight. And the results, if any, will not last. You'll be doing it again soon. Different diet, same system and results.

Business 101 tells me that if I pay you for a temporary, painful—and dieting is painful—solution to my problem, if the solution I am paying for will absolutely set me up for failure, and if I will need you again in a couple of months, then this is not—and I repeat, not—a good investment. When the truth is known—and it is about to be really clear—you will understand that dieting costs a whole lot of money, it is painful and hell to live with, it doesn't work, and it sets you up to fail. When you understand this you will be able to stop the insanity of dieting forever. It's over. There is a solution, and dieting is not it.

A popular woman's magazine recently surveyed 33,000 women and found the following:

50%	Sometimes/often use diet pills
27%	Use liquid diets
18%	Use diuretics
45%	Fast
18%	Use laxatives
15%	Vomit on a regular basis

I find the liquid diet statistic a little low. Everyone I know has used these things—but this is what "the magazine" said, and what "the magazine" says must be true!

As for the fasting (or starvation) statistic—shouldn't this and liquid diets be in the same category? I mean, what's the difference?

And vomit? I have clients who can teach you one hundred different ways to vomit: Jan eats a four-course meal in one of the nicer restaurants, excuses herself, throws it all up without anyone else in the ladies' room hearing her, applies more lipstick, and goes back to the table for dessert.

I never made myself throw up because there is nothing I hate more than throwing up. It makes me cry, and I get scared. But I would have done it, if I could have.

In June 1991 New York City's Department of Consumer Affairs reported that nine out of ten diets on the market today fail to warn us of the potential dangers associated with starvation and weight loss.

No joke. Can you imagine that if just before they took your money, they said:

"Most people gain their weight back." (They'd tell you 98 percent if they were really honest.)

"There's a chance you'll lose an internal organ or two —but just a chance, not everybody does." (People are losing gallbladders over these things—internal organs! Perhaps the advertising should read: "Drink this, lose your gallbladder, and there's a couple of pounds gone.")

"When you diet, you lose mostly water and lean muscle mass." Lean muscle mass doesn't just come back: you have to build it. So when you gain that weight back, it's fat you are gaining, not lean muscle mass. When I would lose 40 pounds and gain back 30 or 35, I always felt fatter. More wobbly. Looser. I thought that it was my imagination—after all, I hadn't put *all* the weight back on, there were still 5 to 6 pounds less on my body —but I felt fatter. The reason was that I was gaining back fat, not lean muscle mass. That's a fact. Take that to your doctor. It is not in your mind, it is in the fat you are gaining back for the lean muscle mass you have lost. So unless you are a part of that lucky 2 percent that keeps the weight off, this diet will make you weaker and fatter. (I have traveled all over the country, spoken to thousands of women, and have yet to meet the 2 percent that keeps it off. They're well hidden—those skinny, starved people!)

With all these new diets on the market you'd think that the average American would be getting skinnier, but the percentage of overweight Americans has grown over the last twenty years. One "weight loss by dancing to the oldies" kind of guy said recently with tears in his eyes that Americans are getting fatter. The numbers are climbing—not literally, because it's difficult to climb when you're in the 200- and 300-pound range—and it's getting worse.

So I asked myself why a leading weight loss expert would say that. If you've spent years teaching weight loss and then you acknowledge publicly that it's not working, something's a little off. Maybe we've been teaching the wrong thing. Maybe what we've been selling to people doesn't work. And if it doesn't work, people have to keep on trying and buying. Now there's a slogan: Keep trying and buying, 'cause it ain't gonna work and you're gonna have to keep on trying and buying.

I know—you've heard all of this. You know the dangers. You know that most diets don't work. We all know that there is no instant cure, *we know*, but we are still all looking for the answer.

Without a doubt, the diet industry ranks as one of the lowest-rent industries out there. There are the promises they throw at you when you are most vulnerable, the prices they charge, and the systems that set you up for failure. The whole scam is pretty disgusting.

STOP THE INSANITY!

I received a letter a couple of months ago from a "Home" show viewer. She put her name, address, date, and time of writing at the top of her letter. It was the "2 A.M." that touched me so deeply. I knew what she was feeling before I read the words.

That was the time that was the hardest for me:

Late at night or early in the morning.

The kids were in bed. Not for long—but in bed.

Everything was done, or not done, depending on the kind of day I'd had.

I was depressed, hating the way I looked and felt.

The only thing to do at that hour then (things have changed—now I will tell you plenty of things that I do at 2 A.M.!) was to watch TV and eat.

That's when it's all splashed at you: the diets, shakes, pills, and promises of perfection that come with them. That's when millions of people pick up the phone and order the magic.

That's when you're the most vulnerable.

That's when they get you.

You may have seen me recently in your bedroom at 2 A.M. I thought it was about time someone stopped selling magic and started telling you the truth.

How many fat people do you see in aerobics classes?
None!
Why?
Something to think about.

The diet industry is not the only industry that you should send your self-esteem therapy bill to. The fitness industry ranks right up there with the get-skinny-quick people.

I write this as an insider. I am an exercise studio owner. I go to the conventions, seminars, and lectures given by the organizations that govern the fitness industry: IDEA and AFFA. They teach minimum physiology and maximum choreography with faster and faster music.

My studio is certified by IDEA, and my teachers are IDEA- or AFFA-certified if they choose to be. But this

14

certification means very little to me. If you need proof of how little certifications mean, I sent a check for $300 to IDEA and they sent me a plaque that states THE SUSAN POWTER EXERCISE STUDIO IS A MEMBER IN GOOD STANDING WITH IDEA AND IS COMMITTED TO MAINTAINING A HIGH STANDARD OF EXCELLENCE IN THE FITNESS FIELD. Nobody from IDEA has ever been to my studio. They have no clue what I am teaching or how I teach it. All it really takes is a little cash to be qualified or legitimate.

The fitness industry caters to 10 percent of the population and ignores the other 90 percent. If you are anything less than brilliantly coordinated and want to be a dancer, very, very fit, and covered in neon, to heck with you! And God help you if you try to do some of the moves without having been in dance class for years—you'll be run over in minutes. If you fit into the other categories, like most of us—average or below average coordination, not fit, fat, a senior, injured or with a physical consideration, or a man (have you ever seen men try to do some of this stuff?)—and don't look good with a neon thong up your butt, you can't come to class. Well, you can if you want to be ignored, run over, made to feel like an uncoordinated whale in the back, tortured and wake up the next day and not be able to move for a few days. Great idea, don't you think?

I have been at seminars where a move is being demonstrated, and I have asked if there is any modification for the move:

"What's the modification for that grapevine with three knees up?" Or, "What happens if you have six unfit people in the room?"

It's always a blank stare and an answer like "You mean like if the person can't do this? . . . Well, I don't know."

"And what if the client is very large and that 'jump up, twist around, and land on one leg from the step' doesn't work for them?"

"You mean too fat to do aerobics? . . . Well, I don't know."

STOP THE INSANITY!

These are questions most aerobics instructors don't need the answers to because most unfit, fat, uncoordinated people don't come within twenty miles of an aerobics class.

Strange. Aren't they the people who need it the most?

The fitness industry feeds the Barbie myth of perfection because they give us nothing else. No modifications, alternatives, or options other than those "special fat woman tapes." It's keep up or get out. Fit in or be humiliated. Perfection or nothing. Kind of like making the bed before the maid comes. Be fit, or close to it, before you walk in, or get ready to die.

Can't take a class till you're fit.

Can't get a job without experience.

I saw a national commercial for a well-known shoe manufacturer that says it all.

A group of people exploring the ruins of Mexico. The group consists of ten goofy-looking, sloppy, badly dressed people *and* a beautiful, well-dressed couple. The ruins they all came to see are at the top of hundreds of ancient steps. In order to get the full view, you have to run to the top.

The goofy, unfit, badly dressed group has to stay at the bottom (because they can't jog), trying to take pictures and appreciate the ruins from below, while the beautiful, fit couple jog up the hundreds of steps to the top, where they, and only they, can appreciate the beauty of the ancient structure. It's hard to believe that they can see the beauty of anything other than themselves.

Believe me, there are other ways to go upstairs besides jogging. There are modifications. It may take you longer, and you may not get there as fast, but you can get there even before you are superfit.

I couldn't have jogged to the top of the stairs when I was 260 pounds. I would have been left at the bottom with the rest of the goofy folks, unable to enjoy the ruins that we all paid the same amount of money to appreciate. I didn't have the cardio-endurance or the muscular strength to jog up there, and there was never a modification given so I could build my fitness level and get to the

16

top of the stairs. It was jog or nothing. And I certainly didn't have the necessary fuel. I was starving myself to death.

Now—no thanks to the diet or fitness industries—I would jog right past the beautiful couple, tell them what I think of them (speaking for all the unfit people who have been blown off by the likes of them), and be loving it every step of the way.

> It is only the first step that is difficult.
> —Marie de Vichy-Chamrond, 1763

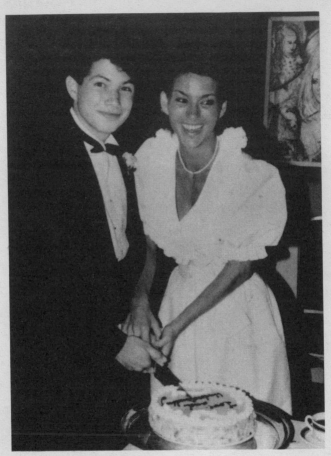

The emaciated bride. Every bride has one thing on her mind before the wedding: "I have to get thin to fit into my wedding dress." I can't tell you how many times I've heard that during the last couple of years, and it's something that I certainly understand. This bride ate lettuce for four months before the wedding. Check out those arms—could I have been any more emaciated than that?

Being Fat

> We are what we repeatedly do.
> —ARISTOTLE

Why are we all so fat?

How did it happen?

Where did we go wrong?

I don't know about you, but I was bribed, manipulated, and rewarded by food for the first ten years of my life. I grew up crunching with "the Captain" every morning— pouring that whole milk all over the cereal. We had a milkman delivering our milk, and the thick layer of cream at the top was considered the prize for whoever got to the door first. I loaded up on the lamb, steak, and pork chops for the protein my growing body needed.

And, OH, the passion I tried to drum up for those starving little children the nuns kept telling me about. They can have my plate of creamed veggies, I thought. If only there was a way to get it to them.

The insanity begins the minute we are born. It started to become clear to me when I was nursing my first son. Breast-feeding and dieting, obviously there's a connection, isn't there? He ate when he was hungry. This was sane. Some days he nursed every hour; some days he'd go hours between feedings. When his body needed more fuel, he'd eat more. Growing a body, developing at the rate a newborn develops, requires fuel—more fuel than you'll ever need again. A newborn hasn't learned to be obsessed with food yet. (We teach them that later.)

So babies eat when they are hungry—unless, of course, they are on that brilliant four-hour feeding routine that pediatricians dreamed up. Who decided that's how often every baby needs to eat? Are all babies developing at the same rate? Do all bodies require the same fueling time? Amazing—these doctors think they know more than God, who designed the perfect body to work perfectly. If a four-hour feeding schedule was the way to go, then your breasts would produce milk only every four hours. But it isn't, so they don't. It seemed a little crazy to me when my doctor told me how much and when to feed my son. So, guess what, I didn't listen.

Every doctor's nightmare: a mother who listens to her instincts and her baby instead of him.

I noticed every time my son would go through a period of nonstop nursing, two things would happen. I'd have very sore nipples, and he would grow. Like a little sprout, he'd grow. It made perfect sense. It was sane.

The same thing happens to my body and yours. Now that I'm fit there are days that I eat nonstop. I have just started taking self-defense classes (no more victim here). Try punching and kicking for a few hours a day and see how much fuel you'll burn—you'll be sore the next day in places you didn't know existed. Now that I've begun punching, I wanted to insure the strength behind the punch, so I threw a little weight workout in. (Yeah, I need to add just a few more things to my schedule, don't you think? How about flying lessons—maybe I'll take up flying next week?) These activities burn fuel. Throw in living my life and running my company, and some days you'll find me stopping every five minutes for food. My body is developing in ways it never has before. On the days it has a growth spurt—metabolically, muscularly, or just in brain power—all I do is eat, and I don't question it. (Did you know that your brain uses 20 percent of your resting metabolic calories? Twenty percent of your energy for the day, without doing anything. Imagine what happens when you are writing a book and actually have to pull from the deepest depths, run down memory lane, and have it all make sense. An incinerator, a fuel-burning hothead, that's what my brain has become thanks to this book. Forget exercise, I'll just write another book.) I don't eat more or less anymore because some doctor, weight-loss counselor, or nutritionist tells me what, when, and how much to eat. I eat when I'm hungry, and just like my growing son, I am developing. Without fuel, my body can't do that.

Getting past the crazy rules about food and eating, the bribery, and the total crap we were raised on is hard enough. It's a wonder we are all still alive—or are we? But when you think about what we eat or don't eat daily, the lack of exercise (running around after the kids may be movement, but it's not the exercise I'm talking about), and the oxygen deprivation that we suffer every day, you'll begin to understand how you ended up looking and feeling the way you do. It's not because you are a lazy slob.

Being fat, for many of us, is simply a symptom of all the wrong advice, guidance, information, and rules we've all been raised on. It's not that there is anything wrong with you.

Being fat is also a symptom of our sedentary life-styles. Convenience is one thing; it's a good thing. But the instant timer remote mentality that exists in our society today creates a couple of problems: one is that we don't have to move very much. You can turn on the TV, record on the compact disc player, and turn on the coffeepot while lying in bed.

I got fat because I ate tons of high-fat food, stopped moving, and ignored my body. That's why 99.9 percent of us are fat. Even the American Medical Association says that a very small percentage, 2 or 3 percent, of obese people are genetically obese.

STOP THE INSANITY!

So you've gotten fat. Let's deal with it. The time has come. It's time to stop blaming your mother, "the Captain," or, in my case, the Prince. When you eat high-fat foods and stop moving, you get fat.

I didn't want to be a 260-pound single mother. I didn't want the life I had. I was depressed. (I had a right to be.) I didn't want to live my life fat. That was my motivation.

Do me a favor, forgive your mother, the Captain, whoever it is you have to forgive, but do stay with me on this Prince thing. I'm not quite ready to forgive him . . . not yet. . . .

This is the story of the white picket fence that exploded. You know the one: your dreams, goals, and future exploding in front of your eyes. The one that leaves you lonely, desperate, confused, and, in my case, 260 pounds.

I married Prince Charming, which is the way I will be referring to my ex-husband from now on—simply, the Prince. We fell head over heels in love, the kind of love that has no boundaries.

The Prince came from a very close, large, Mexican-American family. I came from a small family, not very close knit, and was raised halfway around the world in a Dominican convent in Sydney, Australia. We were miles apart on every level . . . but this was love, and there was no way out from the moment we met.

We met, we married, and we started to set up house almost immediately. The castle (which is what it was to me) had a lawn, trees, a porch, everything but the white picket fence. Who cared? I was nestled snugly in Garland, Texas—you couldn't have told me that at the time; I thought I was on a mountaintop in Shangri-la, but Garland it was—setting up my castle and as happy as any Cinderella could be. (Years later and somewhat emotionally stable, I find that I can't drive within a ten-mile radius of Garland, Texas, without getting hives. Nothing against the fine folks of Garland, but pardon the hell out of me, it is where my life exploded—and, well, call me sensitive, but when I see the old street signs I start to itch and scratch all over, get a little edgy, start to hallucinate, and have to get out of there as fast as I can.) Anyway, my castle had everything—everything but the moat, which would have come in handy later on. We had it all.

We were living the "dream." If not the American dream, the Cinderella one.

Was Cinderella from America?

Was Cinderella real? Where'd this babe come from? Who invented her, and how did she ever get stuck in my head?

Six weeks after our wedding (and what a wedding it was!), I went to a close friend's wedding in New York. (Weddings were my thing then.) Other than missing my Prince so much that I threw up every morning, everything was fine. Call me naive, or anything you want to call me, but I attributed my vomiting to lovesickness.

Remember, this was a love like no other. In fact, throwing up because I missed my Prince so much made me feel all the more that our marriage and our love were bigger and better than most.

Imagine, physical illness from love! It never dawned on me that anything else was involved.

My lovesick symptoms continued during my trip, so the minute I returned to the castle, the Prince and I set up an appointment with my doctor. We went to my OB because that's where I always went when things didn't feel right.

It was touching.

I was examined and told that after six weeks of marriage I was four weeks pregnant. This made me an immediate hero in a large Hispanic family.

I went and blurted out the news to my Prince, who was waiting anxiously in the room full of women. (What a guy, ahead of his time, even then!) We were completing our dream faster than either one of us had expected.

The whole room burst into applause.

I swear this happened.

And the Prince and I left, tearfully, with the new addition to our dream on the way.

To this day, that ride home is one of my most wonderful memories. We were overjoyed, nervous, and confused about what our unique love had produced. A child, our child—nothing could have felt better.

The pregnancy was bliss. The Prince and I had long discussions and made parenting agreements. So very 1980s, don't you think? We discussed my role and his, and being the Cosmo couple that we were, we talked about unity, commitment, and equal involvement in raising and taking responsibility for our child. It was those strong feelings of trust, understanding, and agreement that gave me the freedom to throw myself into being the ultimate pregnant woman, wife, and mother-to-be. The Prince worked overtime (the first fence post was weakening), and we both got ready for the new family.

Our son was born. The first grandson in the Prince's Mexican-American family.

Did you hear that? Grand*son*—"son" being the operative word in a Mexican-American family. If I hadn't been nominated for sainthood by then, I was securing the position fast.

My most humiliating moment in public was when . . .

Someone thought I was pregnant. I couldn't speak for the lump in my throat and just smiled and walked away. I felt so ashamed and embarrassed. Of course—it didn't stop me from eating. *Insane.*
　　　　—Comment from a client

On the surface things could not have been better. However, our beautiful 10-pound boy was born with severe allergies, which kept him awake for days and nights on end. Weeks went by, and all he did was cry. My baby was sick. Finding out what was wrong with him and making him better were all I could think about.

The house was clean, the meals were being cooked, and the laundry was always done, but my focus and attention were on one thing—my baby getting better. The Prince was working overtime and doing whatever he could to help, which usually meant rocking a screaming (and I mean screaming) child when he came home from work so I could get 2 hours' sleep. Picture this in a new marriage. My husband was working overtime; I was totally focused on this sick little person, spending 24 hours a day with him. My baby wasn't sleeping or responding to breast milk or formulas, his constant crying was driving anyone crazy who was around him for more than a few minutes, there were the medical bills and unbelievable stress, and he wasn't fitting into any of the categories that the pediatricians and their charts had set up. The Prince and I were growing apart.

I remember my first Mother's Day one month after our son was born. We had to dress up the new grandson (a prerequisite with my mother—you had to be well dressed at all times) and go to a restaurant that was crowded, hot, and not much fun when your baby screams during the whole lunch. What a welcome to motherhood it was for me.

At this time in my life, my sick, unresponsive baby and my failing marriage were the only two things on my mind. My husband and I were growing apart, and I had a solution: ask my mother to baby-sit so I could go to dinner with the Prince and ninety-eight of his relatives.

I got all dressed up (not an easy thing to do when you're a couple of months postpartum and nursing) and hopped on the back of my husband's motorcycle (a gift I had helped him get to retain some semblance of order and familiarity in his life), and off we rode to meet his relatives for dinner.

If giving birth doesn't knock your insides out, try riding on a motorcycle a couple of months later. It will definitely do the trick. During dinner I was as charming and sexy as the situation allowed. Postpartum, exhausted, squeezing into a dress that didn't fit, sitting with the Prince and his relatives, trying to chat up a storm and appear interested. Then home we went. Apparently my plan worked, or else the Prince just wanted to have sex, because son number two was conceived. My mother said it best: "Oh, they're still handing out that ridiculous information about not being able to get pregnant while nursing." She was a good Catholic woman who had her babies fifteen months apart.

As I said before, the Prince and I come from very different families. In his family, conceiving children that close together means you are a good Catholic. In my family it means lack of thought, no planning, and sheer stupidity.

We met my parents for lunch (my son very well dressed) to tell them the happy news. My father said very little. He gave the Prince a look that can't be described and dubbed him the "Fertile Turtle." I never understood the reptilian reference, but at least the Prince got a title. All I got was a strange look.

From that moment on, my pregnancy was about the Prince's virility (of course I had very little to do with it). We spent months joking about the Prince's manhood while I threw up and dealt with levels of exhaustion that I had never experienced in my life. There isn't a mother alive who doesn't understand the exhaustion and fear that come with having a new baby and then immediately becoming pregnant with the next one.

I had the strange feeling during the next couple of months that birthing back to back was to be my fulfillment. Somehow it was supposed to satisfy me, make me feel complete, and be all that was needed to keep me going.

The losses I felt—MY sexuality, MY freedom, MY marriage, MY energy, MY LIFE—were not supposed to matter. Nobody talked about these things, and when I tried to, I felt ashamed and out of place. But I was totally devoted to our marriage and committed to the joy and love for the son we had and the baby on the way. Still, what was I supposed to do with all those "other" feelings?

My marriage broke up five years ago, leaving me with two babies and a lot of rage. Food has been my solace, my comfort, my friend (my drug of choice) since childhood. But . . . I should know better. You see, I am a physician . . . I feel like such a hypocrite.
    —Comment from a client

The unraveling of our marriage was well underway. I just didn't see it. Well, a word to the wise.

20/20 HINDSIGHT ALERT!!

Here's a big clue that things are not going well in your marriage:

My parents and I took my sick son down to a clinic in southern Texas. There I was, pregnant with my second son, riding hours in the car. I have no idea how far from Dallas it was. I just know it took hours.

What a time! Driving all day, sitting in the waiting room, seeing the doctor, getting the news that my son was very sick and they didn't know what it was yet. Then there was the drive home and being greeted by the Prince and a tall, very thin redhead. They were painting our living room.

Here's where the word to the wise comes in:

If this ever happens to you, do not do what I did. Be smarter than the wife I was, and do what is instinctive: beat the heck out of both of them on the spot!

My reaction was as *Cosmopolitan* as they come. Remember, it was the 1980s, and we were an eighties couple. It was perfectly reasonable for him to choose a tall, thin redhead (whom I recognized as the sleazy hostess at the restaurant he worked in) as his painting partner.

Perhaps she was consoling him. After all, his son was sick, and he must be as worried as I was. She may have been a color expert giving advice; she may have been a professional painter just helping out. The Prince and I were 1980s people—surely there was an explanation for this.

My mother's reaction was totally different:

"Who's the trashy redhead painting with him? This is disgusting! You need to take care of this immediately!"

I calmly explained to my mother that we were from different generations and that marriage today was based on trust, communication, and love. I would handle this my way. Thanks, Mom and Dad, for driving night and day for me and my son. I'll speak with you both in the morning.

The Prince did have an explanation.

See, I told you!

They were painting.

She was lonely, having boyfriend troubles, and he was spending time with her. They might as well work while they were together. Wasn't the Prince brilliant, combining work with counseling? What a man I married!

I put my very sick, sleeping (but not for long) baby in his crib and crawled into bed. I fell into a coma smelling the freshly painted living room.

It may be hard, at this point, for any of you to believe anything out of my mouth from this moment on. How could anyone this stupid give you advice on changing the way you look and feel? How to be in control of your life? It's a little hard to believe that I bought this hook, line, and sinker, but I did. Life resumed as usual. Sure, there were some angry words, a few nights spent in a hotel (by the Prince—could you imagine what would have happened if I'd gone to a hotel for the night?), fights here and there. What marriage doesn't have those?

Someone asked me when I first knew that our marriage was falling apart. Anyone would have known while smelling the fresh paint. I didn't.

Our second son was born and was perfect. I was in a walking coma 98 percent of the time, while the Prince was being congratulated everywhere we went for being able to produce two sons in such a short period of time. He was Supersperm and I was just the tag-along.

I knew things were not right after the birth of my second son. We would go weeks saying nothing more than "Good morning" or "Good night." Physically we were still living together, but there was total separation in our schedules and planning.

The Prince was either working or playing with the kids, but we were never doing it together. Whenever he was with the kids, I stole a nap, did the laundry, went to the bathroom, took a shower—you know, the luxuries!

Our sex life had once been second to none; we had the best sex life on earth. (I'd never thought of myself as a prude. I've always been comfortable with sex—sometimes a little too comfortable. Could you imagine having me as your teenage daughter?)

Now, if we made love once a month, it was planned, talked about, and made to be a romantic experience. That's hard to do when one partner, me, was a zombie.

All of this was normal for new parents. Children so close together will do this to any marriage—even the ones made in heaven. That's what the books said. And I was reading every one of them. The problem was that the Prince wasn't. He didn't know this was normal. The love, attention, and affection that he was missing were just flat out gone.

The first direct sign that I got (remember I was too brain dead to catch on to the living room paint) was when the Prince told me he wanted to talk to me one night. He seemed sad. So I put the kids to bed, cleaned up the kitchen, organized the toys, and sat down to talk to my Prince.

"I need to talk to you. There's something on my mind. It's important." Those are the words I remember. There was some conversation in the middle about feeling separate, lonely, and confused.

Then he said, "I've had an affair and I think we should talk about it."

My response:

Did you say had an affair or had an éclair?

Had an affair or are willing to share?

Had an affair or want to play truth or dare?

What is it that you just said? An affair.

(I'm telling you, it took me a minute to separate a social occasion from a woman.)

Of course you've had an affair. Was it a wedding, a reception, a Bar Mitzvah? Of course, you work in a restaurant.

The Prince had to break down and explain to his zombie of a wife that he was talking about the kind of affair you see talked about on "Donahue." (The millions of other talk shows didn't exist at the time. Donahue was still king.)

An affair. With a woman. Involving sex. Sex that we were not having at the time.

That's how he was feeling. As for me (not that anyone asked, including the Prince), I was desperate for support, love, intimacy, and sex—yes, folks, I needed sex, too. I was lonely, scared, confused, and horny—let's face it, the Prince wasn't the only one not having sex in this little casa.

I thanked him for telling me and being honest. DID YOU HEAR THAT? I THANKED HIM!

I understood his needs, and we resolved to work this out together. I didn't ask him who he had been with—although I was dying to know. Easy guess: the trashy redhead. We went to bed feeling as if we really were that Cosmo couple we'd started out to be.

The Prince was truly sorry. In the Catholic church you do penance for everything. He did his penance. There was more communication, more affection—not much sex, but a lot of hugging and kissing. There was more time to be at home—slow month at the restaurant—and the beginning of a beautiful relationship.

I started reading every "how to get your man back" book on the market. With the little energy I had left, time was scheduled for my husband and me alone. His favorite meals were prepared. I complimented him as often as I could and listened when he came home from work with his worries.

One of the Prince's biggest worries, or insecurities, was his need to work for himself. To not be under anyone's thumb. To feel like a man. This was a big chapter in all the books. A man needs to feel important, needs to feel as if he's accomplishing something important. Funny, they never mentioned anything about the other person in the relationship. I suppose I needed nothing. My self-worth was second to his. And again, like the good fisherwoman that I was, I bought it hook, line, and sinker . . . what in the hell is a sinker?

> There are things that really hurt and even privately humiliate. The times I have gotten warm and actually started perspiring from embarrassment . . . having people look over you, talk over you, almost—no, not almost—being invisible.
> —Catherine, Phoenix, Arizona

My mission, other than taking care of two boys one year apart, was helping my Prince get what he needed to feel important. I helped design, organize, and finance the Prince's own restaurant—his very own that we could build and work on together. It was going to build the respect, intimacy, and togetherness we'd lost.

There are a couple of universal principles in life. One is, don't ever open a restaurant. One out of every two fails. It's a crummy business that requires 24-hour days, presents unbelievable stress, and plants lots of young, good-looking, thin girls at the bar for after-hours discussions.

Could I have been any smarter?

We left the castle and moved closer to his business, so we could see more of each other and begin our entrepreneurial life together.

Part of my plan in keeping my man happy was attending my first exercise class. I wanted to get in shape and look sexy like all the other women I saw hanging around the restaurant and my Prince. You know the type —tall, beautiful, young, dumb as a bucket of rocks. It seemed at the time that the only women alive were those who looked better than me.

I chose the only exercise studio (clubs being too intimidating) that existed in Irving at the time. It was run by an ex–Dallas Cowboy cheerleader.

STOP THE INSANITY!

Good move, Susan.

I don't think I've ever met anyone quite as boppy as the owner of this studio. She tried, God bless her, but she didn't quite know what to do with a depressed trying-to-hang-on-to-her-man housewife who had just moved into the neighborhood. The classes were what you'd expect from an ex-cheerleader, and within weeks I felt so uncoordinated and out of place that I stopped attending.

Walking was a better alternative. It was all I had. I just knew that if I could look better, get skinny, the Prince and I could get back what we'd lost. Getting skinny was always the answer. If only I could lose this weight, then he'd pay attention to me, include me in his life, ask for my opinion, be proud of me, make love to me . . . if only I was skinny. We had the opening of the restaurant, the beginning of our future, our life to come going on all at once, and skinny was the answer to the fights, the separations, and the begging and pleading for love, support, and understanding that were going on daily. Try to forget the past and the other women who had creeped in, put aside feeling as if I were dying—forget it all. I was going to work toward a new body, which would guarantee a new life. We all know that a new body solves everything, doesn't it?

The restaurant opened, and what an opening it was. That night the Prince got the recognition he needed to feel like the succesful, independent man he was. We all, friends and family, worked hard to make this night go well for him. He needed it. Working hard, trying to support a wife and two children so close together. I managed, after total starvation and walking, to fit into a "normal" size (high teens) pink paisley dress. I wanted to look and feel sexy for my husband that night. The young, good-looking entrepreneur and his pink paisley wife. The only thing I felt was pinched to death, but who cared about permanent scars from that side zipper? I had to look good for my man, that's what all the books said.

So the Prince got what he needed, and he was off. Off and running on his new career, operator of his own restaurant. Pride, we got him that; confidence, we got him that also; dreaming of a future, he had that one, too.

My life continued as it had before; add to it, of course, the scarring from the dress, the new town I was living in, a new house to set up with very little money because every penny went back into the Prince's future, the housework, the kids, the laundry, the loneliness, the pain, the sexual frustration, and the separations every other day, and on it went. My life.

The kids were growing, the toys were accumulating, and the how-to books on how to get your man to stay interested were stacking up on the shelves. I had him back (or so I thought), but now I had to keep him interested.

The Prince and I had very different jobs that took us in different directions. But both of them required long hours, and both of them were exhausting. His was owning and running the four-star Mexican restaurant that we had created together. This job included his wearing fabulous clothes and hearing daily what a wonderful job he was doing and what a good-looking young entrepreneur he was.

The Prince had a sense of accomplishment that I was severely lacking. No one was praising me for my days of endless diaper washing, cleaning not only two high chairs, but the walls and floor surrounding them, *and* trying to regain my body after back-to-back births.

The problem was that I just couldn't keep up with the 18-year-olds who were coming into the restaurant for a margarita (or a whole pitcher) and admiring the Prince. Granted, he was something to admire, but he had a family to come home to.

But no matter how hard I tried, it was dying fast. After the birth of our second son, there were hundreds of discussions, tears, attempts at reconciliation, a bit more penance, lots and lots of anger and pain, the restaurant, a few more affairs, and the big romantic trip to San Fran, but it was over. No matter how you looked at it, the white picket fence had been weakened post by post, the dynamite was in place, the match was lit, and POW. The fence exploded.

> *If you are waiting for the fairy godmother of motivation*
> *to come down, tap you on the shoulder, and say:*
> *"You will change your life,"*
> *"You can be as healthy as you want,"*
> *"And it's going to happen now . . . instantly . . ."*
> *It ain't gonna happen. Has the fairy godmother ever*
> *been around when your rent is due?*
> *No, 'cause she doesn't exist.*
> *It's a lie.*

I had a client walk into my studio a couple of years ago. She said she was from Irving.
I mentioned the restaurant.
She mentioned the owner.
I told her he was my ex-husband.
She looked at me in amazement and said, "I didn't know he was ever married."
Bingo!

My most humiliating moment in public was when . . .

I saw my first boyfriend from eleven years ago at a wholesale store. It had been nine years since I last saw him. I felt shame over the 50 pounds and three sizes my body had gained. I wanted this man to remember the old me, the way I used to look when we were dating. I also felt like I had failed at life in some way with my weight gain.

— Lisa, Ione, Washington

I wish I could tell you that I dealt with the breakup of my marriage as a mature, single mother of two sons one year apart. That I picked myself up by my bootstraps and got on with my life.

Kaka!

Nooooooo, that's not what I did. I started eating enormous amounts of high-fat foods and stopped moving—the exercise I had begun to please my Prince ended. I was isolated, angry, lonely, scared, angry (did I mention angry?), eating, not moving, and planning the death of the Prince and his Princess. That's how I spent my days: thinking of ways to ruin his and her life. Well, could you blame me? Our rules were so different. The Prince could come by twice a month, and he was a hero. I stayed awake for days on end, but that was a given. That's what you are supposed to do—you have a uterus. People brought him meals when he first left.

If he could sleep with an 18-year-old, he could cook his own meals—that made perfect sense to me, but not to the friends and family—yes, that's family—who took him food. God forbid he should starve to death.

The Prince's life grew: his business, his list of girl-friends, his social activities—everything. My life faded to black.

One day I woke up out of a fat coma, and I was a mess. I was fat. I couldn't move without feeling exhausted. I had every ache and pain in the book. My self-esteem was in the toilet. I hated the way I looked and felt. I was 260 pounds, and I felt as if my life were over. How did I get into this mess? How do I get out of it? Where do I go for help? Where do I put all the anger and pain that I'm feeling? Lots of questions, not many answers, swirling around in my head, driving me nuts.

There is so much involved in the downward spiral of gaining weight and losing your health. Countless symptoms and traps that shove your self-esteem into corners you never dreamed you'd end up in. Everything changed. The panic attacks began. Shopping for groceries with the kids was too much some days. I'd make it to the checkout counter and suddenly get so scared that I had to grab the kids, leave the groceries, and run out of the store. I'd get the kids and myself in the car and just sit in the parking lot. Scared, not knowing what I was afraid of—just feeling terrified.

STOP THE INSANITY!

Afraid of:

The bag boy.

The people in the store.

The traffic.

The sounds, street signs, traffic lights—all of it was too much for me. How had I gone from a normal person to someone who couldn't go grocery shopping without being scared to death?

My life was falling to pieces in front of my eyes. I felt as if I were losing all control, and I didn't know how to regain it.

Anxiety, fear, and depression. What could I possibly have to be anxious about? Depressed, why would I be? I was facedown in the gutter and had no idea how I'd gotten there, so I went to my OB, right back to where I always went.

Sitting in his office that day, I knew I was in trouble. Sobbing, and I mean sobbing, in a stranger's office, pleading for help, explaining to him that I didn't know how I was going to get through another day feeling the way I did. But it was okay because he had an answer for me.

Praise God, an answer. His answer was a prescription for lithium, an annoyed look, and come see me in six weeks for a follow-up. Six weeks—I didn't know if I was going to make it through the next twenty-four hours, and this man hands me a piece of paper and tells me I'm going to live for six more weeks.

I filled and guzzled my prescription and headed home.

Twenty years earlier my mother had received the same solution, only then it was Valium. They were handing it out like candy to keep all those nervous housewives quiet, and they told her to have a glass of wine at night with her Valium. That made life easier for all of us. Alcohol and pills—what a combo. I spent days sitting and watching the faucets drip. The lithium did keep me quiet. My anxiety lessened. I was the walking dead, so what's to be anxious about? However, that didn't solve any of the problems.

I was still fat, unfit, unhealthy. I still hated the Prince

—I just hated him slower. There were still two children I was 100 percent responsible for—other than twice monthly visits from the Prince—without a break. The isolation, loneliness, anger, fear, starvation (always trying another diet, that's the pattern)—it was just a little fuzzy now, harder to focus on for any length of time, but there nonetheless.

I kept getting fatter. The fatter I got, the more frustrated I got. The more frustrated I got, the more I ate.

Friends and family tried to help me in my hour, or hours, of need. I tried to help myself by joining a women's Bible-reading group. We met in the living room of a friend of mine, who was a mother of three. A couple of her friends joined us. Between us we had about fifteen kids, all needing something at one time or another. I'm not sure if this is what Gandhi did to reach his enlightened state, but I do know that enlightened I wasn't—fat I was.

We did our best to convince each other that since we were mothers now, looking good, feeling sexy, and liking the way we looked were secondary to being mothers. Everyone else in the group seemed to buy this theory, and I wasn't about to ostracize myself from the only social contact I had by standing up in the middle of our Bible-reading group and declaring my sexual needs. So I went along with it, feeling strange and alone, feeling that my needs were wrong, unimportant, and simple-minded. Even if I'd wanted to speak up, the lithium had taken all of the spunk right out of me.

My mother sat me down one day and said, "Look at you! Maybe if you lost some weight and got yourself together, you might get him back." She was talking about the Prince—not my spunk.

Nobody ever asked me if I wanted him back, or if I just wanted myself back. All I really wanted back was me.

Sexuality—ha! I've been in hibernation for a long time.

—Comment from a client

STOP THE INSANITY!

The thought of the Prince and his Princess lying in bed together, making love, made me crazy. It was difficult to live with. *He* had her to tell him how wonderful he was. How smart, how good-looking, how broad his shoulders were . . .

I had a bag of M&M's at 2:30 A.M. and "Love Boat" reruns to comfort me. Lying there, I would think about them making love.

Was he telling her the same things he told me?

Making the same sounds?

Whispering the same whispers?

But that is not what drove me insane. It was difficult, but after months of picturing them in bed together, I got used to it. What really drove me insane, the thing I could not let go of, was the injustice, the inequality, of my situation. I did not know where to put the hurt, anger, and fear that I felt whenever I thought of how different the Prince's rules were from mine. Why—because he has a penis? Why was it okay for this man not to give up his life? If I'd had a couple of affairs while we were married, "Your children would have been taken away from you like that," a lawyer told me as he snapped his fingers at me. "Take what you can get, this is a nonalimony state, little lady. Count your blessings: most women find themselves with nothing."

My goal was never "to take him for all he's worth." We had two babies. If I'm not mistaken, he was half of this—the sperm, and supersperm, and I was the egg. We did this together. Remember, we had all those long 1980s discussions about commitment, understanding, and equality. We had decided together that our children were to be raised at home. And I would stay home with them. Just because the Prince needed to be told his shoulders were broad by someone other than me was no reason to change our children's lives and our commitment to them.

The fight for any support at all was costly and laced with the insinuation that it's the wife out to screw the man financially. Well, I was in no position to screw anybody. I was getting fatter by the day and feeling more and more out of control. It was the Prince and his 28-inch waist that did the screwing.

During one of our many meetings, after a sum of $1,000 a month was mentioned as fair support, I asked a question: "I have two children, twelve months apart, and both still in diapers. How am I supposed to live on 1,000 dollars a month?"

This lawyer, who I'm sure had a wife and kids (and a girlfriend stashed in some apartment around town), looked at me and said, "Get a sugar daddy, darling." Granted, I was sitting in a law office in Dallas, Texas, but he was using a term that hadn't been used since *Saturday Night Fever* was a hit.

Sugar daddy?

Spare me.

Sitting in that office, surrounded by people who saw nothing wrong with this statement, I realized what I was dealing with: the Prince had the money; I had none. He had the rights; I had none. He had the job, so he had some borrowing power, if need be. I also had a job, and a pretty important one—raising two human beings. But it's not very high on the list of important positions in our society.

After months of fighting and borrowing money to fight, I was given $1,400 a month. With the mortgage to our castle $500 a month, nobody could accuse me of living high on the hog. With just the necessities—food, which I required plenty of, insurance, car costs, and so on, I was living below poverty level.

I had become a government statistic.

How did this happen to me?

I found myself grateful that I had a roof over my head. Grateful for the car I had, and scared to death that something would go wrong with it, because I couldn't afford to fix it.

I am painfully aware that $1,400 a month is a fortune for millions of single moms all over this country. I have since spoken with many families living on half that amount. Our government may not know this, but single motherhood is very much a reality, and many of these women and children are living below the poverty level or on the streets.

Imagine my situation with a bit of bad luck (as if I weren't having a run of bad luck anyway)—by bad luck I mean losing my health. Now, granted I was losing my mind quickly, and healthy you couldn't call me. At least I was still walking—slowly—but walking. But if I'd gotten sick and needed to be hospitalized, who knows what could have happened to us?

I tried to make a living. I tried everything. I taught cooking classes. I took in children and baby-sat. I did whatever I could to earn some extra cash. But there sure weren't any "sugar daddies" knocking at my door.

Why wasn't I feeling grateful? I was living up to my end of our deal. We were two intelligent adults who made decisions together that involved two other people, our children. I had not changed anything, but the Prince had, which was why I was paying such a high price.

I understand now that I was lucky. But at that time all I could see was how wrong this was. I was being punished, and I hadn't done anything wrong.

His life was getting better; I was drowning. That's what drove me insane. But rather than go crazy, I threw myself into being a mom.

"So what if we can't afford books, boys, there's always the public library. We'll cut back, and I'll stick to my standards. I'll be a great mom. We'll have a wonderful family, and it will all be okay."

This lasted until the first of the twice-a-month (socially acceptable) father visits.

The Prince pulls up with someone in his car. Both are well dressed, tan, and thin. They're laughing, the "throw their heads back" kind of laughter. (Yes, I was looking out the window—crouching behind a chair is not an easy feat when you're 200 plus—watching them laughing.)

My mind was playing it all in slow motion: those tan, beautiful faces . . . smiling and laughing. S-L-O-W-L-Y their heads are thrown back in laughter. They look into each other's eyes with love and affection. (Wondering how I caught the details of the love and affection in their eyes? Okay, okay, the binoculars were there. What was I supposed to do—not use them?)

Then the Prince gets out of his car, looking back at his beloved one last time before their three-minute separation (which was going to be torture for both of them, I'm sure), and comes to the door to pick up the kids. I am hovering in the corner at the window, sort of stuck between the chair and the wall ("wedged" is a better word). The children are waiting at the door, so excited to see anyone other than the insane wedged woman in the corner as the doorbell rings.

You tell me how I'm supposed to answer the door. Other than being Samantha on "Bewitched," twinkling my nose and instantly looking better than the babe in the car, there was nothing I could do to take away the humiliation, pain, anger, and embarrassment that answering the door was going to cause.

So I didn't.

I just stood there . . . the kids waiting, the Prince standing outside wondering if I'd gone deaf in the process of getting fat, and me frozen. My resolve of pulling myself up by the bootstraps, getting on with my life, and just being a good mom was weakening fast.

I wasn't just a mom. I was Susan, a person, and Susan was dying.

> My husband constantly makes fun of me and says cruel and hurtful things. He likes to make himself feel big at my expense.
> —M. Jane, a client

At one point during the spiral downward, I really went nuts. The Prince was supposed to come for his visit and had to cancel two weeks in a row because he had to work. People, family, and friends would make it clear to me that I was obligated to understand that the manly

STOP THE INSANITY!

Prince had to work. You know—a job. What in the hell everyone thought I was doing was beyond me.

I had been working nonstop for weeks. My job allowed barely any sleep for days on end, lots of bending, picking up, and running around, no social contact, and certainly no time off. The Prince had time off—hadn't he and his Princess gone water-skiing the previous Monday? Nobody was supporting, encouraging, or loving me—and certainly not water-skiing with me. It was a given that because I had a uterus I would stand by the kids, be the best mother I could, and give up dreams and goals without a second thought.

The first time he canceled, I dealt with it. I told the boys that Daddy really did love them. He was very busy, and we must all understand (cursing him under my breath the whole time!).

But cancellation number two was the famous straw that broke the camel's back. When he called to cancel, I told him he needed to come over immediately, it was an emergency of sorts.

I have never been so close to a breaking point in my life as I was that weekend. I pulled a *Kramer vs. Kramer*.

The Prince came over.

I told him I just needed a few hours.

The Prince made it very clear to me that he had to get back to work and could do "this" only until five—it was three P.M.

I watched him drive away with my babies in the back. I turned around and picked up the suitcase I had packed; gathered up the keys, the checkbook, and note explaining that I was gone and put them on the mantel (isn't that exactly where Meryl Streep put everything before she left?); then got in my car and drove to the airport.

Driving to the airport was so painful—the most gut-wrenching experience I've ever had. I have never loved anybody the way I love my children. I needed to be a good mother. I needed to love and nurture them. And I wanted more for them than anyone or anything else in my life.

But I was literally dying.
I could no longer function.
I couldn't breathe anymore because it hurt so bad.
I flew to California.

My most humiliating moment in public was . . .

The first time I sat on an airplane and the seat belt would not go around me. I had to ask for assistance. The stewardess gave me an extension.
                    —Catherine, Phoenix, Arizona

A very dear friend was living on Balboa Island in California. The hippest of hip live on Balboa Island—at least they did in the 1980s.

She had a great apartment on the water, and water being the rejuvenating force it is, my first thought was to drown myself. Maybe I'd feel better. If I wasn't the walking dead when I got there, I was heading in that direction fast.

The phone calls began almost immediately—parents, friends, and what seemed like total strangers telling me what a horrible person I was.

Isn't it interesting how men "leave" their families, but women "abandon" their children?

The Prince hadn't seen his kids in almost four weeks. Nobody called him and told him that he was abandoning them.

Why not?

It was impossible for me to explain to my tall, lean, beautiful living-in-California friend the pain of leaving my children because I could no longer function. She tried to understand—but she needed to figure out which guy she liked most out of the forty who were asking her out. This took some thought.

But she had a brilliant suggestion.

She decided that I needed to get out and get some sun —there's that other healing force of nature. Go to the beach; that's the advice people dying of depression get.

STOP THE INSANITY!

Fresh air and sunshine. The amazing part is that I agreed to go. Did I mention that my friend had the longest, most beautiful legs in the world?

Sitting on the beach, surrounded by tan boys playing volleyball, only reminded me of what my sons would look like in twenty years—except that they would be all screwed up because their mother left them to go to California when they were young. So there we were, the beached whale (that was me) and the mermaid (you guessed it—my friend).

I was embarrassed to walk to the water, so I burned to a crisp.

I was embarrassed to walk to the bathroom, so I almost exploded.

I was afraid to say a word, because I was scared I would break down in tears.

Too afraid to do anything. So I just sat in the sun for hours. We stayed because the beach is fun for a tall, skinny, tanned beauty surrounded by volleyball-playing boys. I was in such emotional pain that I thought nothing could match it until we got home that night and the sunburn kicked in.

My friend tried to console me because she loved me. I tried to explain the millions of thoughts, questions, and fears going on nonstop in my brain. I couldn't sleep, couldn't eat except for the M&Ms, and I didn't know what to do.

Move the kids away from Texas . . . start my own life? But what about their rights? What about growing up without their daddy? I could go back, put them in day care, get a job, and stop being a full-time mom. Or I could stay, do the *Kramer vs. Kramer* thing, get on with my life, stand up for my rights above and beyond anybody else's. Or I could read the books and try to "win my man back" (a thought that made me want to puke). All of this was going through my head, and I couldn't stop it.

After three days I ran home to my kids, knowing I could never, ever, ever live without them. Whatever I was going to have to do; however I was going to make it work; it would be me and the two boys forever, doing it alone.

The Prince was as close to a king as any man could get by the time his irresponsible, emotional wreck of an ex-wife returned to the nest.

"No wonder he left her," they were saying. "He's such a good man, working and taking care of those kids like that for three whole days."

Get the maidens.

Get the horse and carriage.

THE PRINCE MUST RETURN TO WORK!

I live daily with depression and hate the way I look. I am always exhausted and constantly discouraged. Will this ever end?
—M. Jane, a client

I went right back to where I left off, doing the Mom thing. This meant very little sleep, isolation, and no time off.

Finally, one day I woke up. My planned activity for the day was going to the post office to mail a letter—in the heat of summer in Dallas, Texas. I think it was 102 degrees that day. Dallas in summer is hotter than you can imagine, unless you live in Arizona. And when you weigh 260 pounds, 102 degrees feels like 402 degrees.

By the time I got everything in the car—two car seats, two diaper bags, two babies, me at the wheel—I couldn't move. We just sat there. I never left the driveway. Can't you see the headlines: TWO CHILDREN AND FAT MOM SUFFOCATE IN BOILING CAR . . . film at eleven.

We sat for a long time, me sobbing uncontrollably and the kids staring at the back of the head of what was left of their mother. The post office closed, and the letter never got mailed.

With all the courage I had, all the strength I could muster, all the determination, motivation, and control that was in me, I decided to make a change.

STOP THE INSANITY!

> I went to one Overeaters Anonymous meeting. Two
> people showed up. The gal who led the meeting suf-
> fered from anorexia. I never went back.
> —Andra, a client

So what did I do? I did what all of us have done. I went
to the diet industry—the first biggest mistake of my life.
With all the courage, strength, and what little cash I had,
I went on a doctor-sponsored fast program. Along with
my packets of instant food, the doctor gave me pills—
diet pills. Boy, let me tell you, that really calmed me
down. Helped me get through the day. Hormonally nuts,
fat as they come, depressed, starving, and doing diet
pills. A walking time bomb, raising kids.

Did I mention doctor-sponsored?

I was put on an 800-calorie-a-day diet. Shake that
shake, drink that drink twice a day, and somehow figure
out how to eat that "healthy meal in the evening." My
thought at the time was, and still is, If I knew how to eat
those healthy meals, why would I be here? I wouldn't
need you people in your white coats teaching me anything. But who was I? The fat housewife begging for
help.

I shook the shake and drank the drink, and yes, I lost
weight. Here's something to keep in mind: When you
stop eating you are sure to lose weight.

How's that for brilliant?

Pay me $3,500 for that advice!

I lost the weight, and I gained it back: 20 here, 15 back.
Lose 30, gain 28. Lose 70, gain 82—you know how that
goes. As fast as it comes off, it comes back. Boom,
you're fat again. When one fast didn't work (or the way I
saw it, when I failed), I'd try another.

You can buy these shakes in convenience stores now.
Convenient physical and emotional death. That's exactly
what it is.

I didn't care about the physical damage that the old yo-
yo syndrome brings with it. Destroy my body, lose internal organs—who cares, as long as I get skinny; that's all
that mattered. But what was devastating was the emo-

tional damage that went hand in hand with each failure. Every time I failed, it was me that was failing. Never the diet—ME. What was wrong with me? Why couldn't I do what it took to stay on a diet and get back to what I was before all this happened to me?

We all know that fat people lack willpower. Anyone who has been on a diet for more than five minutes deserves a medal as far as I'm concerned. Most women I know have lived with starvation their whole lives. The starvation of three square meals of diet food a day is one thing, the total starvation that comes with those liquid fasts is quite another. If you deserve a medal for dieting, then it's a Nobel Peace Prize you should get for sticking to those liquid fasts.

I did have the willpower (and so do you!). But somehow I always found myself at the fridge door, shoving food in my mouth. At the time I thought I was the only one who couldn't keep the weight off. Something was wrong with me. I began giving myself the old metabolic problem story. That's it, something's gone haywire since having babies and the explosion. My body is incapable of losing weight for any length of time. Something was wrong with me. But I didn't know then what I was soon to find out, the statistics, the truth:

FULLY 98 PERCENT OF ALL OF US ON ANY DIET ARE GAINING THE WEIGHT BACK.

FAILING.

All I knew and felt at the time was that I was failing and that I felt so unbelievably alone in my failure.

My dieting wasn't working. My body couldn't be retrieved. It was over. The Prince's girlfriends were able to stick to diets and be permanently thin. I was incapable.

So forget the diets. They weren't working, and I'd tried every one. I knew then what I needed to do. Since the diets weren't happening and we all know that exercise has something to do with feeling and looking better, I found my answer, the new hope. I'd go to the fitness industry.

Simple concept, frightening reality. If you are out of shape and don't feel well, you turn to the fitness industry.

STOP THE INSANITY!

I always felt like a misfit in my oversize sweatsuit (in navy or black—no decals, stripes, or ornamentation to call attention to myself). It seemed like everyone else in the room was already in terrific shape. I was always the one sweating bullets and huffing and puffing. It was embarrassing.

—Comment from a client

So I walked into an aerobics studio, with two kids in tow at eight o'clock in the morning. The fact that I got there at eight A.M. deserved recognition, a medal, a statue—something. However, what I got was totally different.

After getting both boys (who were perfectly dressed) to the nursery, I went to the front desk to sign in for class. I had to stop for a second and catch my breath because a clone of the Prince's girlfriend was sitting behind the front desk. She was somewhere between the ages of 12 and 18, with big, big blond hair, dumb as a barrel of nails, you know the rest. Looking down—pretending to read. (He didn't sleep with girls who could read.) I could read, and he left me.

I went to the desk and said, "Hi, I'm here to register for the eight-fifteen class." She looked up from her pretend book, held her hand to her mouth, and gasped, "Oh, my God."

Oh, my God?

My first thought was to throw my full 260 across the desk and suffocate her with my huge breasts. Let's show her what 260 can do.

Than I looked around and realized that there wasn't a fat person within a ten-mile radius. The jewelry on some of these women could have paid the mortgage on the castle (okay, the crappy little house in Garland; I was finally seeing it for what it was) for months. And the neon in the place was blinding.

At this point I had three options: Get the kids and run out of there. No, impossible—I couldn't run fast enough. Suffocate the clone—a serious consideration. Or, take the class. I picked number three—I took the class. Big mistake, but one I'm sure I have grown from since. (There's that metaphysical wisdom again.)

I had to do a double, double take when I walked into the aerobics room, because a clone of the clone was teaching the class. They all looked like the Prince's girl-friends . . . they were everywhere.

The teacher was staring at herself in the mirror while her class was assembling behind her. She didn't seem to notice the 260-pound woman who had just walked into her room. So I had to give credit where credit was due, and assume she was

a. visually impaired
b. not very bright
c. totally and legally blind.

I chose c., because that's what you would have had to be not to notice me, a 260-pound woman, walk into your aerobics class. Obvious is an understatement.

Bambi walked to the stereo, picked up the mike, and started her class. The music was blaring. There were 45 people in the room (when you are the only fat, unfit, uncoordinated person in the room, and it's your first class, it feels like there are 145 people jumping around), and she launched into her class.

Screaming and jumping; she kept yelling—yelling and suggesting I do the impossible.

"C'mon and breathe!" was her first command.

Breathe? I thought. You want me to breathe and jump up and down at the same time? How, Bambi, oh, how am I supposed to do that? Can't you see (sorry, I forgot you are blind) that I'm turning blue? How can I breathe, jump, and be blue all at the same time?

"Smile!" was her next command.

Let me get this straight—you want me to jump, breathe, and smile?

Why, Bambi, why?

Will smiling make me skinny?

If so, I'll smile like you've never seen anyone smile.

Will smiling make this hurt less?

Then by all means, I'll smile.

Will smiling make any difference in the pain and humiliation I'm feeling at this very moment?

Then count me in, Bambi . . .

Apparently, if you weren't in the same shape as the clone teaching the class and everyone else in the room, you were flat out of luck. No modification was given for any movement. No option. No choices. Do this or the hell with you!

"Abs in!" she yelled.

This command made me take back all my nasty thoughts about Bambi, condemn myself for my inability to give this "genius" who was teaching the class any credit at all, and think about running to the confessional booth the next morning—even though it had been years since I'd walked into one.

Bambi was going to tell me how to hold my abs in. My abs were hanging halfway down my thigh. Who needs cosmetic surgery when you've got Bambi?

She never got to "how."

She never told me how I was supposed to breathe and jump at the same time.

She never told me why I should smile.

And she couldn't tell me how I was going to be able to hold my abs in.

I never went back.

Remember, fat people have no willpower—that's why they don't stick to exercise programs. Did you know that? It's the lack of willpower and discipline—yeah, that's the problem. Of course, it wouldn't have anything to do with the fact that, other than the insulting "fat people only" classes, there is nothing available for fat people.

There are no modifications being taught.

If you can't keep up, for whatever reason, you are out.

If you're gasping for air . . . oh, well.

If you don't want to be Baryshnikov . . . later for you.

If you have any physical considerations . . . too bad.

And if you are not coordinated enough to keep up, to hell with you, they will steamroll right past you.

I never went back, because my fitness experience left me feeling humiliated, physically hurting, and embarrassed. I ended up sitting in the parking lot sobbing.

Anger is a signal, and one worth listening to.
—Harriet Lerner,
The Dance of Anger (1985)

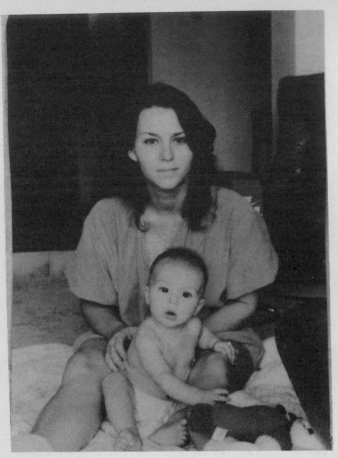

To this day, I look at this picture and cry. My son is six months old. Isn't he beautiful? Look at his face. I'm four months pregnant. Pregnancy didn't make me fat. Of course, I was dying in this shot. Nauseated, tired, not thrilled to be pregnant again. And my marriage was on the rocks big time—not a fun time in my life, but the cutest kid on earth. Hey, look at me with hair, what do you think?

I Quit!

THREE

I have not failed 10,000 times,
I have successfully found 10,000 ways that will not work.
THOMAS A. EDISON

Our society judges a fat woman much differently than it does a fat man. I know this is not news to many of you, and it's not news to any woman who has been or is fat. A fat man is a "big guy" who "probably played some ball in high school"—a redwood of a man who is strong and can hold his own. A fat woman is an undisciplined, lazy, emotional wreck.

The choices, basic freedoms, and everyday life are very different when you're fat. Grocery shopping as a fat person meant that every time I put something fattening in the cart—and there were lots of those (you don't get to be 260 by buying and eating only veggies)—people whispered. I know that I was bordering on a nervous breakdown at this time in my life, and it would be easy for you to assume that hiding food in a grocery cart and thinking people were whispering were part of the breakdown you're going to read about. But I promise you, they did whisper, stare, and give me pathetic looks.

"Poor thing, she can't control her eating."

"Let's drop some 12 Step eating disorder information in her cart." Good intentions, bad feeling, finding that on top of the ice cream.

STOP THE INSANITY!

People do look at the food that a fat woman has in her cart and assume she's fat because she has no discipline. But that redwood of a man "needs" all that food.

"Healthy appetite, that guy."

"What a powerhouse that boy is!"

"Probably playing ball this afternoon; needs that stuff to keep going."

My strategy with the foods that I usually ended up eating in the parking lot—you know, the Ding Dongs, cream pies, and snacky things—was to stick them in the bottom of the cart, where they were hard to get at. Anything to avoid the stares. And I strategically placed all the diet foods and healthful alternatives on top, so at least I got the "poor thing, she's trying hard with all that dieting, and nothing seems to be happening" stare.

How do I know what people were thinking? Well, first, I was the fat woman getting the stares. Now I'm not, and maybe because of what I do for a living—you know, the health and fitness thing—people seem to feel obligated to comment on every fat person they see and what's in their carts.

"Susan, over to the left, there is someone who really needs you—go on, talk to them. Look, look, between the sausage and the ice cream, this person is lucky to be walking around. Give her your card, talk to her." It's amazing how many eating disorder experts there are in this world and how many stories someone can come up with just by looking at another's grocery cart. A person's whole life story told in one cart.

Shopping for groceries now means neon signs flashing —check it out (pardon the pun), look at all the food she's buying and eating within a couple of days. I leave the store with carts full of food, and the flags are waving, the trumpets blowing. And now people look and say:

"Wasn't she lucky to be born with a metabolism that burns fuel at the speed of light?"

"All that food and such a lovely figure!"

"She's one of the lucky ones."

"And what in the hell is the deal with her hair?" (Yes,

let's not pretend they don't think that along with the "lovely figure" comments.)

Luck, of course, has nothing to do with any of it. And discrimination against fat people doesn't end with grocery shopping.

> Food became my mother when my real mother neglected me. Food was my friend. When I get full, I can't wait until I can eat again. Two cartons of Häagen-Dazs—no problem.
>
> —Ann, a client

How do you hide when you're 260 pounds? Where do you go when you see someone who "knew you when" and you can't face another shocked expression on the face of an old acquaintance who's trying not to look shocked?

There's physical pain in this world, stubbing your toe on the way to the bathroom in the middle of the night, catching a baseball with a fingernail (do I have a baseball-catching nail story), birthing a 10-pound baby. And then there's emotional pain. I'd rather stub all my toes while I'm catching the baseball with all my nails, and birth three 10-pound babies at once, than face Harry and Vicki again in the ice-cream store.

Harry and Vicki knew me before I married the Prince. Sure, they'd seen me a little on the heavy side and rail thin (starvation does it every time), but nothing prepared them for what they saw when they walked into the ice-cream store that evening.

My sister-in-law—tall, beautiful, and a professional model—and I had gone to get ice cream together. Going out for ice cream was very different for a professional model than it was for me—260 pounds, severely depressed, wearing the same clothes that the baby had thrown up on hours before (every new mother I've ever met has a little vomit on her shoulder).

My sister-in-law loves and accepts me for what I am, so my physical and emotional state at the time didn't affect her. But Harry and Vicki only knew me "when," so who could blame them for almost falling on the floor of that little ice-cream parlor when they spotted me across the room, licking a double-double rocky road?

I was too engrossed in the double-double to notice them until Harry walked up and said, "Susan, hey, what's going on? . . . You look great."

I looked up, stopped licking, almost died, and said, "Harry, stop lying to me, I'm 260 pounds, eating an ice cream. Don't tell me I look great."

The poor guy didn't know how to respond, because it was the God's honest truth and he knew it, so his gracious wife took over and steered the conversation in a much more pleasant direction, covering everything but weight gain, depression, life in the gutter, and divorce. Women are so good at that, don't you think? Make nice. Mend it. Take over. Harry and I laugh about the incident to this day; however, at the time, my usual quick, funny response failed me. Sure, while we were standing there making nice, we laughed, talked about my sister-in-law's modeling career, said we'd all get together for lunch someday, and said our good-byes. Vicki and Harry simply walked out to their car and into their healthy, productive lives. I left and died.

Died from shame, embarrassment, and guilt—for months. Some may say that's a little extreme—one conversation sending you into a tailspin for months. But you know what the pain and the consequences of an encounter like that are: months of binge eating. Emotionally beating yourself to a pulp. A starvation diet or two thrown in for good measure: "I'm gonna do it this time, no matter what it takes, even if I've got to kill myself to be thin, count me in, I'm there." The failure, more binge eating, more emotional beating . . . and it continues, the cycle that so many of us are caught in. The constant struggle, endless pain, and continual starvation of the insanity.

Oh, did I mention that Harry and Vicki own a clothing store? I shop there from time to time, and it's a whole different world now. When my husband and I have some function to attend—because unless I'm attending one, you'll find me in sweats, jeans, or shorts, depending on the season and whatever's the easiest and most comfortable—I go pick something up at Harry and Vicki's store.

Now buying a size 2, 4, or 6—European styles sometimes run in crazy sizes—is a very different "emotional" experience from getting caught sucking down a double-double rocky road and feeling like you want to crawl (knowing that it would be physically impossible for you to get down to begin crawling) into the closest, largest corner and die.

I don't eat ice cream anymore. I've had a few people ask me over the years, "Don't you miss burgers and ice cream?"

"Are you always so good?"

"Don't you ever cheat?"

"Come on, just one scoop of marble fudge won't hurt."

Well, let me tell you about the marble fudge. First of all, there are plenty of low-fat, creamy alternatives to ice cream. If I want the cookies with the ice cream in the middle just before my period or right after the fight with my husband, I'll have it. If creamy and sweet is all I can think about at the time, then creamy and sweet it will be —believe me, I stink at behavior mod. But you will never see me eating something that will make me fat, clog my arteries, and make me look and feel the way I did when I was fat and unfit. I want to be lean, not fat, and no flavor of ice cream in the world could ever tempt me enough to end up at that ice-cream parlor dying of shame.

None.

Most of my fondest childhood memories center around holidays and other occasions where families got together and ate special foods. In my mind these childhood memories create a comforting feeling surrounded by food. So at times I eat to feel comfort and love.

—Lisa, Ione, Washington

You want embarrassing? How about going out to dinner? I never, never, never ordered big when I was fat.

STOP THE INSANITY!

Haven't you noticed that the larger the woman, the smaller the amount of food she has in front of her? You'll never see a fat woman at a table covered with food, a pitcher of beer in the middle, and another on the way. (You'll see those big guys doing it all the time—but remember, they've got that game this afternoon, and God knows they need the fuel.)

My manager and I were eating at a Mexican restaurant recently, and when I tell you our table was covered with food, I'm talking about almost having to pull tables together to accommodate it all. The pitcher of beer was in the middle, and another was on the way. (One day I'm going to write a "how to have a business meeting" guide, and this particular lunch will be the example used.) There was a woman sitting three tables away who made me want to cry. She was a large woman stuffed into a business suit—from the bow at the top to the panty hose at the bottom—and she looked uncomfortable and self-conscious. Her plate had a couple of enchiladas and a salad on it. Barely any food, certainly not enough to get her through the rest of the afternoon. What she didn't know, and what took everything in my being not to jump in her lap and tell her, was that what was decorating the top of, stuffed inside of, and melted on the top of her food was what was making her fat.

I wanted to invite her over, tell her to blow off work for the rest of the afternoon, get her something big, cotton, and comfortable to put on, give her a beer, and chat with her about the difference between what she was having for lunch and what my manager and I were eating. Don't you think she would have enjoyed our lunch break more than hers? If nothing else, she would have walked away full enough to get through the day.

My worst clothing experience was . . .

Having gotten so big that the size 18's didn't fit anymore.

—Peggy, a client

Still, as bad as it was to order a meal in public, I would rather sit naked, weighing 260 pounds, in a restaurant than go shopping again as a larger woman. When you're fat, shopping for clothes is almost indescribable. It's a horrible experience.

First there are the specialty shops. It's wonderful that there's an alternative. I mean, otherwise there would be a lot of naked fat people walking around, because they sure can't find anything in normal stores. As soon as you get past size 16, you are no longer normal. Now there's a feeling I remember well—going into a regular store and being "outracked," banished from the normal-size clothing wheel. Running out of little white tags to turn to. Size 6–8, in my dreams; 8–10, I'd die for; 10–12 would have thrilled me; 12–14, okay, it'll do; 14–16, surely it would fit; 16–18 . . . I was scared. After not being able to pull the 14–16 over my knees, I was scared to try the 16–18. What would happen if it didn't fit?

I was held hostage in a dressing room in Dallas, Texas, by one of those little white tags. The 16–18 didn't fit. It didn't fit anything. The kids were playing on the floor, the saleslady came by and asked if she could bring me anything else.

A gun?

Some Valium?

Cupcakes?

Anything in the last size left that would make me feel as if I were just a little on the heavy size.

Anything that would make me feel like a normal human being.

Anything that would help me get out of the dressing room.

It was a total surprise to me that I'd grown out of the regular people's sizes. Talk about denial. I had been too busy cleaning the house, picking up after the boys, and hating the Prince to notice that I'd gone back to wearing my maternity clothes. This was not a good sign. And only a few pieces fit. Of course, wearing the same maternity dress over and over again was a sign of efficiency to me. I didn't want to spend unnecessary money. Forget the fact that nothing else fit—yeah, saving money was my motivation.

Besides, looking good didn't seem to matter much to me anymore, being a new mom and all. I was above caring about how I looked; there were children to raise, more important things to get on with. It's much easier to live with reasons like that than to live with the truth. And the truth, and the white tag, held me hostage that day in the dressing room. I was stuck. I couldn't move. Where was there to go?

Back to the house, the same dress, and the fridge for a few more weeks, until I pulled myself together enough to go to a specialty shop and get something to wear.

How about the names of some of these places? Proud Woman. Forgotten Ladies. Big and round, tents all around. We are *fat*, damn it.

I went into our local larger gals store feeling as if I had a sign on my back announcing to the world that I could no longer shop off the regular racks.

The saleslady, who had the tone of a funeral director, suggested some lovely things in my size and brought them to the dressing room for me to try.

God, please tell me why, why, did they make this dress, in this size, in stripes? I looked like a balloon-a-gram when I put it on. Why would I want to announce to the world that I'd hit the low 20's in dress sizes by appearing anywhere in public in a bold stripe pattern? Some man who hated fat women designed the first specialty store dress I ever tried on, probably the same guy who designed panty hose. Find him, I want to talk to him.

As the saleslady brought me things, my mind would play tricks on me. Truly, every item she handed me gave me hope. The dress, pants, top, whatever would look as if it had potential, potential to look normal on me. To make me look as though my mind had me believing I looked—a little bit heavy; sure, I'd gained some weight —but not the way I looked when I put the 20-plus size clothes on. I looked like a fat person. There was no denying these sizes or these clothes. Things may have changed in the last couple of years, but until very recently the clothes that were available for larger gals, and certainly the ones in my price range, looked as if they were made from a carpet remnant sale.

They had elastic waists, special darts, fabric with the ability to stretch a bit, no waists, and those bright, cheery prints. These were special clothes, designed for fat people, and I was in the dressing room hallucinating that every item the funeral director saleslady handed me was going to look good on me and that I could possibly walk out of there with some semblance of normalcy. I was afraid. Are there specialty-specialty shops? Can you outsize yourself? If I could get to the 20's, could I get to the 50's? Is there a size 50? All new questions, all new fears, all new reasons to eat and to hate the Prince.

A friend of ours brought some friends over, and while we were sitting, my pants split apart from the zipper. Luckily no one noticed. I would also wear out the inner thighs of pants before the rest of the pants wore out.

—Andra, a client

Then there is beyond scary. There is the bathing suit.

The dreaded, hateful, torturous bathing suit.

The piece of clothing that was designed to remind women every year that they just can't cut it.

Their bodies aren't good enough to wear it.

The first half of every year is spent dreading it, dieting for it, and hoping that this year you'll look good enough to wear it.

My blue-and-white number caused me unbelievable embarrassment even before I strolled the beach wearing it. My friend, the one I ran to during my *Kramer vs. Kramer* period, was kind enough to pretend that watching a 260-pound woman squeeze into a bathing suit in the fitting room was not an unusual sight. Nothing out of the ordinary for this 6-foot, size 8 beauty.

We'd always gone shopping together, trying on clothes and asking each other's opinions. No difference this time. The fact that her friend was severely depressed, morbidly obese, and dying inside and out was not going to be talked about on this little shopping trip to buy a new bathing suit so we could go out and get that fresh air and sunshine that were going to save my life.

Standing in that dressing room, staring at myself in the blue-and-white number with my friend trying to make small talk to make it all okay—I mean, what could she say?

"It looks nice"?

"The blue really makes your skin look good"? (Helps detract from the bumpy, clumpy cottage cheese–like stuff all over your legs and thighs.)

"Those lines flatter you"? (Even the fashion magazines only have flattering line suggestions up to a certain size. Then they stop, as if the rest of us don't exist. You don't see in those articles, "For that 300-pound bottom, the vertical straight skirt flatters the most. Best line, best look, for all 300 pounds—it will give the illusion of being nothing more than 250.")

The more my friend said, trying to make me feel better, the more I wanted to hide.

Run away.

Pretend none of this was happening.

Go get something to eat to soothe my aching heart.

Murder the Prince. (My murderous instincts always got stronger during moments like this. Clothing stores were very dangerous places for the Prince.)

> I had to face the facts, I was pear-shaped.
> I was a bit depressed because I hate pears.
> —Charlotte Bingham
> *Cornet Among the Weeds*, 1963

One of the most painful reconciliation attempts combined with heavy dieting came as the supersaver attempt for the marriage. I can remember starving for five days in a row, along with drinking that strawberry-, chocolate-, and vanilla-flavored shake. The shake days were considered my eating days—getting ready for the BIG ROMANTIC TRIP.

Like you and millions of our other friends, I had thought that getting skinny ("fit" wasn't in my vocabulary then) would solve my problems with the Prince and everything else. My weight had gone down every time I went on a diet, which was right after the one I'd been on failed. So the Prince had gotten used to the losing and regaining look. Each new diet brought with it that unbelievable excitement of "This one is going to work!" Of course I'd share this with my Prince.

"I'll have more energy when I'm skinny. We can go more places and do more things together."

"This time I'm going to do it! Let's go on a romantic weekend to the beach when I get this weight off. . . ." If I'd known, I would have included his girlfriend . . . God knows he wouldn't have gone without her—can't be away that long.

Hate to keep referring to the babe—why harp on what you already know?—but I could have been Superwoman, with enough energy to topple large buildings, and it would not have solved the problems the Prince and I had.

The Prince wanted to spend some time with his sister. Got to get him what he wants, so the dutiful wife planned a trip to visit her.

Planning.

Starving.

That's what I spent my time doing before the trip.

Organizing the kids. It was the first time I'd left them for more than a couple of hours. It's not exactly easy to find someone you trust and like who will take two babies, one year apart, from Friday to Monday because you need to save your marriage. But I managed.

The kids organized, the house cleaned and ready to come home to, the Prince ready to go, the wife starving to death and worrying about and missing the kids before we got to the terminal at the airport. But I was determined to have a romantic weekend with the Prince—to bring back what had been lost.

I made a hell of an attempt. Emotionally and physically starving while touring the wine country, I could not have cared less, because I knew my romantic weekend wasn't working. The "romantic" bed and breakfast inn I'd booked hadn't gone over that big. "So flowery and fluffy," the Prince commented as we walked up the stairs to our love nest.

The canopied bed, with the heart-shaped pillows, was used for sleeping and very little else. As hard as I tried, I couldn't get my Prince to notice my new, hard-won body. Maybe it wasn't perfect, but it was getting better.

Surely he'd notice how much effort I was putting into regaining a body that he would be interested in.

Give credit where credit is due. Isn't that a universal principle?

Throw me a bone, something.

Make me feel like you care.

Notice something.

Compliment me.

Make love to me.

Act.

Pretend.

Please, do something because I'm dying. Can't you see that?

One of the things the Prince shared with me, on his way out the door for the last time, was about that trip to San Francisco: "Susan, I tried hard to connect with you, but you're just not the same person you used to be."

A couple of hundred dollars in debt, owing my friend my life for watching both my kids (along with her four) so my husband and I could make it all right, more pain inside than I can describe, a broken heart—and again, it was over. No, I wasn't the same person the Prince had met, and I never would be again. My mind was different; God knows my body was different. I was not functioning well. My life was different. I had two babies, a body to fix, a mind to quiet, and a broken spirit that needed fixing. I hardly recognized myself, so I sure as hell couldn't expect him to recognize me.

My dream.

The white picket fence.

It blew sky high, leaving me with the shrapnel from a

life that I thought was going to save me. The rubble after the blast was hard to look at, but it was all I had.

> People change and forget to tell each other.
> —Lillian Hellman
> *Toys in the Attic,* 1960

It is different now. The way people see me, judge me, speak to me, and respond to me is different. It may be unjust, unequal, and wrong—discrimination against fat people does exist, though it may be wrong—but it's a reality.

I like grocery shopping now. Buying clothes is big fun, and going out to eat is almost obnoxious. And the Prince . . . well, we'll get to him later.

How did I finally get there? What happened? When was that magical moment? When did I get motivated enough to change my life?

Never.

There was no magical moment.

You know, the fairy godmother is a lie.

The diet and fitness industries have very little to offer you. I tried the fasts and the aerobics classes, and they didn't work. So I quit. Gave up.

The images that the magazines, TV, and diet and fitness industries offered were obviously far beyond my reach. I was never going to have that all-American, healthy, bring-home-the-bacon look, be the perfect mother, and still have the energy to be a sex goddess at night for the meat-and-potatoes kind of guy. I just gave it all up.

The minute, and I mean minute, I knew that I was never going to be any of those things is when it all began to change. My motivation was desperation. I could no longer live with the way I looked and felt. My body ached. I didn't have enough energy to get out of bed in the morning, let alone get through the day. I hated—hated—the way I looked and felt, and I lived in a black cloud of depression. There was no life left. I was the walking, functioning dead.

But just when I knew "normal" was never going to happen, I started thinking about what I wanted, defining my needs, my goals, thinking about how to get through the day.

To heck with looking better—I just had to *feel* better.

So I went for a walk. There wasn't a fitness goal or physical image in my mind. When I went for a walk I felt better, so I just took a walk.

I got up from the sofa. Took the kids outside. Put them under the tree in my front yard—not the picture-perfect conditions for walking—and went for a walk halfway down the block with my head turned watching the kids.

I wanted to walk forever. Walk away from my life and into someone else's, preferably that of a beautiful model, a successful businesswoman, or one of those women who have children and still fit into their "old high school blue jeans." Anybody's life other than the morbidly obese, depressed housewife's life I seemed to be living in. But I could walk only half a block before one of the boys began to crawl away from the tree. As close as I could to running, I hurried back, picked up one baby, walked another half a block up and back, picked up son number two, went the half block again, turned around, and continued going back and forth, alternating babies until I'd walked 30 minutes.

I should have known enough to call a film crew and tape what was happening, because it was a lot more realistic than any other exercise videotape on the market. But I never knew that someday I'd be teaching health and fitness—at 260 pounds, walking the same half block for 30 minutes with babies in my arms didn't have me fantasizing about being a size 2, teaching health and fitness, or writing a book about choices and changes for women. Talk about an unrealistic goal. We've all been told to keep our expectations realistic. . . .

That half block, 30 minutes a day, made me feel good. Arnold Schwarzenegger I was not by the end of the first week, but instead of being totally exhausted by 2 P.M. every day, the exhaustion didn't hit until 4 or 5 P.M. Not a big deal for anyone who hasn't been there, but who cares about them? If you've ever felt the desperate exhaustion that goes along with being fat, unfit, and unhealthy, then you know that being able to go all the way till 4 P.M. without feeling like you want to die is much more than a big improvement. It's a miracle. Even though I was never going to look good, fit into normal sizes, or have sex again for the rest of my life, I could hope to have energy and feel better, and all it took was a 30-minute walk.

So I kept walking. My strength began to improve almost immediately. It was difficult to move. Let's face it, when you're carrying around that much fat, it's a little cumbersome to get around. But I started to feel something I hadn't felt in years—muscle strength. I didn't need a degree in physiology to know that I'd lost some muscle strength. Living with the feeling that you can't hold yourself up, and the aches and pains that come with lack of upper body, abdominal, and lower body strength made me painfully aware of it every day. Use it or lose it —who said that? Rocky? Arnold? Whoever it was was right. I'd lost it, but I felt it creeping back.

Everyone has a different fitness level. Mine at the time was nonexistent. The nonexistent fitness level is what's kept more than half of America from moving. Unfit? Obese? Senior? Injured? Don't move. Wait until you're fit before you move. There's that logic I love so much. Here is where my passion/anger comes to a head. Don't try until you are fit. Thanks a lot, fellas—that helps.

I was unfit, fat, and had a nonexistent fitness level, so I walked at a very low level of intensity—but I moved every day, six and seven days a week, for those 30 minutes in oxygen.

And since I'd tried every diet under the sun, and none had worked for any length of time, why not eat? Not Ding Dongs—they get such a bashing with me because I love the name; Ding Dongs, have you ever? Whenever I ate junk, and there were days and weeks when that's all I ate, I felt lousy. Good while it was going down, lousy within minutes. Emotionally it was warm and soothing, physically it made me sick. So instead of eating junk, I started eating food. Replacing the obvious high-fat food with lower-fat, higher-quality food. Other than trying to stay away from anything white, creamy, loaded with sugar, and oiled to the max, I didn't think about food anymore. I just ate when I got hungry and drank when I was thirsty. (Remember how a baby eats?)

The scale got put in the corner of the bathroom. Why get on it when I was never going to see those numbers go down? If they did, it would only be temporary. They would eventually come right back up to the 200-plus range. Experience had taught me that, so who cared?

I didn't read one book on nutrition or exercise in the beginning. They all made me feel as if I needed a degree to read and understand them, and it was all so complicated. Complication was the last thing that I needed in my life. I was too tired and depressed to calculate, weigh, monitor, or think anymore about my every food move.

No more.

I didn't get the motivation. It wasn't my digging down deep to an untapped supply of motivation or energy that kept me going. When I combined the exercise—my 30-minute-a-day walk in oxygen—with food, baboom. Energy. More energy than I'd had in years. Eating, breathing, and moving made me feel better. Feeling better was my motivation to keep going. Curious feeling, having energy after living without it. One of my clients described it on the "Home" show as having more pep in his step. That's exactly what started to happen.

Waking up in the morning with a clear head and an ounce of energy is a whole different ball game from waking up wondering how you're going to get through the day. I began to make plans. Take the kids outside and play with them—actually enjoying it instead of playing with a black cloud over my head. Once in a great while I'd feel hope. Excitement that something was changing in my life, that there was a way out.

Motivation was at an all-time high one day, so I decided it was time for me to go beyond walking, learn more about this fitness thing, go to the experts. Off to the video store to get an exercise tape. The privacy of my own home was important after my horrible aerobic experience. Expertise—you couldn't get bigger than this name on the cover; we love her for her acting and aerobics. Motivation, well, that was in the bag until . . . I turned on the tape, ready and raring to go.

The disclaimer: We recommend you see a doctor if you're anything less than perfect. We are not responsible for anything. Good luck and good-bye.

Our famous aerobics instructor/actress was wearing a full-length lace unitard and high-heel boots. And the class! It was a dance—and I mean dance, as in Broadway, Follies, complicated choreography. That's not what it said on the front. "Aerobic workout" was what it said, not "I want to be a dancer more than life itself." With or without boots on, there was no chance. So I got something to eat and sat down to watch. What was I supposed to do to get fit? Motivation was not the problem. Seemed to be a theme in the aerobics industry: no modification of the routines for anyone who was below average in anything—especially coordination. I went from one videotape to another, trying to find anyone who was talking to me. Other than jumping and twisting to some old songs, there was nothing.

The diets had failed, and now the videos were getting dusty on the shelves. Searching for wellness in all the wrong places.

I wish someone would start a gym for people 150 pounds and over. If I had the money, I would. Programs geared for people whose muscles forgot they were ever there. In any other gym atmosphere, people have been taking care of themselves and are usually in pretty good shape. Their programs are not geared to the out-of-shape. Not to mention how embarrassing it is.

—Catherine, Phoenix, Arizona

Consider me temporarily insane—or maybe the little bit of oxygen I was getting was acting like a mind-altering drug—but since the videotape couldn't help, I thought

STOP THE INSANITY!

I'd try an aerobics studio again. Maybe it was a fluke, that first experience. I was a tad fitter now—after all, I'd been walking for weeks, so surely I could keep up.

For months I was the crazy fat lady in the back, lifting my leg once to each of the 50 repetitions by the instructor and her beautiful students. The difference in me wasn't so much the strength I'd gained from walking, but the fact that this time I didn't care. A disrespectful, naughty child was where I was mentally. To hell with them all. I'll do what I can do and get whatever works for me out of this because it's making me feel better. So what if they're making fun of me?

While the instructor jumped, smiled, and yelled her way through class, I would do what I could do—march in place when it was too much, which was every minute and a half, and try again.

Quick story: Years later in my own studio I was teaching a class and this woman walked into the lobby asking for information on the new studio in town, mine. I can see through the window into the lobby as I teach, and I immediately recognized her as one of the ladies in that morning class I had started in so long ago as a fat woman. She had no clue that this was the same Susan. She just knew that this Susan Powter Studio had popped up and was there to check it out.

I ran out into the hallway (yes, I let the class keep moving on their own) and said, "Hi, Mary—it's me, Susan."

Mary almost had a heart attack, which wouldn't have been good for business: WOMAN DIES IN LOBBY OF FITNESS CENTER AFTER TAKING ONE LOOK AT THE OWNER . . . news at eleven.

After the initial "How's everything going?" stuff got out of the way, she 'fessed up: "I've gotta tell you that when you first came into our aerobics class ["our" being the regulars who went every morning to that class], I thought you were fat and weird." "Fat and weird" is exactly what she said. "And now I can't believe what I'm seeing. Look at you, tiny, strong, looking fabulous, what's the deal with your hair, what did you do? I'm so excited, I want to take your class, this is big fun. . . .''

Mary is not only a client of my studio now, she has since trained to teach and—forget the law degree—is teaching women of all fitness levels how to begin to increase their cardio-endurance, increase their upper body, abdominal, and lower body strength, burn fat, and change their lives. Fat and weird, my butt.

Back to the aerobics class. I'm in the back room, lifting my leg once, pressing my arms up in the air slowly and without all that swinging everyone else was doing (it hurts to swing a large limb), just doing what I can do.

I had no clue then, but modification was born. Hey, what should have been the most important new discovery in the fitness industry in the last couple of years? Modification. The way to fitness and health for all levels, the magic, the motivation—I mean, after all, if you can actually do it, you would be much more motivated to, wouldn't you? With modification you can start now.

I knew eating, breathing, and moving were making a difference . . .

When my tight exercise pants were starting to look baggy and my exercise instructor said something about it.

—Lisa, a client

Very exciting, but we'll get to that—now it's on with my story. If it's a cliffhanger full of excitement and motivation you were looking for when you picked up this book, how's this? The most exciting and motivating thing happened to me one morning when I got up and put on my size 16–18 pants and they were loose. Not falling-to-my-ankles kind of loose, but loose enough for me to wonder if the fabric had stretched beyond its limit, finally worn out. After all, they were one of the three things I wore all the time. But they were loose enough for me to float around in on cloud nine for the rest of the week, knowing that something big was happening and I wasn't starving. I wasn't dieting, but my body was changing. The concept was crazy to me at the time, but it sure did feel good. Even if it was worn-out fabric, it sure did feel good to have loose pants.

That was great, but even more fun was the day the kids and I went to the mall. Funny thing, this go-to-the-mall business. It's something everybody told me to do when I was fat. My mother used to say, "Susan, why don't you get out, go to the mall for a while?"

Why, Mom?

So I can look at clothes that I can't fit into and can't afford?

That's going to be loads of fun for me and the kids.

Other than the walking, the mall was not going to do me an ounce of good. But they all kept telling me to go, and you've probably figured out by now that I used to do what I was told to do. So this day I went to the mall.

If I'd had a million dollars to spend, it would not have been as much fun as what happened to me that day, walking with the double stroller, double car seats, diaper bags, high chairs, double everything in my life. Remember, I had been walking in my neighborhood, getting fitter all the while, so my mall walk was a breeze. I was feeling good, loose pants and all, when suddenly it dawned on me.

That feeling I had lived with for so long.

That feeling that's a part of life for anyone who is on their way up the weight ladder.

That stinging, burning feeling that we all live with.

Chafing.

The chafing under your arms, inside your thighs, under the crevices as you lift the fat on your stomach.

The feeling that your bra has turned into a lethal weapon on those Texas hot afternoons. Putting on your panty hose and listening to that *ch,ch,ch,ch,ch,ch,ch,ch* sound that follows you around like an annoying relative.

IT WAS GONE.

MY THIGHS WERE NOT RUBBING TOGETHER.

Gone, as in not there anymore.

My thighs were not rubbing together anymore.

With all the grace my large frame and strong disposition allowed, I bent over and looked between my legs. I had to be careful, because bending over could still cause suffocation. My thighs may not have been rubbing together anymore, but that stomach was still a potential killer.

But when something is this exciting, who can contain themselves?

HEY, EVERYONE, MY THIGHS AREN'T RUBBING TOGETHER!

NO MORE BABY POWDER IN THE SUMMERTIME!

NO MORE STINGING!

IT'S NOT THE FABRIC, I'M SHRINKING!

MY BODY IS SHRINKING. . . .

A million bucks, and I mean it, couldn't have felt better at that moment. I was still large, still shopping in specialty stores, and still tired by five in the afternoon. But my thighs were not rubbing together, and my clothes were getting looser—this was big (pardon the pun) news.

That moment in the mall was not about the end result. It was truly the beginning of the end of fatness for me. Something good was happening, and I wasn't hungry all the time. This didn't take enormous amounts of willpower or behavior modification, and I wasn't walking around feeling like I was going to die. I had given up on ever getting sk—(that word that had disappeared from my vocabulary), but I was shrinking. This felt good, was easy, and made my thighs not rub together. So count me in, what more could anyone want?

Motivation? You couldn't have stopped me at this point. I was an eating and aerobics modification machine, and within six months I couldn't recognize my own reflection. I would stare, waiting for the rest of me to catch up. My body felt stronger because I had used muscles that hadn't been used in so long that any movement made them feel something. You know that flabby, soft, mushy feeling that you live with every day when you're fat? Well, that changes the minute you start using your muscles. It's as if they come back to life. I could almost feel the oxygen and blood pumping through my veins. When I woke up with the energy that oxygen gave me, it was back to class for me. Not much motivation or control involved, simply enough energy to do it. Soon I stopped thinking about the end result.

New beginnings left, right, and center—that's how you could describe my life during those first few months of eating, breathing, and moving. Still poor and definitely sexually deprived. The Prince wasn't the only one who needed to be held, loved, and told he had broad shoulders and a big penis. Well, drop the broad shoulders and big penis and substitute "You're looking so much better, doing so well, could be pretty." Anything out of the mouth of an adult male—now that's desperate—would have been fine at the time. Still, six months into this process I was feeling better than I had in years. I'd left the morbidly obese category behind. Now I was just fat. But I wasn't going bathing suit shopping any time soon. There was more to do and much more to learn before I was ready for a black string bikini.

> For the first time in a long time, there's a light back in my eyes! Actually, the pudge in my cheeks is down and you can SEE my eyes now! They're so pretty!
> —Comment from a client

I had to learn more about eating. A concept that scares the hell out of every woman I've ever spoken to, one that was very, very hard for me to accept.

I'm moving every day, modifying all the way, and then I started to figure out this eating thing. Whenever I went for any length of time without food or when I ate crappy food, I felt lousy.

When I ate, I felt better. Food was fuel. WOW, what a concept.

Fuel . . . and if you really want to get carried away, add oxygen to this mix. Let's pretend for one silly second that you added those two things to your life. Do you think it would affect the way you feel at all? According to the doctors I begged for help, no. Nothing at all, no connection under the sun. Stop being stupid, Miss Housewife, don't pretend that you have a brain in your head. Stop trying to figure it out, take this lithium, and go home.

Eating—food/fuel. Breathing—oxygen. Moving—modification. If it is this simple, why hasn't your doctor, dietitian, nutritionist, weight loss counselor, told you about this? Good question, and one that I started to ask myself as my chafing stopped and clothes got looser.

When I thought of the thousands of diets I'd gone on, desperately wanting to make it work this time, it dawned on me that the first thing we all do when we hate the way we look and feel is stop eating. Diet. Cut back on our fuel. Stop putting gas in the car. But when you go on your diet, do you stop functioning? Do you call your boss and tell him you won't be in for a few months, because you're not eating for a while and there won't be enough energy to work? Kids, husbands, bills, household, relatives—do you stop dealing with them all and just lie out by the lake?

No, I didn't, and you don't, either.

Yee-haaa, here we go. I figured it out. Calories are not the problem. Cutting back on your fuel is the worst thing you can do. IT'S ONE OF THE PROBLEMS, NOT THE SOLUTION. If it worked, one diet is all any of us would have ever had to go on. One, not one hundred thousand. If starvation did what it was supposed to do, there wouldn't be a 98 percent failure rate. None of us would be fat, because we've all starved ourselves for years.

Cutting calories is not the way to go. It doesn't work. Think about what you've just read. Does it make any sense to you? Could any of this have anything to do with how tired, depressed, fat, and unfit you are? Do you think starving instead of eating has anything to do with the level you function on?

YES, YES, YES, it does, Mr. doctor, nutritionist, dietitian, weight loss counselor. Yes, it does. It has everything to do with how you look and feel now.

There is no diet on earth that works.

STOP THE INSANITY!

If there were, I'd be its number one spokesperson, and there wouldn't be a fat person left on earth.

The problem is not your lack of willpower, discipline, self-control, or "eating disorder."

You are not a failure or a lazy emotional wreck. It's not in your mind, it's in your body.

You don't have the problem. The diet and fitness industries have the problem. They have been lying to you, ripping you off, and setting you up for failure. You and I are not the failures, they are.

The first dress size I dropped, I felt surprised. When I went to work that afternoon, I told everybody! It was the most wonderful thing that had happened in a long time. I wore the suit . . . proudly . . . with the skirt almost falling down over my hips.
　　　　　　—Debi, a client

Time travel forward with me—flash to the day at my father's home when I finally got on the scale and saw 114. I almost died and got on and off the scale a hundred times before I believed what I was seeing, but I can honestly say that there were thousands of moments in between the beginning and the beginning that were the best moments of my life.

It was the hope that each stage of getting well brought with it that sustained me. The knowing and understanding that this process would continue and I could take it as far as I wanted to that kept me going. The strength, energy, and shrinking all along the way that made it all worthwhile. That was and is what kept me motivated. And it doesn't stop—there are always new levels of fitness to reach for, so you'll be modifying until the day you die. So let's start now.

My sweet revenge was . . .

Believe it or not—at a funeral. My brother and friends lived about thirty miles away, and I hadn't seen them for *many* weeks. As I walked toward the front where

they were, I heard much whispering. Apparently no one had recognized me until I was right next to them. I spent the rest of the evening stopping by the homes of friends and relatives to see reactions. Fabulous!
—Ann, a client

A birthday is supposed to be one of those landmarks in everybody's life. Let me tell you what it meant to me. I may sound like a completely self-absorbed, shallow idiot right now, but I'm committed to telling the truth, so here goes.

I called my mother up and asked her to throw me a surprise party. My mother had spent years trying to figure me out, and this request only further confirmed that there was something very wrong with me. She tried, tactfully, to explain to me that surprise usually meant that you don't know—unless, of course, the news gets out—and when you arrive at the event, you are surprised.

Before she could finish, I gave her the guest list. Some on the list were people I knew and liked, and some were people I couldn't stand.

She had to tread lightly here. It was obvious to her that I had lost more than weight—my mind had disappeared along with some of the 133 pounds. Mom suggested that I include friends and have a wonderful birthday party and right after it was over make an appointment with a good psychiatrist and deal with new problems that were interfering with my life.

It's hard to explain to anyone who hasn't been there what I was doing and what I was going to gain from doing it. I simply asked my mother to indulge me—after all, it was my celebration—and give me the party of my dreams.

So she did. All were invited, mum's the word, and the big night was days away.

I went shopping for a dress for the big occasion. Normal for any big event, but not for an ex-260-pound housewife looking for that special dress that would prove the point I had to prove that night. There it was. Expensive as hell, hanging on the rack, very tiny, close to obscene, black, and very, very tight. Perfect. Now the shoes. Black, of course, five-inch spiked heels, impossible to walk in, but what was I planning on doing, nothing but standing still and posing all night. Outfit complete, now the coach. I found out early that the fairy godmother is a big lie, so I got my own pumpkin and turned it into a limo. Yep, you heard it right. I arrived at my own party in a limo, wearing a tight, tiny black dress and spiked heels. A little too much, you may be saying, but not if you've ever weighed 260. If you have, you will see this all as perfectly reasonable (and since you are who I'm talking to, let's not worry about what others say—'cause who cares?).

Unfortunately, this story doesn't end here, it gets worse. I arrive, walk slowly to the front door, ring the bell, knowing good and well who's inside, it's dark (what else would it be, it's supposed to be a surprise). My mom answers, I walk into the hallway, and pose—no joke, literally pose—until she turns on the lights. Everyone yells "Surprise!" and the people I didn't like, who hadn't seen me in years, the ones with their mouths hanging— let me repeat, hanging—open were the ones I was posing for. I stood there for as long as it took them to close their mouths, enjoying every second of "sweet revenge"— and let's not pretend it was anything else—and walked into my surprise birthday party as if I'd been a size 2 all my life.

> Feeling and looking better gives me a lift and lots of confidence. I even had someone tell me that I've got a "glow."
>
> —Debi, Dallas, Texas

A couple of months after my white picket fence exploded and the Prince had gone for good, a very dear friend sent me a card with a quote, which to this day I live by.

On the front was a woman in a fur coat with a little poodle. She and the dog were covered in jewels. The card read:

"Living well is the best revenge."
When you opened the card, it read:
"But murder is running a close second."
I don't know who wrote it or where it came from. (I'd give you credit, but I don't know who you are.) But I must say that your card, whoever you are, says it all.

I feel and look sooo good that I actually was confident enough to end a very long marriage that should have ended three or four years ago.
—Cathy, Dallas, Texas

The sweet revenge was mighty sweet. Since then there have been too many moments to mention—such as chance encounters with people who can't believe it's you when they bump into you. You know it's sweet when you have to spend twenty minutes and show them your driver's license before they believe it really is you.

But there are other moments that go beyond just looking good and knowing you've done it. It is really about the lady who waited for me in the airport the other day and told me she had been eating, breathing, and moving for the first time in her life and had never, ever, had the kind of energy and strength she has now.

Then there's Carol Lawrence, the singing, dancing, acting legend who did a segment on the "Home" show and wanted to meet me because she has been following my program and is leaner than she's ever been. I felt like the Sally Fields of the 1990s getting an Academy Award: "You *like* me! It's so nice to know you like me!"

It's really and truly about the housewife in Atlanta who sent me a picture of herself, beaten to a pulp, lying in the hospital. She said, Thank you, Susan, for telling me the truth and helping me find a way out of the fat and self-hatred that were even more frightening than the man who did this to me.

What floors me, tears me apart every day, what makes me so grateful, and what keeps me going are the women who are learning that changing your body, increasing your strength, regaining your choices, and coming back from the dead are not difficult when you do things right. What changes is a lot more than your physical appearance.

Stopping the insanity in your life will give you more than a nice body (although that goes a long way!).

It can give you back a life that may have gotten lost along the way. That's what it's all about.

So revel in your sweet revenge—I did and still do every day—but love and appreciate every step of the process that will give you back your life. The birthday parties end. Bumping into old friends or enemies lasts a few minutes, but your life goes on.

Getting well gives you more control.

I am going to a party tonight, given for me in Hollywood. I asked for a few people I don't particularly like to be invited—not much changes—and guess what I'm wearing? A little black dress along with five-inch black spiked heels.

The true secret of giving advice is, after you have honestly given it, to be perfectly indifferent whether it is taken or not, and never persist in trying to set people right.

—Hannah Whitall Smith, 1902

PART TWO

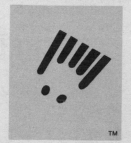

Stop the Insanity!

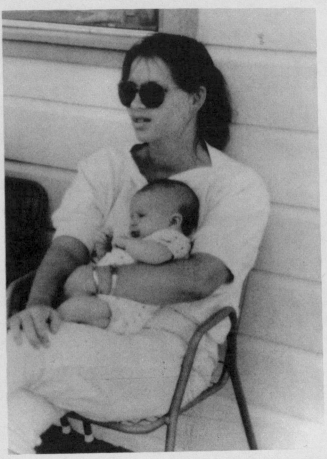

Still not topping 260. Just after the birth of son number two, and it's not so bad. The Prince and I were in a reconciliation period, and I thought the white picket fence was secure.

FOUR

Eating Right

Habit is either the best of servants or the worst of masters.
—NATHANIEL EMMONS

You have not failed, but you've spent years living with the failure of one diet after another. Dieting has been a waste of your time and money, and it's dieting that's made you fat, weak, and too tired to function. And here I am—not a doctor, not a nutritionist or a dietitian—with the nerve to tell you there is a simple solution: Stop dieting—forever.

A simple solution to the pain and self-hatred that you've lived with for years? How about that "compulsive" eating you have learned to live with one day at a time? Yes, there is a simple solution. Before you throw this book against the wall, think about this.

What if I told you to get in your car tomorrow and drive from New York to Dallas, pedal to metal, at 95 miles an hour? Spend today getting ready for the trip. Check your supplies: food, money, maps, kids, husband. (I'm not sure if husbands can be considered a supply— maybe extra baggage, ball and chain, noose around the neck, but supply? I don't know.) Make sure you've got everything you need for your cross-country race.

Now what if I told you that you can take anything you want except gas?

STOP THE INSANITY!

No gas.

Everything and anything else is in, fuel is out.

How does that sound to you? Nuts? Stupid? Insane? Uh-huh . . . see, see, see where the title of this book comes from? What would be your response to a suggestion like that?

"How am I going to drive a car at 95 miles an hour without gas?" Good question. One that you should ask any expert or authority who suggests you do exactly that —diet. Drive without gas or function without fuel. Replace your car with your body, and stay with this theory.

What's your "average" day like? The average day of the average working mother (the phrase *working mother* is beyond redundant, don't you think?). . . . I'm a working mom—let me tell you what my "average" day is like.

Up at five-thirty or six—that's if I'm sleeping late. Kids up and almost ready for school—finishing homework that I was too tired the night before to help them with. Wash the sinkful of dishes (no dishwashers in my house; I'm just too damn organic for that) that have been soaking all night long because I was too tired to do them the night before; organize the house, picking up toys, clothes, cups, socks, socks, socks everywhere in my house of three males, so there is less to pick up when I get home at night; and we're off. Off to school and work.

Drop the kids off, kisses, kisses, finding out about the science project that is due tomorrow that requires construction, materials, and hours of time that I don't have. Drive like a loon because I'm late for a meeting. Teach a class. Run the business, pay the payroll, take care of whatever else is going on at my office, my studio. Work, work, work.

Do the day, then it's back home around five, six, or seven. Tear into the house, late, usually apologizing for something I missed or forgot; throw dinner on the stove while helping with homework, listening to the needs, problems (sibling rivalry for the day), while the first load of laundry goes in (disposable clothing very much a consideration at this point). Dinner on the table; listen to the kids' and husband's day, tell them about mine; finish eating, clear the table with the "help" of a husband and two sons. (Hansel and Gretel could find their way to my kitchen and directly to me.) Washing another load of dishes—you can find me doing that any night of the week. Dinner's over; bath time. The second load of laundry goes in, the kids are clean; bedtime. Tuck and snuggle and story time. (Now I'm showing off—actually, most nights my brilliant, clean children beg for a story and I tell them I'm too tired to see the print. Talk about guilt; everywhere you look someone is telling you that unless you read ten books a day to your kids, they have no choice but to play professional football. Add lots of guilt to this portion of the day—better yet, sprinkle it all through the day.) Finish some of my work, organize for the next day, leave the second load in the washer, too tired to care, lie down on the bed. . . .

It's ten-thirty or eleven, and the husband wants what?

"Why don't you put on that Little Bo Peep outfit, honey, and I'll watch you parade around the room."

Touch me and you die.

Fall into a coma by about twelve-thirty, up again at six. That's my day.

A fair description of an average day for most of us?

To say we run our cars at 95 miles an hour is an understatement.

The race is on from the minute most of us wake up in the morning. Kids, jobs, husbands; seven days a week, twelve, fourteen, eighteen hours a day.

Your car won't run without gas. If you are not putting in the right kind of fuel or enough fuel, not checking the engine, changing the oil, or maintaining it properly, then you can pretty much bet your car is not going to be driving anywhere at 95 miles an hour. So you are with me on this theory. Think about your body and the fuel it needs to keep going—food is your fuel. Yet the first thing you do when you hate the way you look and feel is cut back —how far depends on the amount of weight you want to lose—or reduce your calorie intake. DIET, DIET, DIET

STOP THE INSANITY!

—600, 800, 1,000, 1,200, or maybe that very healthy diet of 1,400 calories a day.

Fine—you've been told to do that. Dieting is the way to lose weight, right?

WRONG, WRONG, WRONG. Take this to your weight loss counselor. Remember the car and gas—you are eating that healthy 1,200 calories a day, and you are running at 95 to 150 miles an hour. The first thing that happens to the human body, any human body, your body, when you take in less than you expend is this:

Your body, my body, everyone's body will crave high-calorie foods. This is not, I repeat, not an eating disorder. This is a physiological response to starvation. It's your body saying "Eat something, anything, because you are asking me to function, but you stopped giving me fuel hours ago." Here's what you do. Get up and go. No breakfast (or you may have grabbed something quick). Lunch is a salad (you are dieting again). You pick the kids up from school, and by four or five every day that eating disorder kicks in (your mother must have ruined your self-esteem at the same time every day), and you find yourself standing at the fridge dealing with your "compulsive eating," feeling like the biggest failure in the world, shoving those cupcakes into your mouth. Sometimes you may last for a few weeks or even a couple of months on that diet of yours and mine and millions of other women, but we all end up at the fridge. Interesting how many of us are suffering from the same disorder?

Get the trumpets ready, I have an announcement to make.

THE FIRST SYMPTOM OF STARVATION IS BINGEING. DIETING IS STARVATION. SO YOU, LIKE ALL OF US, ARE GOING TO END UP BINGEING.

The bingeing during famine, starvation, dieting, is your body's way of staying alive. Eat the cake, try the fudge —hey, here's a bag of chips; eat it, please, please, I'm starving to death, and there are still five more hours in this day.

86

I ate a whole package of orange marshmallow peanuts
—gag, I got very sick. I just couldn't stop eating those
pitiful candies.

—Mary, a client

But that's only the beginning of what happens to all of
us when we take in less than we expend. The second
thing that happens is your body, the brilliant machine
that it is, will slow itself—its metabolic rate—down to
whatever you are taking in. So if it's 800 calories a day,
one of those fabulous doctor-sponsored fast programs,
or 1,200-calorie healthy, applaud-you-when-you-lose-a-
pound-or-two-a-week kind of diets, that's the level your
body will be functioning on.

Tired?

So tired you can't function?

Forgetful, exhausted?

That was one of the things stopping me from getting
my life together. Being so tired all the time, I could barely
function. So tired and depressed that getting through the
day was a big accomplishment. It's the thing I hear the
most traveling all over this country speaking to every
kind of group imaginable.

"I'm so tired. . . ."

". . . too tired to feel motivated."

". . . too tired to make plans."

". . . too tired to reach my goals."

". . . too tired to change."

". . . too tired to get to an exercise class. . . ."

Your doctor will probably tell you it's because your
body is not functioning properly again. It's always our
stupid, perfectly designed bodies that have the problem,
never the doctors. The old metabolic problem, another
thing we all seem to be suffering from. I was told that my
metabolism had changed because I had two children so
close together, and between that and my age, there was
not much hope. Sure, I could lose some weight if I could
find the discipline to stick to a diet—something I just
couldn't do—but to expect to ever look and feel really

good again . . . ''Take your lithium, go home, and get a little realistic.''

How many times have I heard:

''My doctor told me that my metabolism is different from most people's.''

''It's thyroid, that's the reason I'm 400 pounds. I have a metabolism and thyroid problem.''

''Genetic, it's a genetic metabolism disorder.''

''My metabolism has been ruined—it doesn't work anymore, so it's fat for life for me. . . .''

Hi, my name is American Woman, I am clinically depressed, bipolar, suffering from chronic fatigue syndrome . . . the disease of the 1990s. Nothing in my body is functioning properly, and my doctor tells me that's why I am so tired and there is nothing I can do about it. I hate the way I look and feel, so starting Monday I am going on a diet and trying to have the willpower and self-discipline to stick to it this time.

Do me a favor. Go to your doctor (tell him Susan sent you) and ask him if starvation and exhaustion have anything to do with each other. Ask him if dieting slows down or damages your metabolic rate. Ask him these questions just before he recommends the next diet, or puts you on your next liquid fast, or maybe just before that stomach stapling. Yes, there are malfunctions in the body, disease, genetics, and many other things that affect your energy level. But the one thing that directly affects millions of us and determines our energy level is dieting, cutting calories.

Tired? We've only just begun. There are two more things that happen to the human body when you cut back on calories and continue to function.

Number three: The third thing that happens on a diet is that your body will find its own fuel, since you are not giving it enough fuel to function on. The fuel it will use is lean muscle mass. Internal cannibalism. That's what it amounts to. Eating yourself alive. Yes, that's right, folks. Your body will use lean muscle mass for fuel. Now, this is getting old at this point, but you've got to put number two and number three together and imagine what happens. Your metabolism is functioning at a snail's pace, and your body is using lean muscle mass to survive. Lean muscle mass = strength. Energy. With these two symptoms of dieting working together, you are going to end up so tired, you will feel like you want to die. That's a given. Almost a guarantee.

But it's not over. My favorite is the last thing that happens to everybody's body when they take in less than they expend.

YOUR BODY STORES THE FUEL THAT LASTS THE LONGEST IN FAMINE.

IS IT PROTEIN? . . . NOOOOOOOO. IS IT CARBO-HYDRATES? . . . NOOOOOOOO. IT'S . . .

FAT.

FAT.

FAT.

Your body stores fat so that you can live in the famine that you've paid a hell of a lot of money to be living in. Famine, as in starvation. Starvation, as in Third World countries, not America. Starvation, as in death.

Oh, by the way, just for the record. When you "lose" your weight you are losing a lot of water and lean muscle mass, and when you gain back the weight, like 98 percent of us do, what you lost in lean muscle mass you gain back as fat. Your body doesn't just gain back lean muscle mass —you have to build it up, keep it healthy. However, much of the "weight" you lost that was made up of lean muscle mass will come back as fat. That's why those same 40 pounds feel looser, fatter, heavier than they did before. You are not crazy, you are getting fatter and weaker every time you lose weight and gain it back.

I would get into the car at three A.M. to get candy bars andicecream. . . .
— Comment from a client

So let's sum it all up.

Whenever you go on a diet, reduce calories, your body will:

STOP THE INSANITY!

Crave high-calorie foods—instant eating disorder.

Slow its metabolism down—guaranteed exhaustion.

Burn lean muscle mass as a fuel supply. Weak? Don't ask.

And store fat—FAT, FAT, FAT.

The physical, psychological, and emotional symptoms of taking in less than you expend, of cutting calories, range from exhaustion, depression, and decreased self-esteem to losing internal organs and death.

If it's the definition of insanity you are looking for, you needn't look any further than the millions of us who starve our bodies in an attempt to look and feel better—because of information given to us by the diet and fitness industry and the American Medical Association. It made me mad as hell when I found out that I had been set up to fail. There is no way anyone can succeed on any diet out there. Living on freeze-dried, instant, low-cal, bad-tasting crap is impossible. The minute you start eating again, you are going to gain your weight back—you've proved that to yourself—with a little more fat and a little less lean muscle mass each time. You are not "failing" because you are a lazy, undisciplined slob. It is not will-power, motivation, or self-control you are lacking—maybe your mother ruined your self-esteem, but that's not the only reason you are running to the fridge and shoving food in your mouth. There is another reason—this is much easier to understand and a lot easier to work through. There is no way on earth you can live on what they are telling you to live on. Think about this: We are the only nation on earth that not only volunteers for starvation, but pays millions of dollars for it every year.

It makes me want to puke, and that's not an eating disorder, either.

Food doesn't make you fat.

Food is your fuel.

Food is essential.

Food is energy.

Food is what your body lives on.

I've got something for you to cut out and put on your fridge. Check out the back of the next page—it's blank,

Daily Caloric Consumption Predictions for Women

Pounds	Resting Calories "Doing Nothing"	Low Activity Low-Impact Walking or Cycling 2–3 Times a Week	Medium Activity Low-Impact Walking or Cycling 4–5 Times a Week	High Activity Low-Impact Walking or Cycling 6–7 Times a Week
100	1,120	1,450	1,570	1,680
110	1,150	1,490	1,600	1,720
120	1,190	1,550	1,670	1,780
130	1,220	1,580	1,700	1,830
140	1,250	1,630	1,750	1,880
150	1,280	1,660	1,800	1,920
160	1,320	1,720	1,850	1,980
170	1,350	1,750	1,890	2,000
180	1,380	1,790	1,930	2,070
190	1,420	1,850	1,990	2,100
200	1,450	1,880	2,030	2,180
210	1,480	1,950	2,050	2,200
220	1,513	1,970	2,100	2,270
230	1,540	2,000	2,160	2,300
240	1,580	2,050	2,200	2,400
250	1,610	2,090	2,250	2,410
260	1,640	2,130	2,300	2,460
270	1,676	2,170	2,350	2,500
280	1,710	2,220	2,400	2,560
290	1,740	2,260	2,440	2,600
300	1,770	2,480	2,500	2,660

*Individuals running or exercising at high intensities may need more calories.
Modified and adapted from Oliver Owen, "Resting metabolic requirements of men and women,"
Mayo Clinic Report, volume 163 (1988), and "A reappraisal of caloric requirements in healthy women,"
American Journal of Clinical Nutrition, volume 44 (1986) 1–19.

so you can cut it out and look at it every time you go to the fridge.

This book is not about charts and graphs—they never did a thing for me. *Stop the Insanity!* is about your understanding and being able to apply the foundations of wellness to your life so you can change your body forever. Understanding this chart is a great beginning.

The only way to change your body is to eat. You can never get lean, shrink, or be the size you want to be if you don't eat. Follow the chart with me and let's start with line one. We've got weight and activity levels. (Remember the gasoline and the car?) Left-hand side says pounds, as in how much you weigh. Next, resting calories needed. Resting, meaning you do nothing. You get up, shower, and lie on the sofa. Next is low activity. You live your life and take a walk a couple of times a week—that's it, not much more. Medium-activity level: living and walking four–five times a week at a moderate-intensity level. (Level of intensity is a term you'll be so familiar with, you'll be an expert soon—but later for that.) Next and last, high-intensity level: you live your life and you work out six–seven times a week.

Look at the first line, left-hand side. If you weigh 100 pounds (me and half the world hate you—joking, only joking) and you live at a low-activity level, you need a minimum of 1,120 calories a day. Just to get by, remember, that's weighing as much as an ant and doing nothing.

Notice the two things that determine how many calories you are taking in: weight and activity level. Interesting, don't you think?

Let's get real. Let's say you weigh 150 and you do something. Not much, a moderate-activity level. Your minimum caloric intake for the day needs to be 1,660 calories. WAIT JUST A MINUTE! That's way above and beyond any of the diets I was ever put on at 260 pounds—110 pounds more than that 150-pound average person. It's higher than any healthy diet I ever heard of —how about you? Have you ever walked into a weight loss counselor's office, desperate for help (that's not the question, because I know the answer to that part is Yes,

yes, yes, you've been desperate), and been told to eat at least 1,600 calories a day to reach your "goal"?

Why not take this thing further and get a little more realistic? The 150-pound range is small for many of us. Go to 210 pounds and a low-activity level—1,950 calories. That's not seven years before I was born. That's almost 2,000 calories a day. Do you want to know how I went from 260 to what I look like now? The minute I went from the 260-pound column over to the moderate-activity level and started eating 2,300 calories a day. Yep, the second I stopped dieting and started eating, the process began.

> I think I have tried every diet food, packaged meal, and pill at least once. I wouldn't dare say how much I spent on them. But as far as the food goes, the picture on the box would probably taste better. One time I bought a diet frozen veggie lasagna I couldn't get past my nose, so I gave it to my dog, and even she wouldn't eat it—she looked at me as if I were trying to poison her.
>
> —Comment from a client

I had a weight loss counselor from one of the biggest names in the diet industry (you know, the one that is in every shopping center in this country) sign up at my studio for the food and movement workshop, classes, consultation, chat with my manager, a sit-down with me—anything and everything we had to offer, this woman wanted in on. I knew where she was from and had to find out what she was doing in my studio. What could she possibly want from little ole me—didn't Jenny and her friends have all the answers?

Was she stealing my stuff? (It went against everything they teach you before they give you your freeze-dried food for the week.)

Was she trying to figure out what they were doing wrong? (Everything, babe.)

Was she out to steal clients? (Our clients are far too

knowledgeable to fall for the old "cut calories" routine anymore.)

Fat (pardon the pun) chance. . . .

Well, once again my Catholic upbringing made me fully aware that I had just bought another express ticket to hell by judging this person the way I did. She turned out to be a wonderful person who knew she was unqualified to help the desperate women who streamed into her program for help. She told me she was trained to do only one thing—sell, sell, sell the program. Memorize the basic info, hook them, feed off their desperation, get the cash, and sell them as much as she could on the first visit. The more she sold, the more she was commended. She wanted to know more—because of the desperation she saw every day.

The calorie consumption chart is not my opinion. It's fact. The diet industry has known about the connection between activity level and caloric intake for a long time. The American Medical Association knows about it. The fitness industry is aware of it. So why didn't you and I know about it? These experts should be on the front line screaming it to all the starving, desperate women in this country.

Why aren't they? Where has this information been that can change your body, really change it? Why have we been taught to starve our bodies? How come we have had to live with the symptoms of starvation and deprivation with no hope in sight? Good questions. You might want to ask your experts—tell them Susan sent you.

There are two important things that determine your daily caloric consumption: your weight and your energy expended. The more you do, the hungrier you'll be. The more you drive the car, the more gas you use, right? The faster you drive it, the faster you use up the gas—right? Well, the same thing happens to your machine. When you've got the rough day at work, the husband, the kids, the new exercise class (summer's right around the corner, and it's time to starve and exercise your way into that bathing suit), staying awake all night with the new baby, whatever it is that your life requires from you, your body is burning fuel.

95

STOP THE INSANITY!

I understand if you haven't seen or heard anything beyond the calorie consumption chart—talk about a shock. I know what most of you are thinking: HOW COULD ANYONE EAT 2,000 CALORIES A DAY AND NOT BE THE SIZE OF A HOUSE?

I eat 3,500 to 5,000 calories a day. I am a size 2–4— that's not 24—that's a 2 or a 4, depending on the garment.

I don't live in a gym.

I don't eat that much and throw up twice the amount.

I didn't have surgery to speed up my metabolic rate. If there were such a surgery on earth, I would be the first in line and the loudest voice recommending it to the world. There is none.

I eat a lot of fuel because I expend a lot of energy. I have a lot of energy because I eat a lot of high-quality fuel. See how those two tie in?

Going from the insanity to the sanity, getting back in touch with what is normal, is not an easy process. We are so far into the insanity that telling people to eat is dangerous. It is one of the most difficult parts of my job when I'm with a client. But you don't have to worry, we are going to do this together. I wrote this book so you will get all the information you need, but we've got to start right here. You have to understand the concept of fueling your machine, the necessity of eating and what determines how much. And when you do, you're home free.

Eating when you are hungry and drinking when you are thirsty—very sane. The more you do, the hungrier you'll be—very sane. Increasing your daily caloric intake —absolutely necessary if you want to change the way you look and feel. Fact.

The daily caloric consumption chart—or your new fridge decoration, however you want to see it—is only a guideline. You are not dieting ever again, so don't etch these numbers in stone, just look at the calorie range that your weight and life-style put you in, and understand that you should try to take in at least that amount every day. Don't drop too far below that range or you will not be putting enough gasoline into your car. Don't get nuts with the numbers. Understand the concept and get on with eating.

Diets don't work. I beg you—stop dieting forever. Don't ever reduce your caloric intake and starve your body again. If you do, you will get the same results you've gotten every time you've dieted. It's a temporary solution that always backfires and leaves you feeling like the biggest failure on earth and just a bit fatter and weaker. Whenever you have cut calories, has it worked? Does your body look the way you want it to look? No, no, no, and it never will if you continue to cut calories.

It's over forever.

Don't ever diet again.

Believe me, I know what happens to you when I tell you to eat. To increase your calories. I was fat and hooked on diets when I figured this out. Picture this: the kids happily playing in the playroom while I'm sitting reading. Just a little book about fat and health, and I get to this theory about calories.

Energy expended . . .

Weight . . .

2,000 calories . . .

WHAT IN THE HELL . . .

THESE JERKS . . .

WHY AM I ON A 1,000-CALORIE-A-DAY-DIET? ACCORDING TO THIS, THERE IS NO CHANCE IN HEAVEN OR ON EARTH THAT I'LL EVER TAKE THIS WEIGHT OFF. . . .

It made me angry, it frightened me, and it confused the hell out of me. I was still the largest woman in my aerobics class, and according to this, now I also had to be the one eating the most.

Here's where I 'fess up to the splattering of anger. I hit the roof. The money I'd spent. The time and energy I had wasted doing the exact opposite of what this was saying. The self-esteem I'd lost feeling that there was something wrong with me. The doctors I'd begged and cried in front of for help because I looked and felt so bad. The programs I'd gone to for help. Why hadn't anybody told me about this information? I peeled myself off the roof and spent a couple of weeks figuring this out and applied it to my life. My progress doubled. I had energy and I was still shrinking. Eating and shrinking . . . I knew I was really on to something.

> Take away the cause and the effect ceases.
> —Miguel de Cervantes

If you want to get lean, you must start with eating. You must eat to be lean, no doubt about it. If you want to be healthy, you must eat. Food does not make you fat, fat makes you fat.

Fat is what is hanging from your arms, wadded on your thighs, making your butt huge, and dripping from your stomach.

Fat.

I've been through the same brainwashing that you and millions like us have been through. Changing my thinking, clearing up the confusion, was not easy—it's a lot easier for you because someone is talking about it now, yelling about it, pleading for you to understand that it begins with increasing your daily caloric intake and goes from there. Nobody was getting this information out. But that's changed, hasn't it. Help me blow the lid off this stuff.

So, this is it: Calories are your fuel. Reducing your fuel means you won't have enough gas to function. This may be Fuel 101 for some of you at this point, but we are going to start from the beginning, clear up the confusion, and get on with all the other things there are in this world to be confused and worried about. You need to be clear about all this so you can walk into your weight loss counselor's office and blow their minds with your brilliance while you are asking for your money back.

Calories are your friend now, but there is one very important thing that you need to be aware of. Not all calories are the same. They are not created equal.

1 gram of carbohydrates = 4 calories
1 gram of protein = 4 calories
And . . .

One gram of fat—yep, that stuff that looks like cottage cheese on your thighs when you sit down in those shorts —Mr. Fat. Guess how much he weighs?

1 gram of fat = 9, that's 9, calories.

More than twice as much as the other fuels your body needs to live on. Fat, it's big and fat. Ha, just like its name.

Do you know what that means? It means you can eat twice the amount of the other two fuels and still not equal the fat. In other words, more food.

This is where we get to be geniuses. Here is what makes the experts mental. If you need fuel/calories to function and you've got a warehouse full of fat stored, wouldn't it make sense, even to a housewife from Garland, that the obvious thing to do would be to increase the fuel/calories and decrease what you have way too much of already all over your body, FAT?

Call me nuts, but if fat makes you fat, then cut back on the fat. Increase the other two fuels so you get the calories your body needs to function. So what's the problem? If that's all that was involved, then it would be simple. You'd just buy things that are low in fat, something you have probably started to do already, and your daily fat intake would decrease.

Unfortunately, it is not that simple. Step number three is finding the fat. Fat isn't always as obvious as the cream cheese, ice cream, and fatty steaks. You've got to get smart to find this stuff nowadays. You need to become a fat detective and learn how to search out the hidden fat —because, believe me, it's being hidden from you.

Something very interesting has happened in the supermarkets of America. There is no cholesterol in anything anymore. There is no fat. Haven't you noticed? Everything is lean, light, and low fat . . . the buzzwords of the 1990s. Sausage is low fat—I mean, really. Isn't a pig the universal symbol for fat? How could pig mean low fat? Meat is low fat. Potato chips are low fat and cholesterol free. Dressings, sauces, spreads, cakes, cookies . . . everything is low fat.

I have a question. If there is no fat or cholesterol in

anything, why are we all so fat and dying from heart disease? Where is it coming from?

I don't think I'm busting anyone's bubble when I say that manufacturers lie for profit. A lot of those 98 percent fat-free everything labels are a lie, I'm sad to say. I was furious to find out that the brands I had trusted for years had lied to me. The effort that I put into reading the labels trying to figure out the saturated from the unsaturated, the grams of fat from the calories, was wasted. How can they lie? Where are the government agencies that we pay to protect us? American consumers are on their own when it comes to their health. Hey, Mr. FDA Man, how can these companies do this to us?

The loopholes and laws are designed to protect the manufacturers, not you. This could and may be a separate book, but that's not the focus of *Stop the Insanity!* —this book is about getting you the information you need to find the truth, no matter how well it is disguised. Forget what the label says. It's easy to find out how much fat is really in the food you and your family are eating and make the decision that works for you. Not for the food manufacturer's pocketbook.

You may get a little passionate/angry. Go ahead. Write everyone you can write and tell them how you feel. Get it off your chest. Paint the slogans, march the marches, go to Washington, stand and yell, but first let me tell you how to read between the lines. How to figure out the truth, so you can get on with changing your body and getting lean, strong, and healthy.

After I got over the shock of this whole concept of eating and the anger about the lies and deception, I got on with using a fat formula that is worth its weight in gold.

The fat formula. The famous fat formula. This is what you need to figure out where the fat is coming from. If it's a fat detective you want to be, grab your checkered hat and magnifying glass and take your formula to the grocery store.

You need a calculator. (I am assuming you are as mathematically deficient as I am.) And from now on for every single thing you put into your mouth you are going to do two things:

Take the number of fat grams per serving x 9 = X.

Take X and divide it by the total calories.

And that will tell you how much of that serving is fat.

You want to know what percentage of fat there is in that serving you are about to eat.

Is it 20% or 80%?

40% or 75%?

Is it high fat or low fat?

Don't worry if you don't get this right away; it will become second nature even to the most mathematically hindered—take it from me.

Let's read some labels together.

Label number one comes to us from a gourmet popcorn maker. Screaming at us on the front is "one-third less calories, fat, and oil."

NUTRITION INFORMATION (per serving)

Serving size	9.5 g
	(approximately 1 cup)
Servings per bag	18
Calories	35
Protein	1 g
Carbohydrates	6 g
Fat	2 g
Sodium	85 mg

First question is one-third less than what? Would that be one-third less than 100 or one-third less than 40 percent fat—which one is it, Vic?

Popcorn is a low-fat food, so come along with me and we'll do the fat formula together on this low-fat food.

Two grams of fat—see, see, low fat, right? You should be able to eat as much of this as you want. But you haven't even begun the formula, so don't get excited yet.

$2 \times 9 =$ (even I know this) 18.

18 divided by the total calories, which in this less-than-everything product is 35, equals what?

.51.

That's 51 percent fat in every serving—51 percent?

STOP THE INSANITY!

That blank space, my friends, represents silence and shock on the page, and that's what the truth about the fat percentage of our "low-fat" popcorn should create. Silence and shock. Not only are you being lied to, but high-fat foods are being turned into low-fat foods.

Where do these guys stop?

We've got a lot more to go. Follow the labels.

NUTRITION INFORMATION (per serving)

Serving size	1 oz.
Number of servings	5½
Calories	130
Protein	2 g
Carbohydrate	19 g
Fat	6 g
Sodium	140 mg

Label number two is from a "light" potato chip—of course, it has no cholesterol in it, and it's light.

$6 \times 9 = 54$

$54 \div 130 = 42\%$

Even Mr. Potato Head is smart enough to know that there is nothing light about 42 percent fat. These guys are going to get a few feathers "ruffled" when they get the letters from all you brilliant fat detectives.

This is one of my favorite labels because it comes to us from one of the nation's leading professional weight control companies.

NUTRITION INFORMATION

Serving size	3 oz.
Servings per container	1
Calories	220
Protein	11 g
Carbohydrate	19 g
Fat	11 g
Sodium	560 mg

This is a diet morning biscuit. Breakfast is a very important meal, one that should be full of nourishment, high volume for the fuel you need to get through your day, and of course, especially coming from a diet expert, low in fat.

So we'll take the number of fat grams:

$11 \times 9 = 99$.

$99 \div 220 = 45\%$.

If you go to your grocery store and have a look at the size of this enormously high-fat breakfast food, you'll know immediately that it's not enough food to feed your fish, and if you choose to eat it, you can just sit back and watch the "weight" creep back on.

Consider yourself a weight watcher.

Well, look at this. Another label from the same weight control professionals. I'm not harping on any one company, but this is interesting. Watching your weight? Try eating fat as 60 percent of each serving—I wonder what you'd look like at the end of a couple of months. If you think I've lost my mind because you can't understand why any company—let alone a trusted diet brand—would feed you that much fat, just do the fat formula:

NUTRITION INFORMATION (per serving)

Serving size	2 fl. oz.
Servings per container	12
Calories	120
Protein	2 g
Carbohydrate	11 g
Fat	8 g
Cholesterol	5 mg
Sodium	60 mg

$8 \times 9 = 72$.

$72 \div 120 = 60\%$.

Let's pause for another stunned and silent moment. . . .

Moving on.

Quick, instant cheeseburger mix is our next label.

STOP THE INSANITY!

NUTRITIONAL INFORMATION

Serving size	4.8 oz.
Servings per container	1
Calories	400
Protein	21 g
Carbohydrate	35 g
Fat	20 g
Cholesterol	75 mg
Sodium	600 mg

This is from a company that swears by its healthy choices. They have just come out with a whole line of healthful lunch meats and food that you can apparently eat as much as you want of because they are so trustworthy. Isn't it nice to know you can trust a food manufacturer?

Fat formula time:

20 (grams of fat) x 9 = 180.

180 ÷ 400 (the total calories) = 45%.

Carmel with an H, you ought to be ashamed of yourself.

Label number six is a light, 77 percent fat-free sausage. Pork—you know, the other white meat. The stuff that's supposed to be good for you.

NUTRITIONAL INFORMATION (per portion)

Portion/size (1 cooked patty)	28 g (1 oz.)
Portions per container	10
Calories	80
Protein	6 g
Carbohydrates	less than 1 g
Fat	6 g
Cholesterol	30 mg

6 × 9 = 54.

54 ÷ 80 = 68%.

I'm confused. How can something be 77 percent fat free and be 68 percent fat at the same time?

Seems to me that Old Jimmy's got a screw loose. Mr. Dean, what's the deal?

* * *

Light, if it's light you want, then you got it from Philadelphia in the form of cheese. Light, light, light, light. How light? Go on, you know how to figure it out.

NUTRITION INFORMATION

Serving size	1 oz.
Calories	60
Protein	3 g
Carbohydrates	2 g
Fat	5 g
Cholesterol	10 mg
Sodium	160 mg

$5 \times 9 = 45$.
$45 \div 60 = 75\%$.

Light means 75 percent fat? Ring the liberty bell on that one, boys. . . .

Are you getting depressed? I feel the need to call on the old lithium prescription just going over this stuff, and I've gone through it a thousand times. Can you believe the extent of the lying and the amount of fat you've been getting in your diet without even knowing it?

This is a big breakthrough, and breakthroughs are never easy. Consider this a birth. Birthing the sanity in your life and letting go of the insanity. It gets easier, and you keep getting smarter, so you are ahead of the game —what game am I talking about?

Onward. . . .

You need your calcium, and according to the American Dairy Association, the best place to get it is through your daily dairy intake. For instance, a slice of cheese:

NUTRITION INFORMATION

Serving size	1 slice (¾ oz.)
Calories	80
Protein	5 g
Carbohydrate	less than 1 g
Fat	7 g
Sodium	340 mg

STOP THE INSANITY!

So you have a couple of slices of cheese, what harm could that do?

$7 \times 9 = 63$.

$63 \div 80 = 79\%$.

There's your answer. It can do 79 percent fat intake harm. That's a whole lot of harm when you are trying like hell to change the way you look and feel. Ask the American Dairy Association or diet counselor if there isn't a lower-fat, higher-volume slice of cheese. This stuff isn't just plain old fat, it's saturated fat, otherwise known as Mr. Death. One slice for 79 percent of your daily intake as fat—what's that going to do? That won't even give you the energy you are going to need to yell for help when you are having your heart attack. Talk about the exact opposite of what's going to make you lean, strong, and healthy. There are not many better examples of low-volume, high-fat foods than that one slice of saturated fat cheese.

Lunchtime is sandwich time. Sandwich time means some of that delicious 97 percent fat-free ham. At 97 percent fat-free you can consider yourself home free, because that means it's not fattening—right? Fat makes you fat, and this stuff is 97 percent fat-free. Sandwiches on the house. Make 'em, eat 'em, and enjoy 'em. But just in case, let's double-check.

NUTRITION INFORMATION (per portion)	
Portion size	1 slice (12 g)
Portions per container	14–16
Calories	14
Protein	2 g
Carbohydrate	less than 1 g
Fat	less than 1 g
Sodium	150 mg

Less than 1 gram of fat, thank goodness. But what if it were just 1 gram?

$1 \times 9 = 9$.

$9 \div 14 = 64\%$.

Gentlemen, surely you made a mistake on your deli thin label? You would have told us if you'd known that every time I put a slice of this ham in my mouth, I would be getting 64 percent fat from it—wouldn't you?

You stop using butter—100 percent fat is too much for anyone. Margarine, same thing—100 percent fat. But are you coating your pan with cooking spray? Why? Because the cooking-spray people have given you the impression that they are low-fat alternatives to butter or margarine, and you believed them. You know know how far believing these people gets you . . . It gets you fat and unhealthy.

NUTRITION INFORMATION

Serving size	0.266 g
Calories	2
Protein	0 g
Carbohydrates	0 g
Fat	less than 1 g
Sodium	0 mg

Fat formula number ten, let's go.

Less than 1 gram, again. Let's pause for a moment. Less than 1 gram. What does that mean? How much less? Why won't they tell us exactly how much fat is in the stuff? Let's take a little liberty, since they won't tell us how much fat is in each serving, and say 1 gram. I mean, what else are we supposed to do? So . . .

$1 \times 9 = 9$.

$9 \div 2 = 450\%$.

Pam, what's the matter with you? Four hundred fifty percent. That makes a lot of sense, doesn't it? These "less than 1 gram of fat" and "non-fat" labels have been designed to confuse you more, but there is an explanation to clear up the confusion that the laws create.

When a label says there is less than 1 gram of fat in the product, it can mean there is .1 gram or .9 grams, or anything in between. So you'll never know how much, because I guess these guys think you don't need to know unless it's more than one gram. I'd love to be a fly on the wall of these guys' brains (you know they have doodie for brains to make the decisions they make with our dollars), in order to understand how they come up with some of this stuff.

When you look at the label and see that there are 2 calories and "less than 1 gram" of fat, you know the calories have to come from fat. Where else could they come from, the propellant? If you want to confirm this, look at the ingredients again. Canola oil and propellant. (What in the hell is propellant, and what does it do to the inside of my body? Next question.)

If you want to know whether your cooking spray is high or low in fat, that'll answer your question. If you want to know if it's good or bad for you, look at the label. The warning label, that is: FLAMMABLE, MAY BURST INTO FLAMES IF LEFT ON THE STOVE.

Interesting warning—what does that tell you about the product?

When it says 94 percent saturated fat-free, sure it is—canola is free of saturated fat. But canola oil and every other oil under the sun are still 100 percent fat. Since fat makes you fat . . . you decide, it's your choice.

Here I am picking on these guys at the FDA, the food manufacturers, and everybody else connected with this confusion about what the label says and what is actually true. Silly me. It must have been a mistake. Have you heard? They've changed the labels.

The new food labels will clear up the confusion. According to *The Wall Street Journal*, and you can't get much bigger than that, the Nutritional Labeling and Education Act of 1990 (big title, don't you think?) says that all food labels must be presented to the American public in a "uniform manner" (I can relate, Catholic school and all) explaining in more detail what's in the food we are all eating.

Our very own current FDA commissioner David Kessler says, and I quote, the new labeling laws are "one of the most important public-health landmarks this agency has ever engaged in.'' Dave, Dave, is this big news for us, the consumer? This should make it clear to all of us how much of each serving of the food we eat is fat? Because that's what we need to know. Up until now, David himself had ''no idea whether six grams of fat per serving was high, medium, or low.'' And now, Dave, I— Susan Powter, the commissioner of nothing—am here to tell you that you still won't know if six grams of fat are high, medium, or low, and neither will any of us—because, Dave, you guys have done it again. Taken a very simple issue, complicated the hell out of it, and left us— the people buying the products—in the dust.

Let me explain.

Look at the new label. Here's an example.

NUTRITION INFORMATION

Serving Size	½ cup (121 g)
Servings per Container	about 3½
Amount per Serving	

Calories	60
Calories from Fat	5

	% Daily Value
Total Fat 0.5 g	1%
Saturated Fat 0 g	0%
Cholesterol 0 mg	0%
Sodium 180 mg	7%
Total Carbohydrates 12 g	4%
Dietary Fiber 2 g	8%
Sugars 5 g	
Protein 2 g	
Vitamin A	0%
Vitamin B	0%
Calcium	0%
Iron	0%

Calories 60. Calories from fat 5.

Fine start, but it means very little because what you want or need to know in order to reduce your daily fat intake is percentage, Dave. I want the percentage per serving. Continuing down the new label, you'll find Total Fat. In this example, that's .5 grams. Well, we've heard that old story before, that could mean low fat or high fat, depending on the total calories. So let's go to the total calories. Back up to 60. Do the fat formula.

$.5 \times 9 = 4.5$.

$4.5 \div 60 = 7.5\%$.

That's the total fat percentage per serving of this product. Low fat—fine, but my question to you, Dave, is why is it still necessary to do the fat formula, and since it is, how is this label any different from the ones that are on the shelves now?

Dave, let me answer my own question.

You've broken down saturated fat from unsaturated fat —that's good. But we all know that fat is fat; they both kill you—whether it's by clogging your arteries or destroying your self-esteem—but thanks for doing that. Then you've given us the sodium percentage, total carb percentage, protein, sugars, fibers, etc. That's not much different from the old charts, except that it's broken down in percentages of "daily value." But Dave, babe, I still don't know the percentage of fat per serving—but I'll get off that for a moment because I have another question. Above and beyond why you did this and what good it does me, what did it take to get this done?

Dave, your organization estimates that it will cost between $1.4 billion and $2.3 billion to change these labels.

Did you hear that? $1.4 BILLION OR $2.3 BILLION, somewhere between those two figures. I thought my checkbook was unbalanced—that's a lot of leeway, that's like a billion plus, more or less.

The food manufacturers that have to comply with this new bigtime law have 882 pages of rules and regulations that they must comply with. Tons of paper (hope you are recycling, Dave), staff to check and double-check, rules out the yin-yang—and I still don't know what percentage of fat per serving I'm getting in the food I'm buying?

Third and final question, Dave: Who pays for all this?

You know what, guys? To hell with Dave, this is not about him. You and I know the answer to question number three. You and I pay for all this. We pay through the nose, with our money and our health.

Dave, boys at the FDA: You guys need to stop wasting our time and money and listen to what it is we want. We want the truth. Plain and simple. We want to know what percentage of fat we are getting per serving. If you want to break that down into saturated and unsaturated, then fine, do it, but please tell me if the serving of food I am eating is within the healthful fat-per-serving limit or way the hell above. Then, Dave, we don't want to pay a fortune for food and have to work so hard at finding out the truth. See, Dave, you just spent a whole lot of money, time, and energy, and we still don't have the answer that millions of us want.

As a consumer, if you think you are confused now, wait until 1994. You'll be a fat-detective, a fat-formula expert by then, thank God, because you are still going to be doing the same thing. Trying to find the hidden fats so you don't get fat and unhealthy. Not much has changed, for all the cash that's been spent.

> Humans must eat, but corporations must make money.
> —Alice Embree,
> *Media Images*, 1970

It's too much for me to bear. Truly, I'm nauseated. The more you do the fat formula, the easier it is, the faster you learn about the lying food manufacturers out there, and the sooner you'll understand how brilliant and capable you are of making the right choices.

You can have the crackers, cookies, cakes, breads, the snacky things you enjoy. But let's get reasonable. Eating 78 percent fat this, 86 percent fat that, 45 percent fat here and there, and you are eating tons and tons of fat that you don't even know about. That's the point. Cutting back at all will make a hell of a big difference in your life. There is not much sacrifice involved. It's just a matter of bloody (oops, the Australian in me popped out) common sense, and you've got plenty of that. Just like me, you didn't know. Now you do. High-volume, high-quality, low-fat eating is how you get lean. How could it not, if you are drastically cutting back on the fat you are taking in? Where's it going to come from?

Feeling a bit of passion/anger flare up? Put the book down and go to your pantry. Do the formula on everything in there. See all the low-fat stuff you just spent your money on? The frozen diet dinners—high in fat. 70 percent, 89 percent, 50 percent, 90 percent lower-in-fat foods? Flat-out lies. The trusted brands highlighting in red the low saturated fat in their product but forgetting to warn you about the enormous amount of fat you are actually eating every time you eat a serving of their product. Is there a splattering of anger all over your kitchen?

We all know that fat is killing us. You'd have to live in a cave not to know that you need to cut back on your daily fat intake. We've heard about good oils and bad oils —nobody understands this, but we've heard of it. Then you know that it's time to make your heart healthy, and you've been trying.

I felt stupid because I didn't understand what it was all about. It has been presented as such a complicated issue. Surely you need a degree in nutrition to know all this stuff? The low-fat grams are highlighted. The good and the bad have been separated. The labels are pretty and screaming "low fat" from every direction. Surely you, the common consumer, can't figure out all this important information and make better decisions. That's what the manufacturers assume. Yes, you can. Ignore the labels, write the letters, and use your fat formula.

As long as it's labeled, you are okay, now that you know how to use the fat formula. But what are you supposed to do with the chicken that's packaged and sitting in your meat department? That's not labeled, and the butcher won't tell you how much fat per serving there is. So where is the consumer to go?

To *Stop the Insanity!*—where else would you go? Right here in the back of this book is a list of foods with the calories and fat per servings. Consider it a universal label. Look up the food in question, and do the same thing.

Food: chicken.

Take the number of fat grams $\times 9 = X$.

X divided by the total calories . . .

And bingo—you now know how much fat per serving you are eating.

See the percentages? Twenty percent, 60 percent, 50 percent. Now you're asking yourself, What am I supposed to be eating? What's right, what's wrong? Another issue that has been presented as the most confusing on the planet.

Before I figured all of this out, I heard that I was supposed to take in 30 percent of my total daily intake as fat. No more, no less. That was the perfect number presented by the American Medical Association, the people who know the least about nutrition. Why shouldn't we trust them? I was, at the time, quite willing to trust them. I didn't know any better, but there was one problem—I had no clue what they were talking about.

Thirty percent of my daily intake.

What does that mean?

How do I figure that out?

And what does it have to do with my being skinny?

Since it was all too confusing and made me feel like an idiot, I stopped trying and assumed that you had to be one of the experts to know it. Then it fell into place. First, the concept of eating. Then this energy expended/ calories burned thing. Then whammy—the fat formula.

Here it is.

The American Medical Association says that your daily intake of fat should be 30 percent. The easiest way to figure that out is to do the fat formula, and if you see anything above 30 percent, don't eat it. That's how I started. If it said 32 percent fat, I put it down. But being the math genius that I am, the "daily intake" part of that statement threw me for a big loop. How do you figure your total daily intake, when adding two numbers together is a big deal?

Here's my simple solution to that problem. If you calculate everything that you put in your mouth—remember, your daily caloric intake will change every day (are you lying by the lake? do you have an exercise marathon that day?)—and everything is below 30 percent, then you cannot, absolutely, cannot exceed 30 percent of your daily intake.

There is one other way, if you want to do it.

Write down everything you eat.

Total fat grams for the day.

Total calories for the day.

And at the end of the day, do the fat formula on your totals.

Total fat grams for the day $\times 9 = X$.

$X \div$ total calories for the day will give you the average percentage of fat for the day.

But my recommendation is that you start with everything you put into your mouth and go from there. It's easier that way. Adding up your total fat grams and calories for the day is stupid for a couple of reasons. First, it reinforces the diet mentality of jotting down all your food and keeping track like a compulsive whatever. Second, it is almost impossible to calculate fat grams per serving. I mean, if you go out to dinner, how in the hell are you supposed to know if your chicken breast was one or two servings? It's hard enough to get those guys in the kitchen to cook with no oil—try to find out servings and fat grams, and you are liable to have a crazy cook running to the table and yelling at you. (I've pushed them far— believe me, it's no fun.)

Another big concern that a lot of people have dealing with a system this simple is the fear of going beyond the 30 percent accidentally.

Example: You've gone along fine for a couple of days, calculating and making sure you never exceed 30 percent of your daily intake of fat. You look great, your clothes are getting looser, you're feeling in control, then whammy . . . you eat something that is 60 percent fat.

AHHHHHHHH . . . have you blown it? Are you going to get fat? Is it time to run to the fridge and shovel food into your mouth? No, no, no. Don't worry about it. Yes, you have exceeded 30 percent of your daily intake for the day, but so what? Fat burns as fuel. You've been eating below 30 percent for a couple of days, so there's no way to blow this thing. You simply make sure that you stay at 30 percent—or, if you want to go a little wild, go to a lower number for a couple of days. Stay at 10 percent of your daily intake for a few days and balance it out, so to speak. This is not a diet. This is about balancing your fat intake with your energy expended, so your body has a chance to get rid of some of the excess fat you've built up and get leaner.

I have found through my own experience and from hearing about the experiences of thousands of other women that the easiest way to do this is to calculate everything you eat for a while. Then pretty soon you know where the fat is and where it isn't. You can order, prepare yourself, or have a friend bring you the foods you like, the way you like them, and in any combinations you want, according to your tastes at the time—and not think about the fat percentage. Simple is better. You don't need to complicate this. It's easy to live with, and it works.

Before we go on, I've got a few questions for the boys at the AMA.

How come everybody has the same daily fat intake?

Why should someone who has 60 percent body fat eat the same amount of fat a day as someone who has 14 percent body fat?

Should heart patients eat the same daily fat intake as athletes?

When my body fat was 43 percent and I weighed 260 pounds and desperately wanted to lose some fat, should 30 percent of my daily calories have been fat?

Interesting. It's kind of like everybody eating the same amount of healthy calories when they live totally different life-styles. These guys seem to like mass producing health facts, and we believe them. Boys, you shouldn't do that, we are much smarter than you give us credit for.

Could it be possible to eat a lower-fat intake and still be healthy?

Well, Dr. Dean Ornish has a different opinion. Dr. John McDougal has some very interesting news. Gail

STOP THE INSANITY!

Butterfield, Nathan Pritikin, Scott Grundy, Covert Bailey, Georgia Kostas—all these people and many other experts say it is safe and effective to go lower than 30 percent of our daily intake in fat.

You want to hear something? True story. Happened last week. I have a friend who is a dietitian and exercise physiologist. She went to a convention given by the big guys in her field to hear the latest and greatest news in diet and food. After the seminar she questioned some of the keynote speakers who were still recommending that 30 percent of our daily intake be fat. She asked them why they were still standing by that number when all the experts knew that in order to lose body fat, regain your health, or make any significant change in your body, going below 30 percent fat in your daily intake is recommended. Do you know what their answers were?

"We are only recommending what we think the consumer can handle."

"It may not make a big difference in your appearance or your health, but we have to start slow. People are lazy and not ready for the truth."

"We are giving them what they can deal with now, and we'll make the change slowly, when they are ready."

Now I have something to say here. (Surprised?)

First, Mr. arrogant, egomaniac nutritionist, American consumers do want the information that will get them healthy and change the way they look and feel. They can "handle it." Who are you to decide what I or anybody else is "ready to hear"? I have known the American consumer for a long time, and I've seen the women of this country take information, apply it to their life-styles, and dramatically change their lives.

Here's the truth. If you want to make a difference in the way you look and feel, take your daily fat intake down to 15 or 20 percent. What's there to be afraid of? You choose what you want your daily fat intake to be. Anywhere between 10 and 30 percent of your intake is fine. Thirty percent is the high end, so if you don't have much body fat to lose and you are using tons of fuel a day, then go ahead, take in 30 percent. If you desperately want a change and you are not exercising like a rabbit every day, go lower—it will help you decrease your fat supply sooner, and the process of changing your body will be faster. There is one thing most of us don't need to worry about, and that's getting too little fat in our diet.

> If you're eating a balanced diet, it's virtually impossible not to get these essential fatty acids.
> —Covert Bailey, *The New Fit or Fat*

Worried about getting too little fat?

I have had 200-, 300-, and 400-pound people come up to me worried about not getting enough fat in their diet.

You don't have to worry about that. That's not going to happen.

How about being worried about what we have been living, or dying, on? Why haven't we been worrying about the heart attack that's around the corner? The damage being done by the morbid obesity that the huge amount of fat in our food creates for millions? The chemicals and crap in those freeze-dried concoctions that we live on in the name of dieting?

How about what we've been eating? We are all bloody lucky to be alive when you really think about what we put into our bodies and expect them to function on.

The fat formula works.

Eating works.

Calories are important.

Not all calories are created equal.

Fat makes you fat.

You are smart enough to figure it all out and make better choices.

Making better choices will change your body.

Your body does not manufacture fat, it comes from the end of your fork.

You can "Stop the Insanity" in your life by eating.

Good, fine, yeah, yeah, yeah. All of this makes a lot of sense, doesn't it?

Sorry to hear about your picket fence exploding,

Susan. The Prince is a toad. Glad everything's fine now. . . .

I get the part about how my car won't run without fuel. Forget equal calories for the rest of my life. The fat formula and I are connected at the hip.

But please . . . please . . . please . . . just tell me one thing.

WHAT IN THE HELL DO I EAT? HOW MUCH, WHEN, WHAT COMBINATIONS?

There is an answer to this question.

You can eat whatever you want, whenever you want it, and however much of it you want.

Has this book been written to panic the fat off your body? Eat whatever you want and whenever you want it —that statement is enough to panic even the limited dieter, forget about the millions of professional dieters who have a case of the vapors just trying to get past this statement.

The panic you feel is real. It is not caused by your "eating disorder" or your inability to discipline yourself to eat sensibly; it is not your inner child screaming out in protest. It is not your inability to control your hands and mouth that you should be afraid of, it's the zombie reaction we all have to that statement. Your trained response. The panic you feel because you have been trained not to think. You need that program and your weekly weighing and applauding to know that you are doing it correctly. You don't know what eating means anymore. Think about it . . . you are incapable of making the most simple decisions when it comes to the food you are going to eat today and for the rest of your life. Think about how out of control, scared, and confused this decision makes you feel.

I spoke with a woman once who expressed it all in one question. She was 200-plus pounds, desperate, in tears, more than willing to do whatever it took to finally solve the problem and get her body lean, strong, and healthy because she could no longer live the way she was living.

Brilliant, funny, fabulous woman who understood it all. Eating, breathing, and moving—no problem. At the end of an hour-and-a-half consultation, she looked at me and said:

"Just one question. I have a wedding to go to in November. [It was July.] What am I going to eat?"

Well, I had to ask her, "What will you feel like eating in November?"

"What kind of day will you have on November 20?"

"Who's going to be there? Your crazy aunt Lilly, who drives you nuts? If so, you'll probably be shoving that food in. She's driven you crazy for thirty years, so why do you think that's going to change just because you are dieting?"

"Hormonally how will you be feeling?"

"Will you be happy, sad, mad, glad?"

Who knows and who cares what you should eat four months from now?

The diet industry has done a good job, hasn't it? We can't make it without them. Talk about an industry that has created its own need.

You go to your diet counselor and you are treated like a child—no, not a child, an idiot. Sheets of paper telling you what to eat every minute of the day. Dieter's hints—you know the ones—that don't help you one bit when your body drives you straight toward the fridge after a couple of weeks of starvation. The silly suggestions that we've all tried that have nothing to do with your life-style or needs. The constant chipping away at your self-esteem. What this really boils down to is that you do not have the willpower this time to stick with it and get skinny. They imply that you are incapable, and that's exactly what you have become—incapable of making the smallest decisions. (You know the old saying: Tell a child he/she is something enough times, and that is what he/she becomes.)

Thousands and thousands of books have been written on the subject of dieting. The tabloids are filled with celebrity diet hints, tips, and food habits. We hear about food and diets on television, radio, magazines, billboards, telephone poles. (I just saw the same stupid flyer in three different cities on telephone poles everywhere. It said, "Lose 30 pounds in 30 days." Unbelievable.) Everywhere we turn it's diet, diet, diet, food, food, food, get thin quick, lose it fast. The more you diet, the more you lose; the more you lose, the more you gain; then you are right back where you started, and you need them again. The diet experts and programs are waiting. Waiting to take your money, set you up to fail, and make you feel like an undisciplined idiot. We don't question the systems, only ourselves.

My inability to stick to anything was the only thing on my mind every time I failed. My emotional instability, lack of discipline, and failure drove me crazy. It's amazing how deep they get: here is an industry that can reach down into your gut, make you not believe in yourself, make you give them your money without question, and have you give back a thousand times, without ever solving the problem.

The definition of insanity is doing the same thing and expecting different results. I don't know where I heard that, but when I did, my experience with diets was the first thing I thought of. The hundreds of times I thought, This is it. This one will do it. Sure I'll roll in mud a couple of times a day, drink weeds, suck on lemons, drink vinegar, not eat food for a couple of months—what the hell, I'll try it, anything. Maybe this one will work. I think of the fear I see in women's eyes when I suggest eating as one of the solutions to the problem.

It never mattered how much damage I was doing to myself by dieting—if it was going to make me thin, count me in. The fasting programs on the market today, doctor- and FDA-approved, have been connected with irregular heart rhythms; gallbladders being removed left, right, and center; and sudden death. Even when that yummy strawberry, vanilla, or chocolate shake says it's been fortified, it doesn't always have the trace minerals or fuel that your body needs to live. The constant yo-yoing and stress on the heart and internal organs were never a concern of mine. The physical dangers are something we seem to be willing to risk. I sure was.

The physical and psychological dangers of dieting have been documented as early as the 1950s. But we don't have to look for scientific proof to verify the dangers of starvation. There has never been a better or larger scientific study done on dieting than the one done by the millions and gazzillions of women who have tried dieting and failed. The women who live daily with the physical and emotional effects of starvation. You want proof that diets don't work? Go to the mall in any major city or small town in this country and have a look around. Look at all the fat, unfit, unhealthy people walking around.

Let's stop treating the symptoms. Let's solve the problem. I don't require blind faith from you. This is not about dependence, it's about independence. High-volume, low-fat eating will free you from the instant shakes, pills, formulas, and the disgusting frozen, freeze-dried, packaged foods that you've been living on. Once you understand and apply this concept to your life, you will begin to get leaner, healthier, and stronger.

Not because I've given you some magic willpower that you never had. You have plenty of willpower—anyone who has been on a diet for more than five minutes deserves a willpower medal.

Not because the fairy godmother of motivation has come down and tapped you on the head. Remember, she's a lie.

Not because you are following a daily menu with those helpful diet tips included for the stressful, hard-to-handle times.

Not because you have found the way to push that pizza away and enjoy having just one slice. That will never happen—why eat anything that you can only have one slice of? If I can't eat the whole thing, I don't want it. What's the point?

Do you want to have enough energy to get through your day? Do you want to eat more than you could ever imagine—and shrink? How about being able to go to the bathroom without laxatives? If any of these things interest you, then there is only one way to go.

High-volume, high-quality, low-fat eating.

> It's just fantastic to be able to eat until I'm full, snack occasionally, and have energy left to spare at the end of the day. Also, I've definitely decreased the cravings for junk. I'm eating good whole foods until I'm full, and it lasts for hours.
> —Comment from a client

Since we are all ex-dieters, I thought it would make you comfortable if I laid down a rule or two.

Rule number one: Never, never, never skip a meal again.

Breakfast: You don't have to force-feed yourself by a certain time of the morning, but you've got to eat before early afternoon, so let's call that breakfast.

I eat breakfast when I get hungry. Eating as soon as I wake up makes me a little nauseated, so I don't do it, but within a few hours of doing whatever it is I have to do for the day, I am starving. So my breakfast time varies every day. If I am up at five or six, you may find me by eight A.M. at a local restaurant chowing down on an egg-white omelet, with lots of bagels, lettuce, tomatoes, and onions —lots of onions a couple of days before my period, with tons of capers, those salty little buggers. If I don't get up by eight, have someone check my pulse, because it may be I'm dead—that's the only thing now that could keep me in bed that late. But if I am in bed that late, I'll be eating breakfast at about ten.

Here's the plan. When you're hungry, eat breakfast, function for a while, then it's time to eat again. It's called lunch. You are going to need enough fuel to run around all afternoon doing whatever it is that you do all afternoon—maybe that afternoon exercise class, picking up the kids, working at the office—and to carry you through till (yep, you guessed it) dinnertime. Three squares a day. Normal and sane. Just what your body needs to begin functioning properly and give you the energy you need to live.

This is only the beginning of sanity, because everyone knows man cannot survive on three squares a day. If you get hungry during the day, you have to eat. Snacks? I carry food around in my car, so when I'm hungry all I have to do is reach into the bag on the floor of the back-seat and eat. Constant grazing is what I do some days. Get me a feed bag and attach it to my face—it would be easier, that's for sure.

Snacking is fine, but don't let snacking replace a meal. I've had clients who find out that bagels can be low in fat, and that's all they eat for a couple of weeks. Bagels, my friends, are not a well-rounded meal. Bagels alone are not a wide variety of high-volume, high-quality, low-fat food.

A decent breakfast with cereal, fruit, juice, coffee, and the bagels includes a variety of high-volume, low-fat food. Finding those low-fat crackers and living on them is not how it's going to happen.

So, start with your three squares a day and build from there. How do you feel about rule number one? Are you under the table having your first panic attack yet? Don't worry, you'll get used to this fast. It is a hell of a lot easier, much more fun, and it works—you'll feel great, and it's better for you than starvation. All the diets that you've ever been on have you weighing, scaling, journaling, and measuring your food to death to get the answer to the question of how much you are supposed to eat a day. God forbid you go beyond your two 1-ounce portions of whatever it is you've been told to eat—you'll ruin it for the day (a good reason to run for the Ding Dongs). All the dieting I did always had me weighing and scaling for a couple of weeks, doing really well, building hope that this time it was going to work and I wouldn't feel like the fat, lazy ex-wife anymore. Inevitably I ate something that wasn't on the sheet of okay foods, that was beyond the right portion, or that just reached out and grabbed me—and I would die. Convinced that I could never stay with it, I'd run to the pantry and end up sitting on the floor eating cake mix from the box. Starting again tomorrow was always the pledge, and the cake mix was always the end result.

Rule number two: Eat as much as you want.

Don't think about it. Make sure you are taking in at least what your weight and activity level require your body to have so that you have the energy you need. Don't worry about how much you eat at what meal or in what combinations.

All right. That's it.

You've probably had it with me right now. If you didn't think I was a kook before, these first two rules must have convinced you that I am out of my mind and can't be trusted. God help all the eating disorder victims out there to whom I've just given free rein to run wild and shove food into their mouths.

Being the out-of-control, incapable woman that you are, you don't even know when you are full—right? How much is too much? When does emotion take over and hunger end? It's all been so confused by that terrible eating disorder that we all have. And here I am telling you that you must eat whatever you want, whenever you want it, and in any combination you want, depending on something as stupid as your weight and activity level. How could I be so cruel?

Well, you *do* know when you are full. I sure as heck knew I was full every night that I had a huge, high-fat dinner, put the kids to bed, got the bowl of candy, and ate it while I was watching TV. I was full of frustration and pain. I knew I was full when I went into the kitchen two hours later and made six pieces of cinnamon toast with tons of butter to soothe the pain, and I sure as hell knew I was full when I was throwing up and my stomach was aching with convulsions.

You *do* know when you are full. You understand the feeling. All the dieting tips out there that have been designed to fool you into feeling full don't do a thing. Drink tons of water before you eat—that feels good, doesn't it, eating pounds of food on top of an ocean of water? You've done that, I've done that, we all have. Eating wads of fiber before you consume any real food and feeling it explode in your stomach. That's really helped you in the past, hasn't it—swallowing pounds of rope. I am not suggesting you fool yourself into feeling full. I say eat until you *are* full. If satisfaction means too much once in a while, so what? I never learned behavior modification —do I look like someone who has? Look at my hair— does that look like a modified haircut to you? See the nails—fake. When I am frustrated, I eat. I ate when I was 260 pounds and frustrated, I eat now when I am frustrated. A fight with my husband sends me straight to the food. Guilt does it every time, and when you are raising children, feeling guilty is a daily occurrence.

The really big difference now is *what* I am eating. It's not the bag of M&M's. It's not the high-fat, sugary, processed crap that I'm shoveling into my mouth. High-volume, low-fat food fills me up now. I'm still shoveling, just not shoveling sugary, processed, high-fat food. You may not always have a strong hold on your emotions, but who does? Things change when you know you can eat anything except high-fat junk.

> My oldest had friends to spend the night. I bought them doughnuts for breakfast. I knew I would eat them during the night, so I chained the cabinet shut. In the morning, my daughter found only a crushed box and crumbs. I had squeezed through a small opening in the cabinet door. . . . Luckily my daughter had a sense of humor.
>
> —Darlene, a client

I've got a pen theory. It ties right in with diet and deprivation. Suppose I told you that you could have anything in the world—except a ballpoint pen. As long as you live, you can never have a ballpoint pen. You'll see other people with them, relatives and friends will be carrying and using them, but you can never have one.

You'd be fine for a while. I mean, you could have everything else. Who needs a ballpoint pen?

STOP THE INSANITY!

Before you knew it, you'd be angry with me. Who is she to tell me I can't have something? Then you'd get obsessed. Obsessed with—you guessed it—ballpoint pens. Day and night you'd think about ballpoint pens. Every person you see holding a ballpoint you'd want to lunge at, grab their pen, and run. Every situation that you were in would become less and less important if ballpoint pens were involved. A business meeting? Forget what the president of the company is saying, it's the ballpoint pen he is tapping on the desk that you are obsessed with. You may start stealing them and hoarding them in your basement. Pretty soon you'd have to 'fess up to your "addiction" or "pen disorder" and join a 12 Step program for the ballpoint pen–obsessed. And on it goes, a new disorder is created.

The diet industry has created a lot of the eating disorders by telling people that for the rest of their lives they have to live by shuffling cards from one slot to another, weighing and scaling, separating diet foods from real foods. I hate it when they do that, because their diet foods are usually high in fat, loaded with chemicals and total junk, and taste like doodoo—that's not better food. That's not the food that's going to change your body. And who could possibly face knowing you have to live on that stuff?

I am not putting you on special foods. I never will, no can do. If you want cookies, you're going to have cookies. That's not all your body needs, so you can't eat cookies all day long. Eat breakfast, then have some high-volume, high-quality, low-fat cookies. Cake—you want cake? I just ate a huge piece of banana walnut cake the other day with my kids. Did I walk into the supermarket, go to the frozen foods section, believe the 98 percent fat-free label, and take it home and eat the whole thing without having eaten anything else? NOOOOOOO. That's what I used to do, and that's why I got fat. No, I went to a store that makes nondairy, low-fat cakes with real ingredients and ate like an animal and had the best time ever with my kids. Cake, soda, and my kids. I was in heaven.

There was no reason to feel guilty. I didn't "blow it" for the day and have to run home to eat more. I had eaten breakfast, worked all morning, and was taking a break having a snack with the kids before I continued my day. By the way, it was the best banana walnut cake I've ever tasted. I ate mine and part of my younger son's—who could blame me?

You see, this is it. Food is not restricted. If you want to get rid of some of the fat you've built up, you'll have to cut back on some of the fat in your daily intake so that your body has a chance to use the fat you have stored—you know, the stuff that covers your body—as its fat fuel supply. It's that simple. Other than that, the higher the quality of the fuel, the better the performance. The high volume will give you the energy you need, fill you up, and get you your daily calories, and you'll be eating—really eating, instead of nibbling on cottage cheese, a hamburger without the bun (that diet plate still exists—I saw someone eating it the other day—can you believe it?), salad with a teaspoon of dressing. What in the hell is the point of a teaspoon of dressing? You're still eating 60%, 70%, 80% fat—whatever the percentage of fat it is —whether it's one teaspoon or ten. Why have any at all? If you want to guarantee feeling like a social outcast, just say at any dinner table, "No, thank you. I'd just like a teaspoon of that dressing." Listen to the way that sounds. You might as well scream, "I can't control myself! I am a compulsive eater, and this is the ten millionth diet I've tried—maybe this one will work."

It's a terrible position these diet people have put us all in. It's not normal. It's insane. Learning to eat again is as much about getting back in touch with your body and its need for fuel as it is about what kind of fuel you are putting in. We need to respect food and understand the role it plays in our lives. Our obsession and anger with and fear of food have been created by the very industry that wants us so afraid and incapable when it comes to eating. DON'T BE AFRAID OF FOOD ANYMORE.

STOP THE INSANITY!

> It controls me—not quite as much as it used to, but it is the first thing I think about when the depression hits or when my husband says something cruel or hurtful to me.
>
> —M. Jane, a client

I've made some big statements in this chapter. "Don't be afraid of food" is one of the biggest, but if you think that's big, take this one to your dietitian: It doesn't matter what combinations of foods you eat, protein versus carbs versus minerals versus anything else—except, of course, for the fat, which you can find instantly now that you are a fat detective. The rest is something you do not need to think about when you begin changing your body by eating, breathing, and moving.

Nobody knows what's right. The dietitians sure as hell don't know what the right combinations are. They keep changing their minds. We've gone from from the "basic four" food groups to suggestions that milk kills you and your children. Grains have just begun to be acknowledged as human foods. The connection between what we are putting in our mouths and the health of our nation is as foreign to the health professionals as life on other planets. Your doctor spends a couple of weeks max in medical school studying one of the most important factors in determining your health—the foods you put into your body. So if you have a question about the foods you and your family are eating, don't—I repeat, don't—go to your doctors. They don't have the answer.

If you haven't been worried sick about what you and your children have been living on for the last ten years, then why should you start worrying when someone—me—suggests you increase the quality of what you eat and decrease the fat in your foods? What's to worry about? Did you think about the carb, protein, and mineral balance in that fast-food hamburger you ate last week? Why not—because you trust the company that's selling it to you? How about the chemical concoctions we've all been drinking as meals every day for months?

128

Is that freeze-dried stuff that we've all paid a fortune for at the local diet center well balanced? Who's to say?

This stuff is being packaged and sold by people who haven't figured out that you need more than 1,000 calories a day to survive. That's a little scary, folks. We trust them—blindly. "Doctor sponsored" and "FDA approved" mean nothing. These guys have made their bed, now they have to lie in it—they have lied, stolen money, harmed your body and mind, and set you up for failure. They have hung themselves. They will not protect you or tell you the truth, so trusting that seal of approval is as insane as it gets. It's as if they have put a spell on us all. We've hung our brains at the door, walked right in, and bought everything they have to sell. It's worked. All those shakes, drinks, pills and frozen, colored, waxed, chemically beautified foods that we are living or dying on have made us very fat and unhealthy, and we don't feel good. It's time to change it.

Think about it. Sugary cereal for breakfast, hamburger and fries for lunch, and then that balanced meat, milk, and potato dinner. Could we be any more malnourished as a nation? Heart disease, cancer, arthritis, and diabetes run rampant in this country. Most of us are getting way, way, way too much fat, not enough fuel, too much sugary, chemical junk, and too little nutritional value in the foods we eat. There is no better testimony to our brilliant machines (other than the 1960s—how any of us got through that time is amazing) than the stuff we give our bodies to live on and the fact that they just keep right on going.

It's time for a little history lesson. Where it all started.

The insanity started on the walls of grammar school. You don't have to look much further than the "basic four" food chart that we were drilled on. Our parents believed that they were giving us what was best for our growing little bodies because the experts told them that the meat, the milk, the veggies, and the bread were the best things to eat.

EATING BETTER

Hey, Ozzie, hey, Harriet, where are you guys? Will you look at this thing? It wasn't so long ago that we all believed that the chart that was on every grammar school wall was the way to eat.

Whoops—you can't look at it, because it's not there. You know why? I called the National Dairy Council and they wouldn't let me use it. But visualize this, since you can't see it. I love the old definition of the Grain Group. Three slices of enriched bread and an ounce of fortified breakfast food.

THIS WAS THE EXPERT ADVICE THAT WE ALL FOLLOWED WITHOUT QUESTION? HEEEEEELLLLLLLP ME.

Eating enriched bread is like eating cardboard. Actually, cardboard probably has more nutrition. Think about this: They make the food and in the process strip it of all its natural nutritional value, then they put it back in, fortify it. Well, we've already established what happens every time we try to do something better than old Mother Nature—we screw it up royally, and all hell breaks loose.

Guide to Wise Food Choices

Let's go on to some charts that you can see. We've got the old 2, 2, 3, 2, and 6. That means 2 servings of milk, 2 servings of meat—wow, that'll keep you healthy. Remember, we are still keeping T-bone steak in the same food group as fish. Three servings of veggies. Six servings of grains. The only whole grain in there is rice. All the rest are processed. That's enough to clean anybody's colon, wouldn't you say? How about some more whole grains here?

Spend a moment with me on the "other" foods that "don't have enough nutrients to fit into any of the Five Food Groups." They "don't have enough nutrients"??? I love the whole concept of that. This is the new, improved "Guide to Wise Food Choices"? They've taken the old four groups and added another two, so now there are six confusing food groups. But what am I supposed to be eating?

The new, improved, lean, light version is one step away from the cave. Now the experts tell us that there is something called saturated fat. However, in their chart, the chook (that's Australian for chicken) is still in bed with the beef. Protein is still protein. Instead of a couple of slices of enriched bread, the grain section has been expanded. Hey, rice has been included—good job, boys.

The experts still insist that we need oils, meat, cheese, whole milk, and eggs in our diet.

WHERE IS THE FOOD PYRAMID, THE HIGH-VOLUME, LOW-FAT, HIGH-QUALITY FOOD PYRAMID?

Susan's Angle

Okay. Call me big. Considerate, not judgmental, just plain old nice guy. Experts, don't worry. Susan has solved your problem. Finally a low-fat, high-quality, high-volume, balanced, perfectly healthy, versatile, inexpensive way to eat that works with your body and will help you get and stay lean.

Let's start at the bottom—the foundation.

WHOLE GRAINS:

If it's high-volume, low-fat, high-quality food you're interested in incorporating into your life, start with whole grains. Constipation a problem? Eat 10 cups of brown rice and see what happens—throw out the Ex-Lax, pick up the whole grains. A great source of complex carbs, filling—did I say versatile? Cook them up, put them in the fridge, rush home, heat up some sauce, throw in the rice, instant dinner, kids —Mom's a genius.

LEGUMES:

If you want protein without the saturated fat, EAT BEANS. Beans, beans, good for your heart, the more you eat the

Guide to Wise Food Choices

Food Group	Nutrients	Servings			Foods	Serving Size
		Children 2–5	Children 6–10	Preteens, Teens, Adults		
Milk Group	*key nutrient:* calcium	3	3	2–4**	• milk	1 cup
					• yogurt	1 cup
					• cheese	1½–2 oz
	other nutrients: protein riboflavin vitamin D				• cottage cheese, pudding	½ cup
					• ice cream, ice milk, frozen yogurt	½ cup
					• milkshake	10 oz
Meat Group	*key nutrients:* iron	2*	2–3	2–3	• cooked, lean meat, fish, poultry	2–3 oz
					• egg	1
	other nutrients: protein niacin				• peanut butter	2 tbsp
					• cooked, dried peas, dried beans	½ cup
					• nuts, seeds	⅓ cup
Vegetable Group	*key nutrient:* vitamin A	3*	3–4	3–5	• vegetable juice	¾ cup
					• cooked vegetables	½ cup
	other nutrients: vitamin C fiber				• chopped, raw vegetables	½ cup
					• raw, leafy vegetables	1 cup

Fruit Group	*key nutrient:* vitamin C	2*	2–3	2–4	• fruit juice — ¾ cup • apple, banana, orange, pear — 1 medium • grapefruit — ½ • cantaloupe — ¼ • raw, canned, or cooked fruit — ½ cup • raisins, dried fruit — ¼ cup
	other nutrients: vitamin A, fiber				
Grain Group	*key nutrient:* fiber	4	6–9	6–11	• bread — 1 slice • tortilla, roll, muffin — 1 • bagel, English muffin, hamburger bun — ½ • rice, pasta, cooked cereal, grits — ½ cup • ready-to-eat cereal — 1 oz
	other nutrients: carbohydrate, iron				
"Others" Category	They don't have enough nutrients to fit into any of the Five Food Groups	These foods can be eaten in moderation. But they shouldn't replace foods from the Five Food Groups.			• fats and oils • candy • cookies • cake, rich desserts • chips and other salty snacks • condiments • alcohol • coffee, tea • soft drinks

*Serving sizes for children 2–5 should be two-thirds the size of the serving sizes listed above.

**4 servings for preteens, teens, young adults to age 24, and pregnant and lactating women.

SOURCE: *Guide to Good Eating.* Courtesy of National Dairy Council ©

Food Guide Pyramid

A Guide to Daily Food Choices

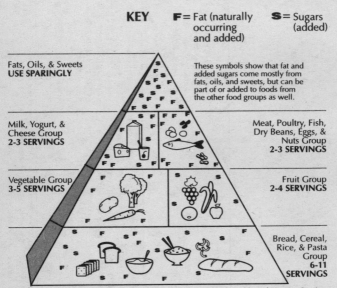

KEY   **F**= Fat (naturally   **S**= Sugars
occurring   (added)
and added)

Fats, Oils, & Sweets
USE SPARINGLY

These symbols show that fat and added sugars come mostly from fats, oils, and sweets, but can be part of or added to foods from the other food groups as well.

Milk, Yogurt, & Cheese Group
2-3 SERVINGS

Meat, Poultry, Fish, Dry Beans, Eggs, & Nuts Group
2-3 SERVINGS

Vegetable Group
3-5 SERVINGS

Fruit Group
2-4 SERVINGS

Bread, Cereal, Rice, & Pasta Group
6-11 SERVINGS

SOURCE: U.S. Department of Agriculture / U.S. Department of Health and Human Services

Use the Food Guide Pyramid to help you eat better every day...the Dietary Guidelines way. Start with plenty of Breads, Cereals, Rice, and Pasta; Vegetable, and Fruits. Add two to three servings from the Milk group and two to three servings from the Meat group. Each of these food groups provides some, but not all, of the nutrients you need. No one food group is more important than the other—for good health you need them all. Go easy on fats, oils, and sweets, the foods in the small tip of the Pyramid.

Susan's Angle
Eating Better Pyramid

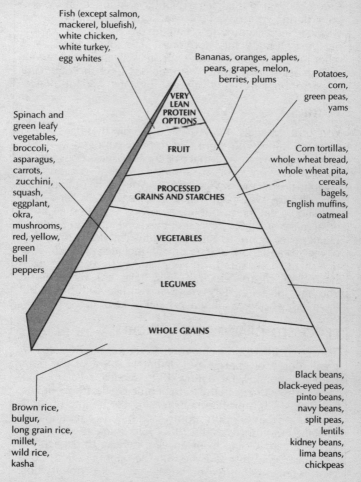

Fish (except salmon, mackerel, bluefish), white chicken, white turkey, egg whites

Bananas, oranges, apples, pears, grapes, melon, berries, plums

Potatoes, corn, green peas, yams

Spinach and green leafy vegetables, broccoli, asparagus, carrots, zucchini, squash, eggplant, okra, mushrooms, red, yellow, green bell peppers

Corn tortillas, whole wheat bread, whole wheat pita, cereals, bagels, English muffins, oatmeal

VERY LEAN PROTEIN OPTIONS

FRUIT

PROCESSED GRAINS AND STARCHES

VEGETABLES

LEGUMES

WHOLE GRAINS

Black beans, black-eyed peas, pinto beans, navy beans, split peas, lentils, kidney beans, lima beans, chickpeas

Brown rice, bulgur, long grain rice, millet, wild rice, kasha

SOURCE: Debbie Workman, M.S. Staff Exercise Physiologist, Susan Powter Exercise Studio

more you . . . I know, gas. Soak 'em, don't worry about the gas—your body will figure it out, I promise.

You can absolutely get enough protein and build those strong bones and muscles without the saturated fat. At any point during your day, if you eat a grain, a legume, and a veggie together, you will get all the protein you need without the saturated fat, hormones, antibiotics, feces, and other junk that comes with your steak. Don't worry about it. Just begin to include this fabulous food in your daily intake for higher-quality calories, lower fat, and lots of gas.

VEGGIES:

You know veggies. Way back in the old diet days, these were the things you were told to carry with you to satisfy your hunger. Yeah . . . that bag of celery sticks does a lot of good when you've been running around all day and are ravenous. The midday salad was your only option, and boy, oh boy, was it satisfying. Yes, veggies are good, and you should eat them, but no, a bowl of veggies does not a meal make. (Call Shakespeare, I've gone into Old English.) Do not ever again, as long as you live, sit down to a bowl of veggies and think of it as a meal. Include veggies in your rice salad, pasta salad, on your sandwich, as a side dish; steam 'em, stir-fry 'em, boil 'em, bake 'em, blend 'em if you have no teeth. Do whatever you like with them, but the midday bowl of salad as a meal is out of here.

PROCESSED GRAINS AND STARCHES:

This is an interesting category. Everyone needs carbs. A great source of energy and definitely, most of the time, high-volume, low-fat eating. But Americans eat most of their carbohydrates in the form of processed carbohydrates, and that's a big problem. Increasing the quality of foods means, for many, going from white bread—that enriched junk the nutritionists in the 1980s told us to eat—to whole-wheat bread. Going from an egg McKaka to a bagel for breakfast. Yes, these are steps in the right direction; however, women can't live on bagels alone. It is not a whole food. Bagels don't grow that way. Have you ever seen a bagel tree? The closer to the original food you get, the better the food and the more nutritional value it has.

Let me explain. Bagels, pasta, instant rice, cornmeal, and whole wheat are all fine and dandy and certainly a hell of a lot better than that packaged Danish in the convenience store. However, these are still processed foods, not the high quality I'm talking about in the high-volume, high-quality, low-fat formula for eating.

When those foods—or any other foods, for that matter—are processed, the tough seeds, flours, and meals that they are made from are lost. A lot of the nutritional value, fiber, and quality of the original food is gone when the bread, tortilla, or cereal is born.

If you eat too many processed grains and starches, you will probably not get the wide variety of foods your body needs to function. Lots of these processed foods have had sugar, salt, and sometimes fat added for taste or texture. So make sure you read the labels—not all breads are created equal.

There is nothing wrong with some cereal or pasta once in a while, but we are not eating these foods once in a while, we are getting most of our carbs in this form and are missing out on the grains that work best with the body and are high in volume, low in fat, and versatile as hell. Eat, enjoy—but it's very important that you understand that the bagel does not stand alone. It should be eaten with other foods.

Hey, how about breakfast? Start with a huge egg-white omelet, stuffed with veggies and loaded with condiments —I love spicy sauces, capers, onions, tomatoes. Then come the bagels, no butter—a little mustard, some lettuce; here's where my tomatoes and onions go—and make your own high-volume, low-fat, fabulous-tasting egg-white breakfast sandwich. Don't eat just the bagel. Eat a wide variety of real food and enjoy.

FRUIT:

Eat some once in a while. Try not to get up, eat some fruit, and expect it to last as an energy source for more than a couple of hours. Sugar is quick to burn, and an apple is not the most filling thing in the world. Include it with your oatmeal, cereal, or whatever you are having for breakfast. Throw in some fruit during your day if you feel like it. If you don't—forget about it.

VERY LEAN PROTEIN OPTIONS:

Top of the pyramid, not the best or first choice, but if it's turkey you want, then make sure it's lean (according to the fat formula). White chicken, fish (not all fish is low-fat— check, check, check), and the old high-protein, lean egg white. There are leaner sources of protein than red meat, beef. There is no such thing as lean beef. It's a contradiction in terms. Beef is a high-fat, low-volume, saturated-fat food, no matter how the beef industry wants you to look at it. Pork, the other white meat—gag me. There is no way around it, even with the millions the meat industry spends on advertising. It's a high-fat food, period. If it's meat you want, these are your lean protein options, but remember, Mr. Bean is stronger, better, and leaner and will cause you less heartache (pardon that pun).

Well, what do you think? Don't you love it? Simple. Just think about it. Don't get nuts and wipe out the pantry and cabinets in the kitchen. You don't need to fill your house with glass jars and legumes, just begin to incorporate some of these foods into your daily eating so that you have less to think about. My view is that the simpler it all is, the better. There is not much fat calculating that goes along with grains, beans, or veggies. Don't think about it, just learn how to prepare these foods according to your and your family's life-style and tastes and include them in your eating.

What can you do with grains and beans? It's endless . . . soups, casseroles, salads, loafs, patties. I make a lentil loaf —I know you want to throw up at the sound of that, but if you tasted it, you'd love it—so good that even the most meat-and-potatoes kind of guy wouldn't know it wasn't the best meat loaf and gravy he ever tasted. Put it in front of him, lie to him, he'll never know the difference, and the whole family will get leaner, stronger, and healthier.

Whole grains. Long-grain brown rice, wild-rice millet, rolled oats, polenta, quinoa, short-grain brown rice—the list goes on. This is the foundation of the chart and should be the foundation of your eating program. Whole grains—with your beans and veggies—give your body the nutrients it needs to be well. They will supply you with the highest-quality fuel your body can get. Low in fat, high in complex carbohydrates, protein, and lots of fiber—that's it, that's how to change the way you look and feel. The easiest and fastest way to change your body is to eat the highest-quality, lowest-fat, highest-volume foods. And you can't get better than whole grains.

Start to become familiar with these foods—there's nothing to be afraid of. If you can pull together that Thanksgiving meal and have everything come out on time and taste good, you can certainly pull together a rice dish—using real rice, not that polished white junk that comes in a box.

Add a grain dish to your skinless broiled chicken dinner. Throw in a grain here and there, and watch what happens to your body.

There are squillions of good grain cookbooks on the market—grab one. If the rice recipes are loaded with butter and milk, don't buy the book, find another. Bean recipes are a dime a dozen, play with them, get familiar with these foods. Eat, enjoy . . . *mangia*.

These foods will give your body the protein, minerals, vitamins, fiber, blah, blah, blah, that your body needs and will help make it a hell of a lot easier for you to get and stay lean, strong, and healthy. The AMA may not be ready to admit the connection between what we are putting in our mouths and the way we look and feel, but I know that the American public is ready and capable of making the changes because we are dying, and there isn't a person out there who doesn't want to improve the way they look and feel and increase the quality of their lives. You'd be shocked at what a huge difference the smallest changes in your eating do for your life. Try it—you may like it. Tell 'em Susan sent you. Good health to you.

STOP THE INSANITY!

As hard as it is to believe, the "basic four" food pyramid is still being used as a guide to healthy living. If it's in your children's classroom, warn them. Tell them the truth so they will know what not to eat and how to avoid the pain and physical harm that you and I have been through as a result of listening to the experts. There is a use for the "basic four" chart. It should be used to teach all of us what to eat to guarantee a heart attack, stroke, cancer, obesity, and hundreds of other diseases. So are you going to be malnourished if you begin to eat high-volume, higher-quality, lower-fat foods? Nope. It ain't gonna happen.

Increasing the quality and quantity of my foods gave me the energy that I needed to get through the day. It made me lean. I'm out of bondage now because I don't think about food other than what I feel like eating. That's going to make a very big difference in your life. It will free you from the food obsession you're living with.

I just got back from going out to Sunday brunch with my husband and the kids. Here's what I ate: a huge salad with vinegar-and-lemon dressing, a nine-layer Mexican bean dip without the cheese and the meat (made with low-fat chips), and a stack of blueberry-and-banana whole wheat pancakes, topped with fresh fruit and maple syrup. What more could anyone ask for? Do you think I'm feeling deprived right now? It's not as if I walked away from the table saying, "Something sweet . . . I'm feeling the need for something sweet." If it's sweet you want, combine the blueberry and banana in your pancakes and add some fruit on top—you'll be gagging from sweet.

Is that what I eat every day? No, usually I leave out the pancakes, because for some reason pancakes are associated with Sunday brunch in my mind. But the salad, the nine-layer dip, and maybe something else would be my lunch every day. (Who can't eat Mexican food every day?) I have already confessed (and you know that's a big Catholic thing to do, confess every thirty seconds) that I failed Behavior Mod 101. Self-control has never been a big asset of mine, either. Restraint isn't in my vocabulary. Does it sound like I have held back in the writing of this book? So far I have three or four major industries planning my death.

EX-FAT WOMAN FOUND AT THE BOTTOM OF RIVER WITH LOW-FAT SAUSAGE TIED TO HER ANKLES . . . news at eleven.

Forget self-control and behavior modification. It isn't gonna happen. Don't you think you've spent enough time trying? Let's get on with something that does work, requires much less effort and energy, and will change your body.

Higher-volume, higher-quality, lower-fat foods in your life. Give it a chance, see what happens. When it clicks, you are in. I've seen the light go on in so many women's eyes. That's it, they get it. The insanity stops in their lives forever.

If you haven't run to the grocery store to use the fat formula, cut out your daily calorie consumption and called a friend over to show her, ripped your pantry to pieces scanning trusted brands for lies, then maybe you need more proof.

Should I really make you mad, get you up and rally you to join the cause? If this doesn't do it, nothing will. Fat to fat comparisons—they'll blow your mind, and it's my favorite thing to do (compare fat, that is, not blow your mind, although . . .).

Fat Comparisons

High-volume, low-fat eating is easy when you understand the concept of fat to fat comparisons, as opposed to the old calorie-counting days. Don't worry about the calories, let's just have a look at the fat.

On the left you'll find some foods you may be all too familiar with. Across the top you'll see five categories: Greens, Legumes, Whole Grains, Processed Grains, and Fruit. Just examples, not the only comparisons under the sun.

STOP THE INSANITY!

Let's go over them, starting at the beginning: 1 chocolate-chip cookie. One, that's all. How many times have you heard this from the diet community: "Learn how to have just one [behavior mod, you know], and then walk away from the table"? Well, that's not fine, even if you are one of those people—and I have not met one person who has this down—who can "have just one and then walk away from the table."

Have a look at this. You can have 1 COOKIE OR 20 CUPS OF RICE. AAAAAAAAAAAAA. Same amount of fat. This is a great example of low-volume/high-fat eating versus high-volume/low-fat eating—you choose.

It makes me nuts every time I think about it. Do you know how many sweet things you do with rice? Soups, casseroles, salads, patties—the list is endless, and you've got 20 cups to work with. One cookie. *One* cookie. Get a life, doctors, nutritionists, and dietitians of the world—why didn't you let us know this? How come I've never been told this by any of the experts? You big jerks. You made me believe that I had this problem because I couldn't control myself. It wasn't me, it was the food I was eating.

Too angry to continue? Not me, let's go. Hop around with me. Snack, you want a snack? How about 1 Hershey's bar? What's equal? 35 cups of popcorn. (Read your label— these popcorn guys are big-time liars. Do your fat formula, or better yet, make your own popcorn.) 35 cups of popcorn for one candy bar? Make your 35 cups of popcorn, salt it up, and enjoy.

Next—I know I'm skipping around, but consider it mental exercise—3 cheese enchiladas or 100 bagels. What do you think you could do with 100 bagels, other than throw up for days after eating that much? If you don't think 100 bagels would fill you up, switch them for the 150 plums that you can eat instead of your 3 cheese enchiladas.

But doctor, doctor, how do I get my protein if I don't eat cheese? Well, 12 cups of pinto beans may do the trick. And then there's that fear—which the American Dairy Association has put into your brain—that without cheese your bones will turn to ash and crumble. You are guaranteed to be hunched over, brittle-boned, and wishing you had eaten

142

more dairy, right? Wrong, wrong, wrong, boys—why don't you tell the American public the truth about osteoporosis? Go ahead and tell them that osteoporosis is not about too little calcium but too much protein in our diet. And while you're at it, why not tell us what's in our food other than calcium—you know the information, the studies have been done. What else we're getting in our cheese: fat, chemicals, coloring, salt . . . You know what? To hell with these guys, they have been lying for so long that they are not about to tell you the truth now. Find out for yourself. Ask whoever it is you get your dietary advice from if 200 cups of collard greens won't get you some calcium.

While we are on the dairy products, follow me to 1 cup of whole milk. One cup of whole milk or 20 cups of spinach. One cup of whole milk or 8 cups of brown rice. How about 1 tablespoon of peanut butter or 20 cups of lentils? Now whether or not it's lentils you like or some other legume, look at the comparison. You couldn't get much lower volume than 1 tablespoon of peanut butter—talk about worthless, and high fat. What's that going to feed?

It's the concept of high volume/low fat versus low volume/high fat that's important to understand, not the food comparisons. But since we are on a roll, let's keep going for a while. Potato chips—10 of them. Now *there's* a reality for most of us. Only in my dreams could I ever sit down and eat 10 potato chips. Why eat 10 potato chips? Well, if you could eat only 10, you could have them—or you could have 40 slices of Italian bread. Surely 40 slices of bread would do more for your hectic day, fill you up, give you more energy, and make you feel full (as opposed to those 20 cups of water you need to drink before your one tablespoon of peanut butter.

I can hardly wait to get to the T-bone steak. Protein? How about those 10 cups of kidney beans? If you cut that amount in half, 5 cups, and include 10 cups of long-grain rice, you've got all the protein you need.

You think I hate meat, don't you? Well, I don't. This is not about vegan versus meat eater. There are lots of unhealthy, unfit, fat vegetarians out there. This is a fat thing.

(cont. on page 148)

STOP THE INSANITY!

Fat Comparison Chart

High-Fat Item	Greens and Vegetables	Legumes
1 chocolate-chip cookie	= 50 carrots	= 10 cups lentils
6 grams fat	6 grams fat	6 grams fat
78 calories	1,500 calories	816 calories
69% fat	**4% fat**	**7% fat**
3 cheese enchiladas	= 200 cups cooked collards	= 70 cups navy beans
75 grams fat	75 grams fat	75 grams fat
1,150 calories	6,650 calories	18,000 calories
59% fat	**10% fat**	**4% fat**
1 piece of cheese pizza	= 30 cups green beans	= 12 cups pinto beans
10 grams fat	10 grams fat	10 grams fat
250 calories	1,313 calories	2,811 calories
36% fat	**7% fat**	**3% fat**
1 cheeseburger	= 80 cups broccoli	= 30 cups pinto beans
30 grams fat	30 grams fat	30 grams fat
500 calories	1,971 calories	7,028 calories
54% fat	**14% fat**	**4% fat**
1 tbsp. peanut butter	= 50 cups cauliflower	= 20 cups lentil sprouts
8 grams fat	8 grams fat	8 grams fat
94 calories	1,200 calories	1,632 calories
77% fat	**6% fat**	**4% fat**
1 bologna and cheese sandwich	= 80 cups Swiss chard	= 12 cups black beans
11 grams fat	11 grams fat	11 grams fat
290 calories	2,800 calories	2,724 calories
34% fat	**4% fat**	**4% fat**
1 cup whole milk or cottage cheese	= 20 cups steamed spinach	= 10 cups lima beans
8 grams fat	8 grams fat	8 grams fat
160 calories	493 calories	2,200 calories
45% fat	**15% fat**	**3% fat**

Whole Grains	*Processed Grains/ Starches*	*Fruit*
= 20 cups long-grain rice	= 6 cups pasta	= 800 grapes
6 grams fat	6 grams fat	6 grams fat
3,242 calories	1,044 calories	1,469 calories
2% fat	5% fat	4% fat
= 40 cups barley	= 100 bagels	= 150 plums
80 grams fat	75 grams fat	75 grams fat
27,920 calories	16,400 calories	6,353 calories
3% fat	4% fat	11% fat
= 10 cups brown rice	= 10 cups pasta	= 15 pears
10 grams fat	10 grams fat	10 grams fat
2,321 calories	1,740 calories	1,469 calories
4% fat	5% fat	6% fat
= 90 cups long-grain rice	= 30 cups whole wheat pasta	= 50 apples
30 grams fat	30 grams fat	30 grams fat
14,590 calories	5,220 calories	4,885 calories
2% fat	5% fat	6% fat
= 8 cups brown rice	= 10 bagels	= 14 bananas
8 grams fat	8 grams fat	8 grams fat
1,856 calories	1,640 calories	1,468 calories
4% fat	4% fat	5% fat
= 40 cups wild rice	= 20 pita sandwiches 1 c. sprouts and tomatoes	= 20 cups strawberries
11 grams fat	11 grams fat	11 grams fat
6,485 calories	1,650 calories	895 calories
2% fat	6% fat	11% fat
= 8 cups brown rice	= 20 cups green peas	= 15 cups blueberries
8 grams fat	8 grams fat	8 grams fat
1,856 calories	2,688 calories	1,218 calories
4% fat	3% fat	6% fat

STOP THE INSANITY!

Fat Comparison Chart, cont.

High-Fat Item	Greens and Vegetables	Legumes
1 cup granola	**= 125 cups zucchini**	**= 35 cups white beans**
23 grams fat	23 grams fat	23 grams fat
420 calories	2,275 calories	8,708 calories
49% fat	**9% fat**	**2% fat**
1 Hershey bar	**= 50 cups eggplant**	**= 10 cups navy beans**
10 grams fat	10 grams fat	10 grams fat
160 calories	1,344 calories	2,584 calories
56% fat	**7% fat**	**3% fat**
1 Snickers bar	**= 30 cups green peppers**	**= 18 cups lentils**
13 grams fat	13 grams fat	13 grams fat
276 calories	750 calories	4,134 calories
42% fat	**16% fat**	**3% fat**
10 potato chips	**= 30 cups sprouts**	**= 12 cups black beans**
10 grams fat	10 grams fat	10 grams fat
150 calories	418 calories	2,700 calories
60% fat	**22% fat**	**3% fat**
1 oz. American cheese	**= 60 carrots**	**= 10 cups kidney beans**
8 grams fat	8 grams fat	8 grams fat
100 calories	1,858 calories	2,248 calories
72% fat	**4% fat**	**3% fat**
1 oz. bologna	**= 25 cups broccoli**	**= 12 cups lentils**
8 grams fat	8 grams fat	8 grams fat
88 calories	616 calories	2,756 calories
82% fat	**12% fat**	**3% fat**
1 12 oz. T-bone steak	**= 150 cups green beans**	**= 60 cups kidney beans**
60 grams fat	60 grams fat	60 grams fat
1,020 calories	6,563 calories	15,286 calories
53% fat	**8% fat**	**4% fat**

Whole Grains	Processed Grains/ Starches	Fruit
= 25 cups barley	= 75 large biscuits Shredded Wheat	= 150 oranges
23 grams fat	23 grams fat	23 grams fat
8,376 calories	6,230 calories	9,236 calories
2% fat	3% fat	2% fat
= 35 cups wild rice	= 35 cups popcorn	= 15 cups raspberries
10 grams fat	10 grams fat	10 grams fat
5,674 calories	800 calories	904 calories
2% fat	11% fat	10% fat
= 42 cups long-grain rice	= 45 cups popcorn	= 40 kiwis
13 grams fat	13 grams fat	13 grams fat
6,800 calories	1,035 calories	1,854 calories
2% fat	11% fat	6% fat
= 35 cups long-grain rice	= 40 slices Italian bread	= 20 mangoes
10 grams fat	10 grams fat	10 grams fat
5,674 calories	3,312 calories	2,691 calories
2% fat	3% fat	3% fat
= 25 cups long-grain rice	= 8 corn tortillas	= 12 cups pineapple
8 grams fat	8 grams fat	8 grams fat
4,053 calories	536 calories	911 calories
2% fat	13% fat	8% fat
= 25 cups wild rice	= 20 cups green peas	= 50 tangerines
8 grams fat	8 grams fat	8 grams fat
4,053 calories	2,688 calories	1,848 calories
2% fat	3% fat	4% fat
= 60 cups bulgur	= 50 English muffins	= 115 bananas
60 grams fat	60 grams fat	60 grams fat
15,045 calories	6,600 calories	12,061 calories
4% fat	8% fat	4% fat

STOP THE INSANITY!

Fat for fat, meat and dairy are about as high as they come. My point is that there are many foods that you can eat without the fat and with the high volume, high quality you need that will give you the energy, nutrients, and vitamins you need to live—and that you DON'T HAVE TO WORRY ABOUT IT. EAT, EAT, EAT, AND ENJOY. Don't wait until you have that opportunity to stop the world, go to school for eight years, do your internship and residency, and then make better food decisions. You'll be dead by then.

It is so easy to begin to include high-volume, low-fat food in your life. Have your skinless chicken and a few veggies, but instead of having that glass of milk, throw in pounds of pasta salad, a rice dish, some beans—hey, maybe if you've got the beans, you won't need the chicken —and eat the food that you can have enough of to be full and not be deprived. Food that works with your body to get it lean, strong, and healthy.

It's so much easier than living fat. It's not food that makes you fat. It's fat. I promise. Read your labels. If there is nothing you can pronounce on the label and it's a mile wide and an ocean deep, put it down. Use your fat formula. Don't ever believe a label again. It's your life they are playing with. They don't care as long as they get your money—it's not their worry what condition your heart, arteries, or body is in. Start eating higher-volume, higher-quality foods. See what happens. The difference in the way you feel will be immediate, the difference in the way you look will not be far behind.

My goal is to make it as easy as possible for you to get lean—not to impose my dietary beliefs on you. There is no opinion or belief involved in this. Look at the comparisons, and you'll understand how you got as fat, as tired, and as unfit as you feel.

The point is that it's not normal to starve yourself. It is ineffective, impossible to stick to, dangerous and guarantees failure. The minute you start eating high-volume, high-quality, low-fat foods, you will be surprised at how many symptoms fly out the window, including your

148

eating disorder. Permission to eat sure does a lot to help eliminate food obsession. You'd be surprised at how those eating disorders can fly. Eating when you are hungry is normal. So is eating until you are satisfied. How much you eat will and should change daily, depending on _____ (fill in the blank). You guessed it. YOUR ACTIVITY LEVEL.

I don't want to end up paralyzed from a stroke or dead from a heart attack. I didn't realize I had so much control.
—Comment from a client

Before I end this chapter, I have to say that I am very aware there are emotional connections to food. No joke, there are emotional connections to everything. People do have food issues that can be dangerous or life-threatening, and getting help for those problems is extremely important. Pretending to be what I'm not is not my style. I am not a therapist, but I do have something to say to the therapist. Here I go again, but speaking is what I do, and I have to speak up here.

I have a suggestion for all the therapists, eating disorder clinics, and 12 Steppers out there. While the people in your meetings are talking about how many times they threw up yesterday, why don't you take them for a walk, get them a little oxygen? How about increasing the quality of foods they're eating? Let's get them away from the processed sugary, chemical foods that we all know are damaging to our bodies and have a whole lot to do with being unbalanced and get some fuel in that helps to heal. Isn't healing what we are all trying to do? Who needs eating, breathing, and moving more than someone who is recovering from whatever?

Whether eating higher-quality, lower-fat foods and getting a little oxygen solves the problem is not the issue. It can certainly help, and we can no longer deny that what we are eating and how we are living are directly connected to how we look and feel, our emotional as well as our physical health. It is very much a part of healing, and since that's what you guys are trying to do, why not include it? Sugar addiction. No joke. Sugar is addictive. Come on, get your heads out of the sand. All these eating disorders everyone is running around with have something to do with the fact that we are literally starving our bodies. Don't they? Our machines are not getting enough fuel, the right kind of fuel, and the engine is so clogged, rusty, and low on oil that it's coughing and choking its way through the day. The old Tony the Tiger engine *ping*ing up the mountain. (Remember that commercial?)

That's how we live. You can't disconnect the mind from the body. The same blood and oxygen that feed the body, feed the mind. If you can worry yourself into a physical problem, an ulcer, then why can't your physical condition affect your mind? Well, without being an expert of any kind, I say it can. I know how much one has to do with the other because I lived through it, and so have thousands of other women. So to hell with the experts who don't want to make a connection. I was so depressed, I couldn't function. I am not anymore. I couldn't get through the day because I was so tired—you can't keep me down now. My body hurt, but it doesn't now—it's strong. I did not work on my brain—I'm still as screwed up as I was then—I gave my body what it needed physiologically to function, and it absolutely affected the emotional and mental. If you have an emotional disorder, join the club—who doesn't? You still have to eat, you still have to breathe, and you still have to move if you want to change the way you look and feel. You may be surprised at how much can change when you add these three things to your life.

I just spoke at the American Heart Association. The fifty-second anniversary. Big gig for a housewife from Texas. These are the guys who made the four-color posters. The target heart rate, 30 percent of your daily intake, all the stuff that none of us understand—these are the big guys who came up with all that stuff.

The speech was held in a beautiful banquet room full of nurses, therapists, doctors, dietitians, nutritionists, and every other kind of expert you could think of . . . and me.

Me, having a chat with all these people. Talking, talking, talking—that's what I did for about an hour and a half. Great speech, big fun, great folks—I must say these American Heart guys are big fun. Lots of information and laughs.

At the end of the speech I said with every ounce of passion I had left:

Please . . . someone in this room tell me that I'm being irresponsible?

Tell me the answer to this complicated, painful problem that millions of women face isn't this simple.

Tell me I'm wrong.

Tell me I'm being irresponsible.

The room was dead silent.

It is this simple. *Stop the Insanity!* is the answer to the problem. No more treating the symptoms. You can do it —this time you are not being set up to fail. It is attainable and understandable.

The American Heart Association has the research, the four-color posters, the experts, and the controlled study groups, but they didn't reach me. A single, fat, depressed housewife living in Texas didn't understand what they were talking about. I didn't know how to apply what they were saying to my life. It was too complicated.

The speech ended, but before I got off the podium, I told the American Heart folks something. What I said was, You've got the research, you've got the theories, you've got the scientists, but you're missing the mouth. Hey, how about you guys hiring me, and we can get this information to everyone who needs it. What do you think? We'll work together to clear this problem up.

I have not gotten the job application yet, but I'm sure it's in the mail.

Business is other people's money.
—Delphine de Girardin Marguerity, 1852

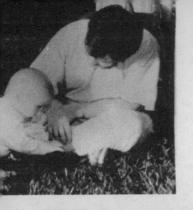
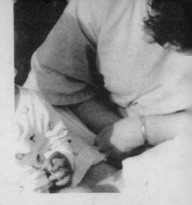
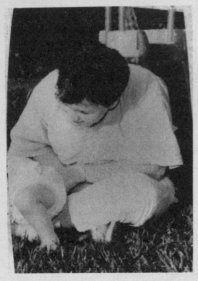

Well, all hell broke loose. The marriage started splitting wide open, and I just kept getting fatter and fatter. My younger son was eleven-and-a-half months old. One year after his birth I was huge. One big tub of lard is what I felt like. It was difficult to move without pain and exhaustion. My hair was getting shorter, my body was getting bigger, my self-esteem was in the gutter, and I was dying.

FIVE

Breathing Right

Without oxygen, you die.

It's time to live.

Not just life as you knew it before you bought this book, but life on a different level. A cellular level.

This, my friends, is unlike any living you've ever done before. Living on a cellular level means living in oxygen. You know, the thing we take for granted. The giver of life. Something none of us can live without.

Without oxygen you die.

By Susan Powter. Don't you love it? I made that up.

There are only a couple of ways to get the "giver of life" into your body. Sure, you know how—breathe. No problem, it's a given.

Not so, fellow soon-to-be good breathers, because none of us has any idea how to breathe properly. It's not just about breathing without thinking. It's about breathing right.

Talk about something we take for granted! Getting enough oxygen into your body requires more than breathing. It requires all of us to get back into the habit of breathing, learning how to do it correctly, and focusing on taking a few literally lifesaving breaths a day.

A couple of years ago my mother died of lung cancer.

153

STOP THE INSANITY!

We could spend chapters on the life-style that killed her, the foods, cigarettes, lack of exercise, and so on. I could write books about the horrors of lung cancer (nasty stuff), but what happened to me as I was helping my mother during her last two weeks of life has a whole lot to do with this chapter.

I watched someone die from a lack of the one thing we all assume is just there—there to feed every cell and muscle in our bodies. That's no small statement when you find out, which you are about to, that there are 75 trillion cells in your body. My kind of number. (Take it further and what do you have—gazillion, squillion?) So you can see that the oxygen you take in has a big job to do, feeding all those cells, plus all your muscles and internal organs. Breathing is more important than any of us understands.

It does happen without our thinking about it—in and out, in and out, lungs work, heart works, and we breathe. No problem.

The problem is that we

1. don't get enough oxygen;
2. never think about or work on improving our breathing;
3. don't use or give credit to a life-giving force.

And the consequences are that bazillions of us are suffering from a disease that I have named Oxygen Deprivation. (Did you know that above and beyond writing books, I name diseases?) Before you can understand the severity of this disorder you are living with daily, you have to have some idea about what this stuff called oxygen is, why we need it, and what difference it makes to us if we don't get enough of it.

You've got your common, ordinary human body. Your body. Inside that body are those 75 trillion cells. Picture this: 75 trillion little birds in a nest, and a huge mama oxygen bird comes along and feeds every single one of them. Without the mama oxygen bird, all the little baby birds would die.

Too science fictiony for you? I understand—that analogy scares me, but you've got the picture.

The first problem with not getting enough oxygen is that your cells and muscles don't get the one thing that they live on. Can you imagine what could happen to cells that haven't gotten enough oxygen in years? Now if you throw in tons of body fat, weak muscles, an unfit cardio system, and a sewer for a blood flow, do you think disease could set in? Maybe the cells could begin to mutate, not respond properly? Immune systems could begin to shut down? All right, I've taken this whole thing too far by even suggesting that oxygen could have anything to do with any of these things. After all, the AMA hasn't said so, and here I am again . . . Pardon me, I'll get on with it.

Breathing is not a mystical thing. Metaphysics has very little to do with it. As far as I'm concerned, India is not the ideal place to live, and sitting on a mountain on a bed of nails breathing is not my idea of fun. (Do you think I could get any more stereotypical than I just got? Wow, I wonder which TV program in my youth instilled that sick picture in my mind?)

Learning how to live on a cellular level and understanding oxygen means learning how to use it right here and now, in the U.S. of A., in the 1990s. The nineties version of the guru will have a cellular phone in her hand —how can anyone live without these things anymore? You don't need candles, incense, or flowing robes, and it's not necessary to meditate in order to get enough oxygen to live. Feeding every cell and muscle in your body is much more tangible than most of us could ever imagine. Getting your body the oxygen you need is easy, but first you might like to know what this stuff is.

The first and most important fuel.

The ultimate energy. The most vital ingredient in wellness. The feeder of the internal fire. Get the Olympic flame, I'm going for the gold here. . . .

The golden fuel.

The big cheese.

The finest fuel in the land.

Exaggerated? Not at all. True, true, no description could do this stuff justice.

Here's how it works. As oxygen feeds the internal fire

of the 75 trillion cells in your body, the product or fuel this fire produces is called adenosine triphosphate, or ATP. Without ATP there is no energy, there is no life. (No small statement.) Pretty important stuff, this ATP. Those birds in the nest? Forget about them without this stuff. ATP provides the energy you need to lift your arm, the energy you need to feel, the energy you need to think. Interrupt the output of ATP and you'll have symptoms ranging from exhaustion to the onset of serious disease.

Like mutating cells? Not getting enough ATP? Mutating cells? Cancer? It's all just too farfetched, isn't it?

Back to breathing. "Autonomic" is the official term used to describe breathing. Every time you take a breath, the diaphragm and the intercostal muscles (I have no idea where they are and don't really care, but I do know that they are somewhere between the ribs) automatically do what they are supposed to do—they expand, then relax to release the air. Autonomic and automatic—very, very close. Automatic, meaning "without thinking."

Breathing is automatic, thank God, because if it required any thought, we would have wiped ourselves out. As we've established, we take it for granted. I find it fascinating that oxygen is something we never talk about, don't teach the importance of, and totally ignore in our society. Could this be the beginning of dysfunction for all of us? The ultimate dysfunction, a whole country not speaking about the one thing that gives us all life. The bigger the problem, the greater the silence—or, you are only as sick as your secrets. No wonder we all have the same eating disorders. We are all dysfunctional. Well, consider that all changed from this chapter on. No more silence about the big cheese. It's over, I'm coming out of the closet with my oxygen banner waving, going to Washington, and yelling at 'em all. This has to stop right here and now.

I wish I had known any of this when I weighed 260. It isn't difficult to find out how oxygen fit you are. I would have had encased this number in gold and framed it. Do me a favor. Figure out your unfit number and then check it out a few months later. Big fun.

Here's how you find your breathing range. You'll need Granny's tape measure (a very handy piece of equipment that needs to come back into style), your chest, and this simple formula.

1. Take your tape measure and wrap it around your chest.
2. Exhale fully.
3. Measure the circumference of your chest at the full exhale point.
4. Take a huge breath.
5. Measure your chest at the height of inhaling. Hang on to that number.
6. Take the difference between the two numbers and divide it by the number your chest was when you exhaled.

I'll do mine with you: My husband, husband number two (yes, I did it again), wrapped Granny's tape measure around my exhaled chest. I swear it was the closest thing we've had to sex in weeks—who has time to make love between the job, the kids, the house? If you have found a way to manage all these things and still be the sex queen, write to me and tell me how, because I'm failing miserably in that department. Anyway, here are the results. My chest measurement after exhaling is a full 35 inches. I take my big, deep breath in, and my chest expands to 38 inches, fully impressing that husband of mine. The difference between the two numbers is 3. I run for the calculator because I can't divide. The calculator divides 3 by 35 (the original chest measurement). The calculator says 8.9 percent, close enough to 9 percent for me. So let's just call it 9 percent so I'll get a more impressive reading, and go straight to the numbers—the low, the high, the normal—that the little men in white coats sitting in laboratories have spent years figuring out.

There is the brilliantly fit range, the normal range, the low end, and—no expansion rate at all.

No more oxygen.

No more ATP.

STOP THE INSANITY!

No more life.

You're a goner. . . .

Drumroll—I'm about to be categorized.

Brilliantly fit? Competitive athletes have a 15 percent expansion rate.

In my dreams.

Heart patients and people suffering from respiratory problems can have as low as a 2–5 percent expansion rate. It looks like I'm above that. (Thank God, me being a fitness expert and all.)

Based on my test results, I have concluded that normal is a 5–10 percent rate. So I'm at the high end of normal.

You know by now that I'm not big on tests and statistics, but anything this cheap and easy to do is worth doing.

Considering how I felt when I first began to change my body, I can tell you that I was close to the heart patient category, because taking a deep breath was something I never ever did, and a strong cardio system is something I definitely did not have. Since I don't have the numbers to compare, we'll never know. But now you'll have the numbers to compare your unfit self with your soon-to-be new and improved model.

However, there's more to breathing than ATP, chest expansion measurement, and my theory about the 1990s guru. The heart and lungs play a big part in the process. Consider them the head honchos of the body's oxygen distribution system. They get the oxygen into that bloodstream of yours and distribute it through your body. But the oxygen drama doesn't end here—there are more players. The arteries that the blood flows through also play a role in maintaining the health of the internal organs that receive all that blood and in making sure that your cells and muscles get the nutrients they need to stay alive.

So don't be fooled into believing that all you have to do is walk around without thinking and do what comes naturally and you'll get what you need to live.

Don't assume that your birdies are being fed what they need or that there isn't a malnourished one among them. It takes a bit more than doing something without a second thought to feed 75 trillion (just ask the government of India), but nothing too complicated.

There are only two ways to get oxygen into your body. One: You can carry around an oxygen tank and suck from it every few minutes. When I found out how important oxygen was and how much it affected the way I looked and felt—yes, that skin, those eyes, that healthy glow, are all directly connected with oxygen—I seriously thought about the oxygen tank option. But it didn't work for me, because carrying myself around with the two kids and the grocery bags was tough enough—add an oxygen tank and I would have been down and out of the game. Who's to say, however? What's wrong for some may be right for others. So if the tank works for you, go for it.

The only other way to get oxygen into your body is through movement. Exercise. That oxygen tank is sounding better and better, isn't it? Why do you think I even considered it? When I heard about option number two, I was running—well, walking fast—toward the surgical supply store.

The worst part is that most of these "counselors" have never been overweight a day in their lives. How could they possibly know what an overweight person is going through?
—Comment from a client

Exercise. A simple concept, but a very scary reality for most of us. Let's do some word association together, shall we? Exercise.

Torture.

Pain.

Humiliation.

Exhaustion.

Being beaten and made to feel like you want to die.

You know it's supposed to be good for you, that in order to have a "healthy heart" you've got to do it. You may have heard rumors about those endorphins that are waiting to burst onto the scene and make you feel higher than you've ever been. As good as that stuff they give you in the hospital after surgery? I doubt it. You may have even tried it once in a while—exercise, that is, not the stuff they give you after surgery. If you have, I know you joined in the word association, because you probably experienced the torture, pain, humiliation, and exhaustion when you went to the class, gym, fitness warehouse, or wherever it is you went to do this simple, all-important thing they call exercise.

So far you know that you've been right about a lot of things, and you are right again. Exercise is essential to life and it is supposed to make you feel better. Your body needs movement every day to be well, to get the oxygen it needs to live. Above and beyond that, exercise does a couple of other important things. You know that metabolic disorder you have? When you ask your doctor about the connection between dieting and your metabolism, ask about exercise as well. "Doctor, doctor, what guarantees a screwed-up metabolic rate?"

Your doctor will reply, if he knows, "Not eating and not exercising."

Then you ask, "Doctor, doctor, what heals, increases the efficiency of, or improves a screwed-up metabolic rate?"

Your doctor will reply, if he knows, "Why, the best way to increase a metabolic rate is to eat and to exercise."

Fine, fine, fine. But this book is not about being healthy. This book is about getting leaner, and it's time I told you what oxygen has to do with losing some of that fat hanging from everywhere on your body. First, fat burns in oxygen. Big important realization for anyone interested in losing some fat.

As I've said over and over again, there is only one way on earth to change the way you look and feel. You must eat—you've got that down. You must breathe—you're there (or here, however you want to look at it). And you must move. Mix that right in with breathing in this chapter—slide in the exercise part. They are connected. Breathing and moving are both very important in the process of burning off some of your fat supply, making sure it doesn't come right back (your new whippersnapper metabolism and this whole new food angle will take care of that), and ensuring your body gets the one thing it can't live without.

The diet industry is not the only industry that has lied to you and stolen your money. The food manufacturers also hold a place of dishonor, and next to them is the fitness industry. Let's not leave these guys out. God knows they've done their share of damage.

Give me some room here, because I have to clear something up. Since this is my book, I can take as much time as I want on any given subject, right? Well, I've got to say this, and if there were a way to create a banner on the written page, this would be on a banner. (Graphics department, let's get creative.)

The aerobics industry has raped the word *aerobic*. (Darker letters—that's creative?) In order to burn fat through exercise, you have to understand the definition of the words *aerobic exercise*.

Jumping around like an idiot? Tons of choreography? The loudest music, the latest moves, neon, neon everywhere? (The look is changing—after all, it's the 1990s— and the look in L.A. right now is grunge. The last teacher I had out in L.A. was wearing black combat boots and her father's boxer shorts, and she looked as if she hadn't bathed in years. I'm not sure which is worse—the old Barbie image or this new look.)

It's important to the future of your body that you are clear about the real definition of aerobic. (Call in the graphics department again.)

The definition of aerobic is any movement under the sun for 30 minutes or more in oxygen. Any movement. Jumping up and down for 30 minutes in oxygen while picking your nose in your living room can be an aerobic activity. Walking can be a fabulous aerobic activity. Jump, row, hike, bike, swim, do whatever it is you enjoy—but if you want to be aerobic, you must be in oxygen, and if you want to burn fat, it's got to be for 30 minutes or more in oxygen.

It's hard to believe that anyone could screw that up— but they have.

STOP THE INSANITY!

How many memberships to health clubs do you have? Have you spent years paying them off after going only three times? Or are you like me—do you consider it more important to make them call you every month and beg for payments? Then at least they have to work for their money. How many times have you committed, with every ounce of determination in your body, to an exercise program—only to stop a couple of weeks later? If we could recycle all those stationary (stationary being the operative word here) bikes that sit and stare at us as we get dressed in the morning, we could build a mosque to exercise in every city in this country. Ode to Exercise, we could call it.

How many aerobics classes have you walked out of feeling like the walking dead? I took a class in New York a few years ago at a very exclusive studio with lots of dancers and some very beautiful people. I invited a friend who wanted desperately to get fit—and who better for her to go with, to begin her life of health and fitness, than the ex-260-pound, know-it-all-about-fitness Susan Powter? On the way to class I explained the concept of oxygen, the 75 trillion cell theory, the importance of control and focus, the strength thing, the fat-burning thing—I explained them all. My friend was all ready to feel those endorphins running through her brain, to get high on movement, man (I just had to add "man" at the end of that statement—it sounded like Linc from the "Mod Squad," didn't it?), to burn body fat and change her life forever.

Halfway through class, she left.

Rehydrating, I thought—brilliant.

I had not told her about the importance of rehydration when you are moving. But right to the water fountain she went. My friend was doing better than I thought she would for a first-timer.

Twenty minutes later she hadn't come back. Maybe she was stretching? Cooling down a bit, another important concept she'd grasped without my mentioning it —overheat and it's over, better to cool down early than end up dead. Not to worry, she'd be fine.

After 40 minutes I began to worry. I went looking for my friend, stopping first at the water fountain (not there), then the locker room (not there), then all over the studio (not there, either).

I found her sitting on the steps leading up to the chic studio, smoking a cigarette. This was not a good sign.

She hated the exercise class. There was no endorphin rush—there wasn't time; she had only been in class a few minutes. No fat burned—again, we are dealing with time here; I mean, not much gets burned in 5 minutes. Strength built? No chance. Commitment for life? I doubt it. As for rocketing into a life-style based on this stuff, you could have placed a big bet that it wasn't going to happen and been sure of winning. My friend was not thrilled. It hurt her, not emotionally—although there was a bit of that going on: embarrassment, humiliation, feeling like a goon—but physically. The exercise hurt her. She had no chance of keeping up. She felt out of place and didn't know what to do. But smoking made her feel good, so she'd come out to have a puff. Why wouldn't she prefer something that felt good over something that didn't? Very normal, very sane. It wasn't my friend who had the problem sitting on the steps of the chic studio—it was me. What kind of a teacher was I?

The modifier of all time had forgotten something.

Had I forgotten where I'd come from—the ex-cheer-leader's class, the clone of the Princess at the front desk, the 1 leg lift to the whole class's 50? . . . The 75 trillion cell theory and those endorphins couldn't have done my friend any good if she didn't know how to stay in oxygen for 30 minutes or more and maintain her aerobic pace at her fitness level for long enough to have all that stuff happen. I forgot to tell her how to do that.

I sucked.

You may have found yourself in the exact same position as my friend and me (before I experienced temporary amnesia that day) the thousands of times you've tried to exercise. Unable to keep up, too unfit to exercise, and feeling like an idiot. When I was exercising in the class that finally accepted me as the crazy fat woman in the back doing her own thing—you remember, 1 leg lift here, 2 arm lifts there—a funny thing started to happen. The fit, "normal"-looking women started to ask me questions about what I was doing, because my body was changing dramatically, while theirs stayed the same.

Why are you moving your arms that way?

Does marching in place do something different? Because you sure do a lot of it.

Why do you refuse to do the grapevine-with-three-knees-up move—is there something wrong with that move?

Why is your body changing so fast?

What's your name? (The first time, I might add, that anyone had asked me that question.)

What was this world coming to, when people were asking the fattest woman in the class questions about aerobics? Well, modification was born during those classes, and it does work, but it needs to be explained—something I left out on my fitness excursion with my friend that day.

When I modified within my fitness level instead of trying to keep up with someone else's fitness level, a funny thing happened. I woke up the next day with more energy than I had had in years. Sounds strange, a cure for the exhaustion within twenty-four hours, but that's exactly what happened. I also woke up every morning with hope. Hope that I was really on to something and that this time, by working within my fitness level, I was really going to be able to change the way I looked and felt.

Here's what you are going to do. First, understand the concept of taking in oxygen. (Understanding concepts is a big theme throughout this book, because once you understand what it's all about and how to apply it to your life, you're home free. And that's what this book is all about—being free from all the insanity). For now, your normal breathing will do—we will get to advanced breathing later. Then, to get that blood pumping oxygen to every cell and muscle in your body, we are going to condition your heart, lungs, internal organs—the whole kit and caboodle—so that you are bursting with energy. Fair enough?

You are going to start changing your body by exercising within your fitness level. Fabulous—how do you feel? Better already, most probably—or maybe not, because you still have no clue how you are supposed to get up from that sofa and move, because you are too unfit to move. Never mind. The solution is modification, not motivation, and it's time to begin.

> To think I even have a fitness level is a true accomplishment in itself.
> —Cathy, a client

Let's begin with facing your fitness level—one of the hardest things you will ever have to do when it comes to exercising. Facing how unfit you are is one of the reasons people never begin to move. It ain't easy. So let's face it.

It's real easy to let this cardio-endurance thing slip by for years without thinking about it, but when most people start exercising and get winded within 30 seconds of moving, they tend to back off, because they are afraid that continuing the movement for more than a few minutes will kill them. It doesn't feel good to be gasping for air 5 minutes into an exercise class, knowing you've got 55 minutes to go.

But I walked into many a class thinking and feeling I could at least keep up with the rest of the class—just as I walked into clothing stores believing I could squeeze into a size 16. Same illusion, or do they call that denial?

The truth is, when you weigh 260 and are cardiovascularly and muscularly weak, there's no chance of being able to keep up with anybody. One or two arm lifts and it's over. So it was time to modify until I could do the next set or two. It was embarrassing and discouraging, but I was alone in all this—you are not alone.

Facing your fitness level is about 'fessing up to the fact that you can't move without getting out of breath. Okay, that means you need to modify within a few minutes of moving. Big deal. You are not a weenie, you are simply starting your exercise at a low level of intensity because you are cardiovascularly unfit. Anyone can build a fitness level, and that's exactly what you may need to do. So face it. If you need to modify a thousand times during your exercise routine, that doesn't mean there is anything wrong with you, except that you must make your heart and lungs stronger so they have more endurance. When you deal with that and modify your aerobic activity, you will be able to stay in oxygen for 30 minutes or more, no matter what your cardiovascular fitness level is . . . and that's great, isn't it?

Hey, do you know what that means? It means fitness for everyone—any age, any weight, and any physical consideration. That old knee injury flaring up? Well, modify for it. Degenerative disease? Modify for it. Too much body fat—hard to move? Modify for it. Haven't moved in years and smoke like a chimney? Well, MODIFY FOR IT. If you are at the non-existent fitness level, have no fear—that's where I was, but not anymore. Getting out of breath when you move anything is a good sign of a beginning fitness level. Carrying a bag of groceries and feeling as if your arms are going to be sore the next day is a good sign of a bottom-line fitness level. Defining your aerobic activity as going to the fridge for more food is not a good indicator.

But don't stop here, we've only just begun. There is another step you need to take to be on your way to the fitter you.

Step number two is defining your fitness goals. Everyone has a different fitness level, but that is no longer a reason to exclude yourself from the fitness crowds. Everyone also has a different fitness goal—something the aerobics industry completely ignores. I have clients who want to lose tons of body fat, increase their strength, and end up in a bikini. I also have clients who just want more cardio-endurance. Their fitness goal is to be able to walk up a flight of stairs without sucking wind. Then there are the people who are looking for strength, muscular strength, so that the aches and pains they have lived with for years go away. There are the arthritic patients who feel better when they get a little oxygen to their joints. The recovering heart patients who are fighting for a new chance at life—a very different motivation and goal from the bikini. There is the woman who wants to recover her pride and self-esteem and regain the control in her life she feels has been lost. The client suffering from depression who couldn't care less about the way she looks— she just wants to lighten the black cloud that follows her around. I have seen as many different fitness goals as I have met different people.

Years after my Bambi experience, I found out that she wasn't any better than me just because she could do all that fancy jumping and strutting. Bambi wasn't any smarter—as a matter of fact, and let's put this on the record, she was as dumb as a bucket of rocks. There was a difference between the two of us—thank God, there were many differences. We had different fitness levels, and we had different fitness goals. I needed to build a fitness level; she already had an advanced case of fit. I just wanted to be able to get through the class and maybe someday look better than the Prince's girlfriend; she wanted more than life to be an aerobics star (is there such a thing? A hell of a lot of people I've met in the fitness industry are striving to be aerobics stars. What does an aerobics star do? I need to find that out), and she was using the class I was taking as her springboard to stardom.

"Keep up or get out." That sign should hang over the door of every aerobics class in every mass-production fitness facility in this country, because modification doesn't exist until people like you and me start doing it. There is only one person you should be concerned about keeping up with. The most important person—you. Your fitness level and fitness goal are the only things that you should consider in order to increase your strength and go to your next level. When you do, you'll not only use that membership and come back for more, you will be able to exercise long enough to get that all-important oxygen bursting through your whole body and have the opportunity to reap the rewards of movement rather than getting beaten to a pulp, walking out blue in the face, and going home to bed for the rest of the day. It's a whole lot more motivating to be able to function within your current level and build to the next than it is to be made to feel like the biggest goon in the room.

Hey, anybody out there from the industry reading this —did you hear that? Let's try motivating people by giving them a way to exercise—modification—and then let's help them build whatever fitness level they want. How about that—instead of motivating them with whoops and hollers, loud, obnoxious music, fancier and fancier steps, and a whole lot of smiling. You'd be surprised how well these "fat," "lazy," "unmotivated" people respond when they have some clue about what in the hell they are supposed to be doing and how they can keep up.

As I moved my limbs, used my muscles, and got stronger, I could do that leg lift more than a couple of times. A thought for the aerobics industry: You can't do the lifting if you don't have the strength. It's even harder when you have a very large limb and no muscular strength yet to lift it with. You'll know because the teacher makes you feel like a jerk if you don't, so you try to do it anyway.

This is the beauty of modification: you work within your fitness level. The limb gets stronger, the fat begins to burn off—because you are staying in oxygen for 30 minutes or more and burning fat—and bingo, it's a breeze to go to the next level.

A thought for the reader. If your arms feel as if they are going to fall off, they are. You have gone beyond your upper body strength level, and it's time to modify. When you are so out of breath that you are hating every moment, even though it's only the first few minutes of your aerobic activity, it's time to modify. If the move that is being presented by the wannabe aerobics star is too complicated, it's time to modify. Can you modify a move? Sure you can. You can also watch the aerobics star flip out when the fat, unfit woman has the nerve to modify a move of hers . . . or his. March in place until you get it all together—it's okay.

Recently a friend of mine—unfit but getting fit, very aware of modification—was taking a class from a guy who is known around town as an arrogant boob. He was doing a move that involved two steps with a clap in the middle of the move. (That clap was certainly doing a lot for everyone's fitness level, don't you think?) Well, my friend was having a hard time keeping up with all the fancy two-stepping and chose to modify the movement just a bit and leave out the clap. In the middle of the class, in front of everyone, the instructor marched over to the stereo, turned down the music, and said to my friend (glaring, I swear he was glaring), "This clap is not an option; it is a part of the move. I am the professional here and will decide who needs to do what in my classes."

A true, true, true story.

I took a class last week in Los Angeles after doing the "Home" show, and the teacher was doing a move on the step called "around the world." It is the dumbest move ever, because it does very little cardiovascularly. It is complicated, it is about choreography, not fitness, and my feet hurt when I turn and twist too many times—especially when I am turning and twisting on an 8-inch-high bench. So I modified it. This teacher got so mad, he —yes, it was another man; I'm not picking on men, it's just that a lot of them are boneheads and there's nothing I can do about it—yelled above the music (don't ask how loud he'd have to be yelling to be heard above this stuff), "At least try to do my move—put some effort into doing it!" I yelled back, "What if I am modifying because of an injury?" Remember, this heated debate is taking place while the whole class is going "around the world" on benches and the music is roaring. Didn't he know that I was the queen of modification?

"What am I supposed to do if I can't do the move?"

"What happens if this move confuses me, and I would rather do something else?"

"What if I just don't want to go around the world with you?"

STOP THE INSANITY!

I asked him these questions, and he didn't have any answers.

Is your aerobics ego more important than my injury? Shouldn't *you*—you worthless piece of crap—be modifying for *me,* the client who paid fifteen bucks for your stupid, worthless, badly cued class?

Me, the person who came to work out?

Me and millions like me who have no interest in going around and around on a bench, especially when we understand enough to know that 25 minutes into the class we should be in high cardio, not doing some dumb move that has our heart rate dropping by the second—all because you are such a bad instructor that I couldn't follow you around the world even if I wanted to.

Answer me, moron.

I got a little mad. I admit that. But it struck a nerve. It hit too close to home for me. I was screaming for all the women who have told me stories, worse than my Bambi experience, about the humiliation and physical pain they have suffered trying to go around the world with idiots like this instructor. He walked away calling me a bitch. But who cares? We get called bitches for a lot less than that.

> I was always the one sweating bullets and huffing and puffing. It was embarrassing. . . . I always felt I was working out for everyone else but me.
> —Comment from a client

Does defining your fitness level mean running to your doctor, having a battery of tests run, getting involved with hundreds of charts, formulas, and calculations? I am very aware that every exercise tape you rent or buy, every fitness program you watch on television, and every audiotape you listen to tells you to check with your doctor before beginning. My audio and video programs do, too—the distributors forced me to include a warning, but they almost had to tape my mouth shut, tie my hands together, and put me in a padded room for a couple of days. It is not easy to force me to do anything, but if I want to get this information to you guys—and I do—then

I have to put that label on the front of everything I do, except this book. (My publisher is having a heart attack over this—Simon may be the only one left; Schuster may die over this, but here goes.)

Hang on to your hearts, boys.

YOU DO NOT NEED TO GO TO A DOCTOR BEFORE YOU BEGIN AN EXERCISE PROGRAM.

Moments of silence again. Time to regroup and get on with our cardio conditioning and aerobics modification.

If you are under a doctor's care for heart disease or some other condition, don't go for a jog today, full speed at high noon when it's 102 degrees, have a seizure, and tell your doctor that Susan Powter said you didn't need him to tell you whether or not you could jog. What I said is that you must be in oxygen while you are moving for 30 minutes or more, that you always have to make sure you are working within your fitness level, never above, and that modification is the key.

Most of us don't need a doctor and a stress test to determine our fitness level because most of us are very, very fat, unfit, and unhealthy. Do you need a doctor to tell you that? Something much cheaper and more accessible than a doctor is a flight of stairs. Walk up one and see what happens. Are you sucking wind? If so, you are cardiovascularly unfit. Lift your arms up and down a few times. Do they feel like a ton of bricks? You don't have much upper body strength. Do a couple of sit-ups (if you can get on the floor)—is it impossible to lift your chest by using your abdominal muscles? Do you even remember what an abdominal muscle is? Are your boobs suffocating you? Then you don't have much abdominal strength, and you have too much fat in the middle. Walk around for a while. Do your legs throb and swell? It's time to build that lower body strength and burn some of the fat that your legs have to sit under all day, every day, for your whole life. What is it we need from the doc? Do we need him (slip of the sexist tongue) to tell us that we are unfit?

STOP THE INSANITY!

The average American is pathetically unfit and fat. Most of us can't walk up the stairs without gagging. Forget about bending over, or we'll pull something. We live with the aches and pains and exhaustion that go with being unfit and fat. Most of us don't have a healthy cardio system or enough muscular strength to call ourselves fit or flexible. So it is safe to say that millions and millions of people are at a nonexistent, beginning, or just above beginning fitness level. Fair enough? You don't need a stress test to tell you that.

What difference does it make to me if you go and spend a lot of money on some test? Let it go, Susan. Don't rock the boat. Keep your mouth shut. It's safer and easier for me to just say what everybody else does. But I can't. Never could, never will be able to. It just doesn't happen. This is something I've lived with all my life.

Here's why I'm carrying on about stress tests. Thousands of people have told me they can't afford a stress test (remember, not everyone in this country has the privilege of medical care), and that's why they have not begun exercising. They are afraid. But this is just another case of "Without me, you can't do a thing." The AMA has the same attitude as the diet industry: "Don't think, darling, and don't ever try to do it without me."

This is about as illogical as it gets. I'm dying, inside and out. I look and feel horrible. I'm suffering from ten million symptoms of being unfit and fat. I am on every medication under the sun—partly because I am unfit and fat—and I can't begin to solve the problem until I go to the doctor, which I can't afford, and spend more money, which I don't have—so I will need more medication, will feel worse, and will eventually . . . die.

If you want and can afford a stress test, or you just like taking them, go ahead. If you can't, do not put off one of the things that can truly begin to solve the problem—exercise. Until you can afford that stress test, just be smart. Listen to your body—and modify, modify, modify. I did not have my doctor's approval before I started to walk. I didn't need any test to tell me I was dying. I lived with the feelings of slow death every day, and I had to do something to change the direction I was heading in. So if you are as unfit as I was, or worse, and can't afford that stress test, don't worry. You are going to move at your fitness level, for 30 minutes or more, burn the fat, and increase your strength and cardio-endurance. So what is the big deal?

If it's a test you want, I'll give you one right now. You can get an immediate indication of what sort of condition you are in by determining your resting heart rate.

Here's how you do it. The minute you wake up tomorrow morning, before you move a muscle, lie there and take your pulse for 1 full minute. If you get a reading of 80 to 90 or 100, you are barely alive. You are extremely unfit. If your resting rate is 60 to 80, you are in the normal to high-normal range. And if you have a resting heart rate of 40 to 60, you are very fit.

One more time:

Very fit	40 to 60
Normal	60 to 80
Half-dead	80 to 100

Now you've got a couple of numbers that will be a thrill to compare before and after: resting heart rate and breathing range. Not bad for someone who thought they didn't know much about fitness. I'll tell you what—trade in your damn scale for these numbers, they will do you more good, won't cause you as much pain, and are truly an indication of how your body is changing.

See how unimportant that scale becomes when you begin to understand skinny versus fit and how to monitor fit? You are going to be amazed at how many ways you'll have to monitor internal and external changes in your body as you get fit. Who knew we were capable of doing all this stuff, being our own experts, defining our own fitness goals, and managing our own lives? Who knew?

Your breathing range and resting heart rate are good numbers to have and to compare later, for a couple of reasons. The most important (and the biggest fun) is getting proof positive, a couple of months down the line, of what I always say—that the internal changes you are making in the first couple of months are what make the external changes permanent. What better indicators of internal changes than these two simple numbers? Another very important reason to know your resting heart rate is to impress yourself and your friends with what an aerobics expert you are. And the third important reason is to show the aerobics industry how little is involved in being an "expert"—before you finish this book, you'll understand more than your aerobics instructor could ever dream of understanding.

So take your resting heart rate, remember it (because it's gonna improve), and let's keep getting cardiovascularly fit, getting some oxygen, and distributing the hell out of it.

What do you think you need to determine your cardio-endurance level? A monitor? Your doctor by your side while you are exercising? How can you possibly tell if you have gone beyond your cardio-endurance level without placing yourself in grave danger?

Again, the answer is simple. Get back in touch with your body and monitor your breathing. That's it. A damn good cardio monitor. You don't have to bother with straps or beeping devices. The minute you are out of breath, you are no longer burning fat—you have gone beyond your cardio-endurance level. And you are not in oxygen, you are out of it. Put this statement on every aerobics room wall in the country. When you are sucking wind, blue in the face, and panting for breath, you have gone way beyond your cardio-endurance level and it is time to—that's it—MODIFY YOUR AEROBIC ACTIVITY IN ORDER TO BURN FAT.

But isn't there more than just checking your face color? What about that famous chart on the wall of every exercise studio in the country to help us monitor our aerobic efficiency? What about those NUMBERS, 20 to 25 minutes into your aerobics class?

NUMBERS, NUMBERS, EVERYONE.

During my humiliation, beating, and torture—my class with Bambi at 260—I was clueless when all of a sudden everyone held one arm in the air, walked around the room (the first movement I could actually keep up with), and proceeded to shout numbers at Bambi: "17!" "21!" "26!" "19!" The only number I ever thought or cared about, after having two kids one year apart, was the date of my last period—so that's what I gave her. You should have seen Bambi's face as I walked half-circle, arm in the air (with no idea why), and yelled, "12/15!"

Poor Bambi. I was already a challenge to her—fat and in her class. Now she had to worry about my sanity while everybody else, after calling out their numbers, checked the black and red chart on the wall of the studio.

After I'd given Bambi the date of my last period, she wanted one more thing from me that I didn't understand.

Anyone over 30?

Thirty what, Bambi?

Thirty pounds overweight? I win hands down.

I raised my right hand because my left was already in the air like everyone else's, and poor Bambi got the fear-of-God look on her face—I didn't know it then, but a 260-pound woman in an aerobics class who has a heart rate count over 30, 25 minutes into class, is heading for the emergency room. I think Bambi was afraid she'd have to do CPR on the crazy fat lady in the back. Could she weed her way through the crowd and get to me in time? Would she have to put her mouth on mine? Was she sure what CPR was? Questions racing through my leader's mind as I told her I thought my number was 130–140, I couldn't figure it out. With 130–140, there was a good possibility of a heart attack or stroke. What was Bambi to do? How could she possibly hear me dying over her loud music? Oh, God, that meant she had to turn her music down—where would she get her motivation from? Poor Bambi had had it with me. I was truly too much of a challenge for her. Why was I in her class, not the 9:30 class? I had the craziest answers to her simple questions, I was walking around with both hands in the air, yelling numbers like 130–140 that don't exist, requiring her to worry about my health and my sanity, and all she wanted to do was lead an aerobics class and stare at herself.

STOP THE INSANITY!

I have to spend a minute on this target heart-rate chart, because if it's useless you want, it's useless you'll get.

Monitoring your aerobic effectiveness by taking your pulse, walking around with your arm in the air, and referring to the target heart-rate chart is out. No good. Never really has been, never will be, the way to monitor yourself.

The aerobics experts have come up with this thing called target heart-rate zone. The thing we strive for. The numbers that determine whether our aerobics workout has been effective or a waste of fat-burning time. We are told that the best fat-burning zone is 60–80 percent of our maximum heart rate. Maximum is the highest you could safely be before you drop dead. They have based this on your age, the only factor they have taken into consideration.

Big question. What about fitness levels?

What about medications?

How about length of time since you've moved?

Injuries?

Disease?

How about the hundreds of other factors that determine your efficient heart-rate zone? None of these are considered, because we are all averaged out. The experts have told us what range we should or shouldn't be in, based on our age—and that's that, damn it. The 60–80 percent zone is where you want to be after you've done your counting with Bambi, gone to the chart, looked up your age, and compared your count with their definition of effectiveness. If you are within that target zone, you've done good. If not, keep trying, babe, maybe someday you'll make it.

One of the biggest flaws in the experts' numbers, calculations, and charts is that the 60–80 percent range of effectiveness applies only to relatively or moderately fit people with an already low resting heart rate. If an unfit person were to exercise, something the aerobics industry obviously doesn't consider, and try to work within the 60–80 percent target heart-rate zone that the experts recommend, here's what they would run into.

1. They wouldn't last for more than a couple of minutes.
2. They wouldn't ever get to the point of burning fat.
3. They would always be out of oxygen.
4. They would be exhausted and blue in the face.
5. They would never be aerobically fit.
6. And like the millions of people who do, they would walk away feeling like they wanted to die and never want to go back the next day and do it again.

There are a couple of enlightened human beings in this field of aerobic target zones who agree with me and are trying to get this point across to the other experts. One of these is Mr. F. A. Kulling from Oklahoma State University. F.A. suggests that we should encourage and teach people how to work at 46 percent, not 60–80 percent, of their maximum heart rate. According to F.A., working at 46 percent will burn more fat than the old 60–80 percent standard, will allow you to go at a lower level of intensity for a longer duration, which gives you all the benefits of aerobics conditioning, certainly includes more fitness levels, and is a whole hell of a lot better than what has been used in the past. (My words, not F.A.'s.) Sally Edwards also has a new book out. She has a whole bunch of different ways to figure out your maximum target heart rate.

Until brilliant women like Sally and gallant men like F.A. spoke up (not that it's done much good; the industry still stands by its old chart), the only option you had was to walk into an aerobics class, be made very aware of the fact that you were unfit, uncoordinated, and unable to keep up, do your best to try to reach that 60–80 percent range, always striving for it while feeling like the biggest failure on earth, or do whatever the teacher was suggesting for 30 minutes, no matter how blue in the face or how out of breath you were, so that you could be in the 60–80 percent zone when you finished and feel as if you got a "good" workout.

You now have another choice, thanks to *Stop the Insanity!* and F.A., our friend in Oklahoma. There's another formula that you can learn lickety-split that will help you walk down your path to aerobics expert land.

Formula number three. Start with the Karvone formula —the old way to figure out your target heart rate. But let's do it the new way, the O.K. Oklahoma way. . . .

Take 220.

Minus your age.

Minus your resting heart rate.

Multiply by 46 percent (in the old days, it was 60 or 80 percent).

Then add back your resting heart rate, and bingo, you've got it. The number that will be much closer to reality for most of us. You will not find this zone as the acceptable zone on any target heart-rate chart in the country. But you could stir up a whole lot of trouble by explaining this concept to your aerobics instructor and asking him/her to show you your zone based on 46 percent instead of 60–80 percent.

Just as I did with the AMA boys and their 30 percent daily fat intake, I have a question for the aerobics scientists. Where did the old Karvone formula come from? Did they include any unfit people in their testing before they decided on a standard for us all? And where are the new charts that can really help us all—all fitness levels and all physical considerations—get fit? You better get your printers cranked up, boys, because there are a hell of a lot of unfit people who are getting really smart and are about to go out and get fit. We want the answers and the results, don't we? So get ready, boys, because we are walking in by the millions to every aerobics studio in the country.

I've got great news for you. You don't even need to do the formula if you don't want to. I didn't, and I don't use it for myself or any of my clients. I have a better way for you.

Here's a way to check and monitor your aerobic effectiveness, and it's called perceived exertion. This method of monitoring requires you to be very much in touch with your fatigue level throughout your class and to stay in constant touch with your oxygen/breathing. It allows you to modify constantly so that you can stay in oxygen for 30 minutes or more, reach the ultimate fat-burning level without anybody's charts or graphs, and have a very effective aerobics workout every time you exercise.

You'd think, based on all that, that this would be a widely used form of monitoring. But have you ever heard of it? Do you have any clue what I'm talking about? There's a reason why you don't. It seems that the guys in the aerobics labs have been chatting with the guys in the AMA labs, and they all decided that we don't want anything that requires us to take any responsibility. We may not be able to handle being in charge of our own fitness levels and effectiveness, so they better give us guidelines that are easier to understand, as if they were, and instant answers, even though they are so standardized that they don't apply to half the world.

Is that 220-minus-your-age formula supposed to be easy? I never, ever understood it, I have never, ever used it, and I am "in the industry." The experts can call me stupid—or they could stop and hear that I, like millions of other people, didn't understand what they are saying.

But now there is a way to monitor yourself, and I know you are capable of understanding and applying it and getting more for your money out of it—perceived exertion. Here's how it works. You stay in touch with your breathing, and the minute you are out of breath, you modify, bring your intensity level down, and continue moving at a lower level of intensity. You also stay in touch with your fatigue level. Staying awake all night with the baby may make you a bit tired during your 8:00 A.M. aerobics class. So you modify. Have you had enough food? (God forbid you've been dieting. If you are dieting, do not—I repeat, *do not*—exercise.) Have you been traveling and only been able to get on-the-road crap for food? Then you may not have the high-octane fuel level that you normally have, so modify. Fatigued for a million reasons? Who cares why—this is why you'll be modifying for the rest of your fitness life. The reason why is, there will always be something to modify for, and the best way to monitor it is by using perceived level of exertion.

STOP THE INSANITY!

Not much has changed in the last few years—well, besides the 133 pounds I've lost; the cardio-endurance I've gained, the muscular strength and flexibility; the business I've built; the national TV I do; the speeches, the seminars, the book—it's still the same. When I work out I modify, every day for every kind of reason imaginable, and I always work within my fatigue level. Walking up and down the street at 260 pounds for 30 minutes in oxygen, always working within my level of intensity and always modifying, reducing my level of intensity every time I was out of breath—that's what I did then and that's what I do now. The Bambis of the world and I are just working at a higher level of intensity. Oh, gosh, did I just put myself in the Bambi category— HEEEEEELLLLLLP ME, SOMEONE, HELP!

I was dealing with a few physical considerations during those early walks. The stinging, rubbing, chafing all over my body. Any movement made me feel like the Michelin Man, rolls and rolls rubbing together. The back pain. My famous excuse for a long time for not working out.

I can't move, I have this backache—after having two babies so close together, it's inevitable, my O.B. said to me. (Hey, that could be a country-and-western song: "My O.B. Said to Me"—call Nashville, let them know.)

If I exercise, I may hurt my back.

Oh, thanks, I'd love to come to that aerobics class with you, but there is this one thing I have to think about— my back.

But there was a little something that my O.B. left out when he was explaining the constant ache I had in my lower back. The fat that was hanging halfway down my thighs on my stomach. The abdominal muscles that were so weak after years of not strengthening. Do you think all that could have had something to do with the ache he told me to live with? Oh, doc—the answer to the problem was much easier and less expensive than the prescription you gave me for muscle relaxers. My prescription had no side effects, and I solved the problem. I burned the fat off my stomach. Increased the strength in the lower, middle, and upper sections of my abdominal wall. I got lean, strong, and healthy. How about that, doc? Impressed? You should be.

The anger I felt for the Prince? Where was that taken into consideration on your target heart-rate chart? It absolutely affected my workout. Focus requires energy. Many mornings I'd get up, get ready for my walk, and then get a phone call from the Prince about the late check I'd called him about, or his "visit," or whatever we were disagreeing about at the time—and every ounce of energy would be instantly zapped from my body. I'd fall right into the "What's the use of trying when his girlfriend is a size 0 and I'm a cow?" way of thinking. The old tapes would start playing like an orchestra inside my head, and emotional fatigue would set in. So, more often than not, just getting out the door meant I was already fatigued. I'd have to start walking slowly, because every step I took, my seven other personalities were screaming, "Don't bother, you'll never get fit." "Look at you, you've got years to go—do you think this little walk is ever going to change those thighs?"

But after a couple of minutes, long enough to get that life-giving oxygen into my blood and running through my body, all of a sudden I'd get some energy—oxygen, sweet oxygen, it does wonders for the mind and heart—feel a bit better, and start thinking about other things. Before I knew it, I would have walked my 30 minutes or more in oxygen, burned some fat, increased some strength, and taken one more step toward my goal.

TO HELL WITH THE PRINCE, I'M GETTING FIT.

GET OUT OF MY HEAD, YOU SEVEN OTHER PEOPLE, I DON'T HAVE TIME FOR YOU.

YOU MAY BE A SIZE 0, YOU SLEAZY PRINCESS, BUT I'VE GOT A PERSONALITY, I CAN READ, I HAVE TWO BEAUTIFUL CHILDREN WHO LOVE ME, AND YOU CAN'T FINISH A SENTENCE WITHOUT SAYING "OH, MY GOD" . . . I HATE YOU!

I still get tired—very, very tired. There are still nights without much sleep. It may not be babies keeping me up, it's book writing and deadlines, but what's the difference? The Prince still makes me mad—he is a bigger part of my life now than when we were married. (You better believe there is an explanation about that on its way. A whole chapter, as a matter of fact.) The job, the bills, the PMS—it's all the same, and it all still makes me tired, anxious, afraid, nervous, angry, tired—did I mention tired? And it all still requires me to modify my workouts, monitor my oxygen and fatigue level, and increase or decrease my level of intensity according to my fitness level, my fitness goal, my perceived level of exertion. Fat or unfit people are no different, no matter what the aerobics industry says.

> If I miss a day of activity, I feel less energy—I've noticed the more you move, the better you feel.
> —Jennifer, a client

You know why you are going to modify for the rest of your fitness life—so that you stay in oxygen, burning fat and increasing cardio-endurance. You know when you are going to modify—for the rest of your fitness life. The minute you're out of breath, whenever your arms or legs feel as if they are about to fall off, whenever you're hormonally whacked out, tired, injured, and on it goes.

The only thing you don't know yet is how to modify. In the last couple of pages, the phrase *level of intensity* has been rearing its head. You may have been too enraptured by the concept of modification even to pay attention to it, but level of intensity it is—the key that unlocks the golden door and gets you in to see the big cheese, oxygen.

Understanding how to increase or decrease your level of intensity during your workout is the only thing that will keep you going. Your mind will be the first thing to start whispering, "Hey, let's blow this pop stand and go watch some TV—who needs this sweaty workout gig anyway?" It will not be your determination and willpower that keep you going when the first 3 minutes of exercise have you searching for an ache or pain that could justify stopping and running home to bed. It will, for the rest of your fitness life, be your understanding and your ability to increase or decrease the level of intensity of your movement that will get you to the point (and it always happens) of being in oxygen long enough to clear your brain, begin to get your body moving, and get those endorphins rushing through your body so that you can get that high and complete your workout.

In all the years I've been doing this, I have never ever, ever, ever heard anyone who left a workout saying, "Gee whiz, I wish I hadn't done that."

Thousands of times I've heard, "I'm so glad I did that —I feel so much better."

Or, "Boy, I never thought I'd get through that today, but I'm sure glad I did."

Or, "I expected to have one of the worst workouts because I didn't want to do it and wasn't into it, but it was one of my best."

I've got every reason under the sun not to work out every day. Let's start with the fact that I'm already fit and like the way I look and feel. So what's a day or two of not working out? My thighs are not going to get big, so blow it off. There is always the busy schedule excuse, and I can back that up in a big way. The kids—gotta go to that baseball game, so I'll work out tomorrow. See? Not much has changed. I still have to get myself up, modify my workout until I'm ready to increase my level of intensity, and get myself going—and I always feel 100 percent better than when I walked in the door. It never fails. I taught a class the other day, and after 1 hour of focused, energized, fabulous fat burning, I looked at the class and said, "Isn't this the best? Exercise is the cheapest, best high out there—it feels sooooooooooo good."

Anyway, you have to know how to increase or decrease your level of intensity before you can get that sooooooooooo good feeling every day.

Increasing level of intensity means making it harder. Decreasing level of intensity means making it easier.

There is no difference between beginning, intermediate, or advanced fitness levels, except the level of intensity they are working in. An advanced level means doing the movements correctly in oxygen for 30 minutes or more and modifying for physical considerations. That's exactly what a 400-pound person who is just starting out should be doing, so what's the difference? There is none, except that the brilliantly fit person should be working at a higher level of intensity. Not because they are "better" than the 400-pound new-to-fit person. Simply because they have built the muscular strength to do the moves, have less fat so it's easier to lift that limb, and have the cardio-endurance to sustain the movement at a higher level of intensity for the same amount of time.

The very fit don't have anything you don't have, they have just conditioned what you have yet to condition. They are no better, just more fit. You are going to start at a low level of intensity so that you can build the fitness level you need to go to the next, and the next, and the next level, until you look in the mirror and love what you see and feel, and then, bam—you maintain what you love.

IT'S SO SIMPLE. HOW DID THIS FITNESS THING GET SO SCREWED UP?

That's a scream on the printed page.

The how to's of level of intensity are simple. (Maybe I should call this book the simple book?)

There are a couple of things that can increase or decrease your level of intensity instantly. I am going to use walking as an exercise example, but this applies to all movement, and I'll be throwing in other examples as we go along.

Let's start with pace. Pace is one way to increase your level of intensity.

You are walking down the street—it's a breeze, and you start to think that walking is for wusses. How about increasing the pace? Try walking at a faster pace. You can go from a slow walk to a faster walk to a jog, if you want. I am not suggesting jogging, and I never will, because I hate jogging. And you don't need to jog, because there are plenty of ways that you can take that little old walk and turn it into the highest-intensity walk you've ever had. Have no fear, there are lots of ways to challenge yourself. If swimming is too easy, swim faster for the same 30 minutes. If that treadmill is too easy, turn up the speed. Has bike riding become a breeze? Pedal faster.

Another surefire way to increase your level of intensity is to increase your range of motion.

This is a pet peeve of mine because I can't tell you how many times I've been in aerobics studios and seen the superfit women up front sighing and raising their eyes to heaven as if there were nothing in this world—no move, no step, no class—challenging enough for their exceptional fitness level. But during the class, their arm and leg lifts look as if they have a lock at the elbow or knee. They are all bent up, swinging their limbs all over the place, and their range of motion (a term any exceptionally fit person should be very familiar with) is for doody.

Your range of motion is determined by how far you reach up, or out, or under. How high you lift that knee or press your leg out. The longer the range of motion, the more difficult the move and the higher your level of intensity. Increasing your range of motion uses more of the muscle you are working and includes other muscles to do the movement. Activating more muscles means burning more fuel. Burning more fuel means you reach your fitness goal sooner. Until you increase your range of motion, it is hard to understand how powerful an inch higher in that press-out or lift-up can be. I think the athletes who understand this best are dancers. Watch them lift and press and extend and hold a move. When you know what's involved in doing that, their strength, endurance, and level of intensity are something to be worshiped. (Worshiped? I may have taken that a bit too far, but you know what I mean.) It truly is amazing.

So you are on your walk, have picked up the pace, and it's still not enough. Add a bigger range of movement. Instead of swinging your arms by your side without thinking, pump them, using long movements, long range of motion. Also, while maintaining your pace, increase the range of motion in your legs—don't leave out the lower body. Bigger steps. Longer range of motion. Is that swim getting easy, even with the faster pace? Reach farther, as far as you can—you'll be feeling muscles all the way down your side. You can feel it right now with me.

Put the book down and reach your right arm up in the air. Just reach up while sitting on your chair. Don't lock your elbow, because that does nothing but cause injury, and it does nothing to build strength. So always keep a soft elbow—but a long, lifted, extended arm—and reach. Now, keep your arm up, think about pressing your right shoulder down—you want the reach to come from your muscles, not from crunching your neck up to your ears—and reach an inch higher. Shoulder down, arm up. Keep it there if you can, or modify the move by bringing your arm down, shaking it out, and then going back up. (You are modifying for an endurance level that you have not built yet, but soon you'll have more endurance and strength, and you'll be able to hold your arm up for longer and longer. So don't sweat it—well, do sweat it, just don't worry about it.) Next, think about your fingertips being alive (they are, you know), and reach right through them, sending your energy to the ceiling. Arm up, shoulder down, elbow relaxed, and reach all the way up and through your fingertips.

See what you've done? You've made a move efficient, because you've used more muscles than that superfit person in the front row who throws her arms up and lets them swing down.

Using a fuller range of motion you can make a squat torture. Just press an inch lower or lift up—no locked knees—an inch higher.

> It is wonderful how quickly you get used to things, even the most astonishing.
> —Edith Nesbitt, *Five Children and It,* 1902

Another day, another trick. If you want to increase your level of intensity even more—because no pace is fast enough, no reaching could be high enough—then here's another element. Try adding some resistance. Resistance adds resistance—brilliant, don't you think? And pressing against something, or walking through something, or lifting up or pressing down against something is a hell of a lot harder than swinging or flopping your arms and legs around like the ladies of the front row.

Fine, but what do you press against? Do you need equipment? Is there some resistance device out there that you haven't heard about? Well, I got your resistance for you—mud. All you gotta do is think mud. Yep, mud.

You're walking. Your pace is good, your range of motion is long and extended. Now add some mud. Think about your arms pressing through mud. Your legs walking through mud. The thicker the mud, the more resistance.

During your swim, you don't need to add mud, because water is the best resistance you could get. I read an article the other day about a new fitness breakthrough: walking in a pool burns more fat than walking on land. This article went on and on about walking in water (not *on* water—there's only one person who can do that—*in* water) but never told us why. I'm sitting on a plane screaming in my head, TELL THEM WHY. EXPLAIN RESISTANCE TO THESE PEOPLE. TELL THEM THAT THEY CAN GO DOWN TO THEIR LOCAL Y AND GET FIT WITHOUT ALL THOSE STUPID AEROBICS CLASSES. TELL 'EM, TELL 'EM.

What the article left out was *why* it was more effective, and *how* you can apply it to your life in order to change the way you look and feel. This seems to be what they always leave out.

You can add mud without ever adding mud. It doesn't end in the mudhole. I've got a few more resistance tricks up my sleeve.

On a treadmill? Try a little elevation. Yep, lift that sucker up a bit and walk at the same pace with a wide range of motion in your arms and legs, and you'll be sucking wind faster than you could imagine.

Go for a walk around a track and add some stadium stairs. Walk for a couple of laps and then take the stairs just once—no need to run, walk up them—then walk down and continue your walk for a couple more laps.

STOP THE INSANITY!

Stairs, walk, stairs, walk—you wouldn't believe how much that can increase your level of intensity.

Increase, increase, increase your level of intensity. What about new-to-fit readers? Have I just blown them away like a bad habit? Sold out, catered to the already fit who want more, more, more? What the hell has gotten into me?

Gandhi, or some other wise man, said that everything has a purpose. I've explained how to increase your level of intensity first for a reason; there is a purpose. (Right in line with the wise men, there's where I like to be.)

Here's the reason: If you can increase your level of intensity, you can also DECREASE your level of intensity. The same thing applies in reverse.

If you are walking and dying for air—remember, it doesn't matter if it's only 3 minutes into your walk; you're building that cardio-endurance level, so don't worry about it—then you can decrease your pace, bring your level of intensity down a bit until you catch your breath, and then increase it. If you're doing an aerobic activity and you are sucking wind, decrease your range of motion in your arms or legs. Shortening the range of motion requires less from the muscle you are using, doesn't include all the other muscles, and thus decreases your level of intensity. You have a lot of other choices. You can take your arms into shorter presses through mud, and if you're still out of breath, you can take your arms out altogether. Yes, you heard it right, it is okay to take your arms out of the movement until you regain your breath, and then put them back in.

This is it. The golden key. The secret that can unlock the mysteries of fitness and throw at your feet everything you need to get fit. Understand this concept and you are free. Free to get fit. Free to burn fat. Free to build strength. Free to slap the hell out of the next instructor who insists you do something that you know is stupid and ineffective and has nothing to do with building or strengthening anything. Free, free, free at last. You haven't just seen the mountain, you are about to be able to walk right up that mountain, no matter what your fitness level is . . . yipppeeeeeee!

Excited? See how many choices you have? See how much of an expert you can become overnight? See how you can get fit, no matter what fitness level you are starting at? See how fitness is for everyone? See why I can't stand the aerobics industry? They didn't tell me any of this. You didn't know it, either. We didn't have the opportunity to get fit, because nobody ever explained how to do it. You are not lazy. You are not lacking motivation. You just didn't know what you were supposed to do or how the hell you were supposed to do it. Neither did I. When I found out, I did it. Motivation? Self-esteem? Willpower? What do any of those things have to do with it? When people don't know how to move, when to move, what to do—or even that it's possible—they won't do it. Why are we wasting our time talking about all this other crap and blaming the lack of physical fitness in this country on low self-esteem and willpower? I've seen it thousands of times—unfit people getting their hands on this information, understanding it, and running (pardon the pun) with it. Getting fitter than they ever imagined they could be. My story is one in thousands—it is not unique. You can have the exact same before-and-after story if you learn to move within your level of intensity, always working at your fitness level and building to the next.

I've got a resistance bike story for you. It happened to me a couple of months ago in a class on stationary bikes. Spinning, it's called. A lot of bikes in a room, loud music, and lots of pedaling.

I'm in pretty good shape. Fair enough—biking has never been my thing, but if it's cardio-endurance it requires, it's cardio-endurance I have, so no problem. We start biking, warming up slowly, and the pace increases as we get into the aerobics section of our class. Then this teacher starts doing things I have never in my life seen another human being do.

Resistance? Let's start by turning up the resistance on the knob so that mud seems like cotton candy. This felt more like quicksand. Then add a little more—what the hell, stand up while you're doing it. Then as if this weren't enough, while you're standing, increase the pace at the same resistance level on the knob.

What are you, nuts?

Get out of here.

I'm gonna puke if I stand and do this.

This isn't exercise, this is bionic stuff.

This teacher—and I use "teacher" respectfully in this case, because she acknowledged my friend and me when we walked into the room—asked if we were new spinners. I liked that title, new spinner, and I very much appreciated her acknowledging me. She checked my seat height, and made me feel welcome and comfortable. She was one of the rare breed of teachers in the aerobics industry. Above and beyond that, she was also superhuman.

I'm telling you, I've seen lots of things in the last couple of years, but this kind of strength, endurance, and cardiovascular fitness level I've never seen the likes of—don't even ask how perfect her body was, I mean the kind of perfect where you can see every muscle, toned, tanned, and lean—but I'm sure you and I have better personalities, so who cares? Well, anyone would feel out of shape next to her, and I was no exception. First I had to accept the fact that I was one big weenie next to this woman—not easy to do when you are a "fitness expert" blasting all over TV and are kind of recognizable. That was a bit of a blow to the old ego, but I got over that fast, because I was too busy modifying everything she did throughout the whole class so I wouldn't heave all over her. Talk about embarrassing. Can't keep up and puking? Hey, check out the big fitness expert passing out in the corner.

Taking that spinning class for the first time felt exactly the same as my first walk or my first time picking up a weight. And there will be many different beginnings in your fitness life. Modification—increasing or decreasing your levels of intensity—never ends, so start now, and keep it going.

I am now feeling fabulous . . . eating all the time, getting leaner, and fitting into clothes I have not worn in two years. HURRAY! In short: I'm eating; I'm breathing; I'm moving. It works—it really works!
—Comment from a client

Let me tell you about Bill.

Bill had a couple of obstacles on his fitness path. He was 400 pounds, lived an hour and a half from my studio, had a night job that required him to stand during his eight-hour shift. The morning classes were the only ones that he could get to.

Bill's life had become impossible. He had no energy, was too big to do anything, was always uncomfortable, and almost died when he heard his daughters' friends laughing and snickering about how fat their daddy was.

Bill was a proud, beautiful man. One day he broke down crying in my office—telling me that his weight had destroyed his life. He explained that he was physically unable to take care of his personal hygiene. His wife had to help him clean himself because he couldn't reach around his own body anymore. Watching a proud, beautiful, loving human being break down because of fat—you want to know what drives me, that's it right there. Bill and I started working out together. He worked within his fitness level, modifying all the way, burning fat, increasing strength, increasing cardio-endurance, and coming back to life.

He was loving it. Smiling, laughing, feeling better every day, and realizing that he had to do what I did, what everybody has to do who wants to change their body. Eat, breathe, and move—there is no other way.

One day Bill called me, very upset. He had hurt his knee at work and couldn't walk. It was not the cost of the emergency room visit, the injury to the knee, or the fact that he wasn't able to work for a few weeks that was upsetting him. It was the interruption of the one thing that was making him feel better, his exercise class.

Stop exercising just because you can't walk? Bill, Bill, Bill—you oughtta know me better than that. I had a couple of questions for Bill:

STOP THE INSANITY!

Can you walk to your car and drive here?

What time can you make it over?

And do you have any small weights at home?

Yes, 2:00 P.M., and yes were Bill's answers. Then he laughed and asked, Is there any way out with you? If a busted-up knee doesn't get me out of this exercise thing, what would? Bill, unless you are in an iron lung, you can move. If you can move anything, you can get some oxygen. There is a modification for almost everything, so come on down, big guy (pardon the pun)—we've got some fat to burn.

At 2 P.M. that afternoon we worked out. Bill sat on a chair doing the class with me, using his upper body, holding on to 1-pound dumbbells. You want to know if you can get your cardio up while you're sitting? Do what Bill did. You'll be sweating and burning fat in no time. He left the studio dragging his bad leg behind, covered in sweat, upper body thoroughly worked, and feeling great.

Like most things in life, I learned by doing. Living through it and talking about it seem to be the way it happens for me. This "you gotta experience it before you understand it" way of living isn't easy for me or anyone around me, but it sure lends itself to some great stories. Let me explain. You see, I could work out with Bill injured and on a chair because that's exactly what I had to do myself for months. If it's wheelchair fitness you want to know about, give me a call.

I get my life together, change my body, start teaching aerobics, and what do I do? Fall and smash both feet to pieces. Two casts, two sons—easy to raise the kids when you can't walk—wheelchair, walker (on a good day), and there I am going through experience #1,000,076 in my life and wondering what in the hell this one's about.

After the break, after the surgery, and after the Demerol wore off, what do you think I was concerned about? Feeding the kids? Paying the bills? Keeping the house running? Nope. The one and only thing I could think about was getting fat again.

The fear of regaining my weight was much more painful

and frightening than any surgery or busted-up feet could be.

Ram Dass, this spiritual guy (with a name like that, what else could you be? Certainly not in construction, you'd be beaten to a pulp), said it best: If you are busy pushing something away, you are not free; it still has you, because you are busy not doing it. I'm not sure if that's exactly how he said it (do you go to hell if you misquote a guru?), but that's what he said.

You see, the weight still had me. I was very busy pushing it away—and doing a very good job, I might add—but it still had me. My body was lean, strong, and healthy, but my mind wasn't.

After the surgery I was put on one of those morphine drips. The IV is in your arm, and whenever you feel pain, you push the pump, and a couple of drops of morphine mix into the IV. Within seconds you are happy as a clam. The more I thought about getting fat again, the more I pushed that pump. Thinking and pumping—that's what I did for the first day or so after the pins and things were placed inside my body. Numbing—a constant theme in my life. And what better way to jump right into "everything's going to be okay land" than with morphine? Unfortunately, I recovered enough to leave the hospital and face my fear of getting fat again, because as hard as I tried to convince them, they would not let me take the morphine drip home with me.

You see, the problem was that I knew too much to go back to starving to keep the weight off. Eating—no problem, I'm great at that. Breathing—fine, what else am I going to do all day? But it was the moving part of the equation that had me stumped. I knew a lot about fitness at that point, and I could make someone fit, but making someone walk again—the only person I know who's done that is the same guy who walks on water, and moving to me at that point meant walking.

I explained my fears to my doctor and asked him what I could do. He made me feel like an idiot. A worrying woman. So I fired him. You should have seen his face—a crippled, ex-260-pound woman in casts firing him on the spot. It felt great for about 30 seconds until I had to face the reality of still being afraid of getting fat, having no answers, having both legs in casts, and having no doctor.

First I had to figure the fat thing out—you can find a doctor on every street corner. Here's what I did. On Wednesday, two weeks after surgery, my regular day to teach my men's conditioning class, I got up, got myself in the car, drove to the facility—my doctor would have had a heart attack because he'd specifically told me not to drive, but that didn't apply, since I didn't have a doctor, so I drove—got myself out (it took me forever), wheeled into the building, right to the door of my aerobics room, where the substitute teacher was teaching, thanked her very much for filling in for me for a week, and told her I was fine and wouldn't need her anymore. The men in the class expected nothing less from me, but you should have seen the expression on the face of the sub, who'd never met me. Bald, in a wheelchair, and telling her I was fine and wouldn't need her. . . .

I taught my class by doing all the upper body movements and having someone from each class come up and demonstrate the moves as I called them. If this fitness thing didn't work out, I could have gotten a job as a square-dance caller anywhere in this country—after a couple of months I got pretty damn good at it.

Until you are faced with a disability, you never think about it. I became very aware of bathrooms that weren't facilitated for the handicapped, curb cuts in the sidewalk that were nowhere to be found. People who were not handicapped parking in handicapped parking spots. No ramp? My wheelchair can't go down those stairs—how am I supposed to get in to teach my aerobics class?

Well, I did gain some weight back. Fifteen pounds, to be exact. I had gone from teaching five classes a day to sitting on a chair, teaching classes on Demerol. (Pills are nowhere near as strong as the drip, but they did the trick.) My metabolism was in warp mode. That's why I gained some weight back. I continued to eat, breathe, and move, and my body continued to develop. I worked on different things when I couldn't walk. My upper body got stronger than it had ever been, and stretching was a breeze, because once I was down on the floor it was as if I were anchored—those leg casts should be available in every stretch and yoga class.

My broken-foot experience comes in handy every day. I know so many people who are working with so many different physical considerations, and I tell them what I just told you. Unless you are in an iron lung, you can get fit. Grab a chair and let's work out. If you want to increase your level of intensity—get some weights. All you therapists, counselors, physicians, and wannabe experts on the habits of the unfit, come to my studio any day of the week and have a look at what's going on. Watch how hard these people work when they are given the right information and understand how to apply it to their fitness levels. Watch the focus, the concentration, the effort that these "lazy," "undisciplined," "unmotivated" people put in. And then watch them come back to life, change the way they look and feel, regain their choices, and empower themselves.

I have never met a lazy person, and I've met a hell of a lot of people during the last couple of years. I've met a lot of angry, scared, confused, skeptical people, but not lazy people. It's not discipline these people are lacking, it's information. Nobody has a clue, because the experts have made it so damn complicated.

It isn't laziness that's kept you from using your club membership. You—like the millions they cattle herd into these places—are left having no clue what to do or how to do it. What are you supposed to do, keep going back day after day, clueless? Unfit people, fat people, seniors, people recovering from illness, the less coordinated, anyone dealing with a degenerative disease—all of them need oxygen, strong muscles, and a healthy percentage of body fat. You have to do all the same things I did, and anybody else does who wants to get lean, strong, and healthy.

Understanding how to work within your fitness level and modification are the way to do it, and I haven't met an exercise yet that can't be modified. Increasing or decreasing your level of intensity is what will keep you going and take you to the next level. Fitness is for every-one. Fitness is attainable, and fitness is simple, not com-plicated.

If the double double back flip doesn't work for you, modify, modify, modify, but don't stop moving.

HOW TO BEGIN

Here's what you need to know to begin. First, breathing. Oxygen. Giver of life, remember? Tired? Try one of these breathing exercises instead of the cup of coffee. Ready to kill someone? I've got a deep-breathing exercise that will help you get over that. But we have to begin with one thing —getting back into the habit of breathing.

Getting back into the habit of breathing requires you do just that—get back into the habit. The best way to do that is to breathe 100 times a day.

There is the Susan Powter breathing exercise.

One hundred times a day, stop, think, and take a breath.

Don't worry about technique, form, mountains, chants, anything. Just breathe. In through the nose. Out through the mouth. Again, in through the nose, out through the mouth. Again, in through the nose, out through the mouth. Again. . . .

A hundred times a day.

ABDOMINAL BREATHING

If you want to take it one step further, try this. Abdominal breathing is simple and powerful. It requires you to breathe from your belly instead of from your neck and throat, which is where you are probably breathing from now. To make sure you are breathing from your belly, you should

Sit on a chair.

Place your right hand on your chest and your left hand on your belly.

Inhale.

If your right hand rises more than your left, you are breathing through your chest. If your right hand was around your throat, you'd really see it . . . but here's what you want.

Oh, yes, exhale.

Inhale again, concentrating on your left hand. Make the left hand rise with the inhale. It feels odd at first, but try it a few times and see how quickly you become an abdominal breather.

I've got the same thing in a lying-down version with a telephone book—options, options, options, that's me.

Lie on the floor.

Book on your belly.

Inhale.

Make the book rise.

Exhale and feel the book lower.

Pretty soon you can blow off the telephone book, because you'll be so used to abdominal breathing that throat breathing will be foreign to you.

How often: A couple of times a day. Morning and night would be nice, but don't get nuts—this is not a schedule set in stone. Do it whenever you can and as often as you think about it. Oxygen is the most vital ingredient in wellness, so the more you do, the more you get; the more you get, the faster you get well.

Where: Anywhere you can. In the car on the way to work. Turn the radio off for 2 minutes and breathe. Who cares what you look like? We pick our nose in cars and pretend nobody can see us, so why not breathe and pretend nobody can see?

Anywhere you can find a minute or two to breathe, do it.

DEEP BREATHING

This is the martini or Valium of breathing. When you feel like you are about to explode, do this instead. Deep breathing is a stress buster. The martini or Valium may seem stronger, easier, and more effective in the beginning, but after a few sessions with Mr. Deep, you'd be surprised at how effective it is. It's definitely cheaper, has a lot fewer side effects, and it works.

Exhale completely.

Do your abdominal breathing, but take it a bit farther, releasing all the air from your abdomen.

Inhale, filling your abdomen with air, keep inhaling, filling the chest and the collarbone, all the way to the shoulders, with air.

Keep inhaling until you are filled with air—remember the telephone book, it's rising.

Now exhale.

Slowly, in reverse.

First, collarbone.

Then chest.

Then abdominal wall—upper, middle, and lower—slowly contracting the abs, pushing the last bit of air from your body.

Exhaling is relaxing. Think about the last big sigh that you took. Maybe it was a nice relaxing sigh while you were sitting on a balcony overlooking the ocean as you were being served breakfast, but if your life is anything like mine, it was when you finally hit the bed last night.

The breathing experts of the world say that you should take twice as long during your deep breathing exhale as you should during your inhale. Take the time to sigh that breath from your collarbone to your abs.

How often: Whenever you feel tired, stressed out, at the end of your rope, or just want a moment to yourself and there isn't one available. As often as you like. Deep breathing is a luxury that is at your disposal—you can have it whenever you want it.

Where: Anywhere. Just be careful. This technique feels so wonderful that you will find yourself closing your eyes in relaxation and pleasure—and that doesn't work in a car or anywhere that seeing is imperative.

You may as well throw in some mind re-taping as you breathe. Think about redefining exercise.

Exercise means energy.

Movement burns fat.

It increases strength.

It increases your metabolic rate.

Exercise will make your body lean, strong, and healthy.

Take a moment to think about this while you are breathing. Why not put two tools together? It will only help you change your body.

EXERCISE

When do you exercise? Whenever it works for your schedule.

What do you do?

Any aerobic activity that works for you for 30 minutes or more in oxygen.

How often? Five to six days a week if you've got some fat to burn and some changes to make.

Three times a week if you want to maintain what you have.

Four times a week if you want to increase your metabolic rate just a smidge.

How in the hell do you exercise if you are unfit, fat, or have a gazillion physical problems? By always working at your fitness level. Always staying in oxygen. Decreasing and increasing your levels of intensity throughout every workout, as many times as you need. Thinking about what you are doing while you are exercising.

You are moving to get oxygen to those 75 trillion cells and every muscle in your body.

You are moving to burn fuel and fat, and you are moving to change the way you look and feel.

You are not competing with anybody.

You are doing the exact same thing that everybody who wants to get lean, strong, and healthy has to do.

And it works.

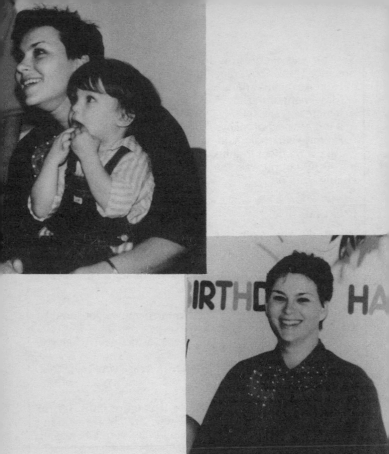

The fashion queen. If it's birthday party fashion you want, I would have been the one to call back then. You know it's bad when the birthday hat band chokes you. . . .

SIX

Moving Right

It is never too late—in fiction or in life—to revise.
—NANCY THAYER

You are a cardio machine. You know how to stay in oxygen for 30 minutes, no matter what your fitness level is when you start.

That may be enough for the first few weeks, but pretty soon you'll be screaming for more.

You'll want to build that fitness level you know is under all that fat, and the best way to do that is to learn as much as you can about moving correctly.

This chapter is about moving right, and correct movement is the difference between a crappy workout and an effective one. Those ladies in the front row of the aerobics class need to listen up here.

Exercise is not about just going through the motions every day, day in and day out. It's about using movement to change your body, and the only way to do that is to apply form, resistance, control, and extension to every move you make.

Modification was my big find as I was changing my body. Resistance, the mud theory, was icing on the cake —then came form, control, and extension. Wow, what a difference it made in my exercise. I've seen the most beginning of beginners, who didn't have any cardio-endurance to speak of, apply form, resistance, control, and extension to their modified movements and get further, faster, than the people in the room who were at much higher fitness levels but were jumping around like idiots.

You want to be the road runner of fitness? Then you've got to get moving, using correct form.

Form is about the way you do a movement. Correct form simply means using the muscles that you are working to do the movement, and not bending, swinging, or throwing yourself around like a loon. Incorrect form is all over the place in the aerobics industry. Teachers and clients alike are swinging around like monkeys, jumping, hopping, bouncing—using no form at all, which is fine if you don't mind a big chance of injury and movement that doesn't do much to change your body and if swinging like a monkey is a goal of yours. It never was a goal of mine, so I began using basic correct form every time I moved and got on with changing my body.

One of the best ways to define form is to give you some examples of the worst form you could imagine.

Sit-ups—here's where you see lousy form almost every time. The old head and neck pull is what you see people doing who are trying to do abdominal exercises. This is a great example of an exercise done without correct form that results in very little abdominal strengthening and a whole lot of incorrect movement that doesn't do much to change your body. I see people pumping those abs, lifting high, grunting and groaning, and not using one section of their abdominal wall.

Have a look around your health club at people working out on those machines. How about that StairMaster? The machine that everyone clamors to get on at the health club. On they get, pumping up and down—great for the legs, good cardio, then you get to the upper body. Most people on these machines are slouched over, huffing and puffing—way beyond their cardio-endurance level, not in oxygen, not burning fat, and because of bad upper-body form completely disregarding the upper body. Why not use as much as you can? Include the upper body, have it working for you while you are getting your cardio. Get as much as you can out of the movement. The only way to do that is to be aware of basic good form while you are moving and apply it every time you move. Get on the StairMaster and stand up. That's it, put down the book and stand up. The first thing you need to think about as you are standing there is pressing your shoulders down. In order to understand what that feels like, lift your shoulders all the way up, up, up, up to your ears—shoulders up, shoulders down, which is it, Susan? Shoulders up for now, all the way. Now press the half circle down and back. All the way, feel that feeling? That's what it feels like to have your shoulders pressed down. Remember that, you'll be using it a lot.

Next—lift. Abdominally lift, that is. To be lifted is to be using correct form. You're standing with shoulders down. Now think of your abdominal area, and lift it up. Don't worry if you don't feel anything because your abdominal muscles have atrophied beyond feeling—you'll get that strength back, just concentrate on lifting. Shoulders down—when you first start doing this, the immediate reaction will be to lift through your abdominal wall by raising your shoulders. That is a good example of what it feels like to do a movement by using other muscle groups and tension and not activating the muscles you are trying to use and strengthen. The tension in your shoulders that you create by hunching them will never help strengthen your abdominal wall. You have to require the abdominal wall to do the lifting, activating the abdominal muscles and strengthening them.

So you're standing with your shoulders pressed down, lifting through the abdominal wall, abdominal muscle doing the work, and breathing—another thing that tends to go right out the window when you tell people to lift. We all lift and hold our breath. You need to lift and breathe.

Next, soften your joints. Perfect form requires soft joints. Locking the joints does not build strength, burn fat, or help your workout. Locking an elbow or knee can create injury, and who needs that? While you're standing, shoulders down, abdominal wall lifted, breathing, soften your knees. Make sure they are not bending forward—that is never a good idea—just soft. The final step in creating good form is shifting your weight onto your heels, so you are sort of sitting back. Your body weight should be back on your heels, knees soft, pelvis slightly tucked, abs lifted, shoulders down, and you should be breathing like a dragon. There it is. Comfortable? Well, you are not just going to stand there—you are going for a walk, just like that. Walking in correct form is much more effective and will change your body ten times faster than the way most of us walk. We walk briskly, but you can bet the shoulders are hunched, stomach flapping, arms swinging, and there's no form in sight. What a difference your brisk walk will make when you are lifted, shoulders relaxed, knees soft, and you use the rest of the info in this chapter. Same person, same fitness level, totally different walk.

Think about doing the same thing when you swim. Or when you ride your stationary bike—that's where I see some of the worst form ever. People are bent all the way over, sleeping on the handlebars while pedaling like mad. Good workout, huh? Try using some form on your treadmill. Abs in, knees soft, shoulders down, body lifted, lifted, lifted, and breathing. You are not going to apply all this on your first walk, so don't expect to. It's a lot to think about, but you'll get it—an ab lift there, a shoulder press there, all add up to a much better workout and a fitness expert in the making.

Walking, treadmilling, swimming, or whatever your aerobic activity is—using correct form is a good beginning, but only a beginning. It's a time to throw a little mud into your aerobic activity.

Mud equals resistance, and resistance is what's going to help you increase your level of intensity when you feel the need for a challenge. Resistance is also a big part of the mighty four that make a workout work. . . . Oh, I love that, making a workout work, that's cute. Think mud, think quicksand, think water, think anything you want—just think resistance. Your arms are not swinging by your side during your walk, they are pressing through quicksand. And it isn't just your arms pressing forward and pressing back through the resistance, it's your legs. Your torso is pressing against quicksand—think of the air around your body as quicksand. Walk against resistance and in perfect form, and you'll see how much the level of intensity of your exercise increases without changing anything else. Same walk, same person—it's getting harder and more effective by the minute.

Important note here. Notice when I was talking about your arms moving through quicksand, I mentioned the press forward and the pull back? This is a big fitness secret that most teachers in the industry either don't know about or just forget to tell their class every time they teach. There are two parts to every movement. There is the press forward and the pull back. There is the lift up and the press down. Right back to the crappy sit-ups most people do. They jerk their heads up and then fall back down, causing a couple of different results. Number one, they are barely using any of the abdominal muscles to do the lift up—more often it's the hands pulling the head and jerking forward, so there's not much muscle being used. And number two, they are completely eliminating the other half of the move—the press down —making it about as effective as lifting your index finger to increase the strength in the abdominal wall. And you can pretty much guarantee that they are annoying, pulling, and in some cases injuring the muscles in their necks and shoulders.

If you want to get the most out of every movement, try doing both parts of the movement, against resistance and with perfect form. It's amazing how effective some of the most simple moves can be when they are done correctly. Hey, aerobics industry, did you hear that? How about eliminating all the stupid choreography you've got us doing—which doesn't do a damn thing, other than confuse the hell out of most people—and get back to some simple, effective moves that people are taught how to do correctly? Then you could have more than one fitness level working out in a room, because the moves wouldn't eliminate half the world, like they do now. . . . Oh, then there'd be another problem that would be bigger than the one you've already created—the teachers would have to teach. Boy, would that be a lot to ask.

If you are going to take moving correctly all the way, you need to add some control. That's right, control yourself.

Controlling a move requires you to think about it. Flipping and flailing your arms around is out of the question for you at this point, and covering your arms with mud certainly cuts down on the chances of that happening. But control is how you ensure that will never happen again in your fitness life.

To control, you have to slow down. Another big problem with most fitness programs—between the speed of the music and the lack of cuing or teaching, it is impossible to control anything they are asking you to do. Hey, aerobics industry—why don't you slow the hell down? You know that increasing the level of intensity in a class has nothing to do with speed. You know that the better the form, and the more the resistance and control when you do any movement, the harder and more effective it is. And you know it is impossible to complete the range of motion, or control the move, when the music is so fast. Slow it down, slow it down, slow it down.

If you think about a movement or the muscles you are using while you are doing the movement, you will automatically make it more effective. Do you have to memorize a muscle chart before you can do that? Be an aerobics expert instead—you already are, so don't worry about it. I only know the basics when it comes to muscles. Biceps, triceps. Abdominals—that's a hard one to figure out. Quads, the big ones on the front of your thighs. Glutes—your butt. Who cares about every muscle in the body—like math, you're never gonna use it, so don't bother learning it. (Oh, God, every math teacher in the country is burning this book at this very moment.) You know what I mean—the only thing you need to do in order to think about what you are using is to think about what you are using. Where are you feeling it? If the muscle you are using is underneath your arm, then think about underneath your arm. It is not necessary for you to know the official term, the triceps, or the shape and size of the muscle—who cares? Legs—think legs. And on it goes until you become more familiar with your body.

It may have been a long time since you've even considered your muscles. Eventually you will become familiar with the names of muscles, exercise terminology, and all the hip phrases used in the fitness world when you start eating, breathing, and moving, and getting lean, strong, and healthy. You don't even know yet how much you want to know. You may end up studying the human body and becoming a muscle expert—or, like me, you may want to know just enough to be sure you are using the right muscles and to be safe and responsible, be able to identify some of them once in a while, and get on with getting fit.

You may never need to know what every muscle looks like or what muscle you are using for each move. One arm lift may involve chest, shoulder, and back. You'll know that because that's where you'll feel it. It does not have to be complicated or completely understood before you do it, but it does have to be done with correct form, against resistance and with control.

While you are resisting and controlling like you've never controlled, try adding extension. Reach as far as you can without locking the joint. By the time you use form, resistance, and control and then throw in extension, you will be doing whatever aerobics activity you choose better than most people out there. That's my goal —well, not my only goal. Yes, I want you to get the most out of your movement, but I also want you to impress the hell out of everyone you meet in the aerobics industry with your brilliance. . . . Call me selfish, but it's true.

Extension: You push out against mud and pull in against mud, always resisting. Your shoulders are down, abs lifted, knees and joints soft—form, form, form. And then you extend. Extending an inch or two makes all the difference in the world when you are doing any movement. When you walk, extend your legs as far as you can. Don't just step, extend and step.

What are you doing? Using more muscles, you are screaming back at me. Press those arms up to the ceiling as far as they can press. What are you doing? Yell with me, USING MORE MUSCLES TO DO THE MOVE-MENT. (That's yelling in print.) Think about this. No, don't think, just do it. Step side to side. Right now, put the book down and step side to side as if you've never heard of the concept of extension. Nothing to it. Just a regular step side to side. Now extend the movement. Step one inch farther—or, as I say every day in my studio, one plank wider. You see, I have a hardwood floor that cost me a fortune, and I'm gonna use if for everything it's worth. Because of what it cost to lay the damn thing, I get on the floor in the middle of class, point to the next plank, and ask my clients to step on the next plank, please, when they are stepping side to side, so I can justify the cost.

This does two things. First and most important, it makes me much more comfortable with the cost of the floor. Second, it requires the person doing the move, and hopefully the whole class, to extend, using more muscles and reaching their fitness goal sooner. See the harmony involved? Cost and effectiveness combined . . . a perfect marriage. A perfect marriage. That depresses me. I haven't been able to find that balance yet . . . will I ever? I try, God knows I try, but I continue to fail. Well, I'll keep trying with this marriage, because it's worth it—I should say he's worth it, because he is. This is not a marriage manual, because if it was, I'd be thrown to the wolves for even attempting to write it, so let's stick with exercise—because that I can do.

After understanding the high-volume, low-fat food concept and the "I want to live in oxygen for the rest of my life" theory, if what you want to know is how to exercise, and be safe and effective when you do it, you're got it. It's done. Believe me, you now know more than most of the superfit ever know. Form, resistance, control, and extension are the ways to make movement effective, use more muscles to do the movement, and be safe and effective. The stuff works. Apply what you can, when you can. Be patient with yourself, and don't ever expect perfection—because it's never gonna happen. One step at a time is a good theory. Building one brick at a time is another one, and I can't think of any others, so we'll just stay with those two and pretend they are the only building-block theories on earth. If you apply resistance and control but blow off the extension and form, big deal— it's never all or nothing. It's as much as you can do, and doing better next time makes more sense and makes it all happen. These are new concepts that don't soak into your brain overnight. They will enter your dreams, though. A client of mine had a horrible dream that she had to tell me about. She was running, scared to death, chased by a madman. Don't you have those "running with someone right behind you" kinds of dreams? Anyway, she was running for her life, but she was running in form, resisting all the way, controlling, and extending. She was worried she was going to get killed but also worried she wasn't doing the movement correctly and wasting her workout, all at the same time.

Some aerobics experts may say that I have asked a lot of you guys, maybe too much, but you know better. It doesn't end here. There is something else you may not know about that will catapult you to your next fitness level.

> I've never considered strength as a benefit. It's a new idea for me.
>
> —Comment from a client

STRENGTH TRAINING

Don't be afraid. It's okay. I know more than anyone that the last thing you need right now is more bulk. If anyone had suggested that I pick up weights when I was 260 pounds and start a weight-training program, I would have thought they were the cruelest person on earth, that they were out of their minds, and that steroids had obviously warped their sense of reality for them even to think that strength training was for me. But I would have been wrong.

Strength training is exactly what I should have been doing from the beginning, and it's exactly what you should start right away. Include it with your cardiovascular conditioning. If you do, you will get the results you want faster than you would by just doing your aerobic activity.

How?

The myths and fears surrounding weight lifting are amazing. Women are desperately afraid of looking like the ladies you see in the weight-lifting magazines. Who could blame them? With all due respect to the ladies of bodybuilding, you guys look awful. It ain't pretty. That's not what I want to look like. No massive lean muscle mass, low-body-fat starvation diets, loads of body oil, or funky poses for me. I just want to look and feel good, thank you, and unless weight training can get me there I'm not interested.

Let's cover the health issue of lean muscle mass versus no lean muscle mass first, and then get on to the more important issue of looking good.

Your muscles need to be strong and well developed, and get the blood and oxygen they need to function and do all that you require them to do every day. Every move you make, every inch you move, every function of your body, requires muscle. The stronger, more developed they are, the better they function. That's a fact. The healthier the muscle, the better it functions.

Muscle maintenance is the same as any other physical maintenance. It requires the same things as cardio maintenance—correct form, resistance, control, and extension—done consistently, in oxygen, over a period of time to get the results you want. You have to define your fitness level and your fitness goal with strength training, just as you do with cardio training, and the internal changes you make at the beginning are what make the external permanent, included in the end result. Same process: getting as lean, strong, and healthy as you want to be.

I got a clue of what strength training could do for me when I started reading books written by some of the leading contenders in bodybuilding. They never referred to larger women, of course, and certainly didn't give modifications for the sets or reps. I mean, after all, who the hell ever considers a fat, unfit person doing anything that has to do with exercise? But I started doing some of the things they were suggesting anyway—call me rebellious —and the results were amazing.

I didn't know something very important at the time. (Don't you love how all this stuff I'm telling you to do happened by chance for me? Expert by experience— that's what you can call me.) What I didn't know then I can share with you now that I'm a "fitness expert"—that lean muscle mass burns fuel. A lot of fuel. It isn't a quick burner—it burns fuel slowly. But it burns it for a hell of a long time, and one of the fuels it burns is . . . fill in this blank, because I know you know the answer . . . FAT, FAT, FAT.

Increasing lean muscle mass by lifting weights does a couple of things. It increases your fat-burning, which is your goal in life at this point, and it makes your life easier. Those grocery bags you lift once or twice a week (depending on how organized you are) get a hell of a lot easier to lift when you have strong muscles to lift them with. The babies that you have on each hip—no problem. Give me more—if it's more babies you need call the Fertile Turtle, he'll help you get them, no problem. Lower back pain? Try increasing the strength in your abdominal muscles and see what that does for your aching back. Leg pains? You wouldn't believe how much difference strong leg muscles make in the way you feel.

Notice I keep saying increase strength, not build bulk. Building bulk is something you never need to worry about, unless you are willing to train like an animal and lift hundreds of pounds of weight. Do you know what these women go through to get the bulk they have that makes them look like they do? Hundreds of pounds of weights. Constant training, as in living in a gym. Diets you couldn't imagine. If you think you and I should have medals hanging from our living room walls—these women would have a house decorated with nothing but medals for low-fat dieting and starvation just before their competitions. There's no need for you to go through all that to build enough strength to look great and get through your day and help make your daily activities a breeze.

This is about getting leaner, and since lean muscle mass burns fuel, increasing it will help you burn more fuel, so do it. There is another advantage. As you are burning fat, you want to make sure there is muscle being developed underneath the fat, so that when your fat is burned off, you are left with a nice arm, a good-looking leg, or a tight butt—as opposed to a lot of loose wobbly stuff on your limbs and having to live with no strength.

> There is more definition in my arms, legs, and waist. Now I look forward to the next day. Anything is possible!
>
> —Linda, a client

One more little secret that will thrill you. Tell your weight loss counselor this when she is putting you on that 1,000-calories-a-day diet. One pound of lean muscle mass weighs the same as 1 pound of fat. They weigh the same. When you go on your 1,000-calories-a-day diet, you are losing water, which you can gain back the second you take the next drink, and lean muscle mass. And what you lose in lean muscle mass, you gain back as fat. Take this one to your doctor or weight loss counselor. This will shock the heck out of them.

Say you weigh 150 pounds and are 25 percent body fat. You hate the way you look, and you go on a diet—1,000, 1,200 calories a day . . . you know, starvation. Let's say you have the willpower to stick to it long enough to lose 20 pounds. Bravo. You've lost 20 pounds. If, like 98 percent of us, you gain that weight back, within six months you are back up to 150 pounds, you miserable failure—

but this time around, you are 26 percent body fat. Do it again, you are 31 percent body fat. Again . . . it keeps on going, because you don't gain back lean muscle mass—you have to build that. Once more: What you lose in lean muscle mass, you gain back as fat. Isn't that amazing? Each time I gained my weight back I would feel flabbier, heavier, looser, and I thought it was my imagination. Me —I'm the one with the crazy body and mind. Unbelievable.

If you decide that what I am saying makes any sense at all and you choose to lose body fat instead of dieting and to spend your time increasing lean muscle mass, you'll end up reducing fat and building lean muscle mass. Back to the point: 1 pound of muscle weighs the same as 1 pound of fat, but the really big difference is that 1 pound of fat takes up *5 times* the volume in the human body. Fat just lies around taking up space—a lot of space.

So, stay with me here—you lose the fat by not dieting and by decreasing the fat in your daily intake. Then you increase the lean muscle mass by weight lifting—and you'll end up littler and leaner than you've ever been or ever thought you could be. Remember, the muscle mass continues to burn fuel. You will be a fat-burning machine without even thinking about it.

I get up in the morning as a lean, strong, healthy person and burn more fuel than I did when I was working out at 260 pounds, because my body is a more efficient machine. I have much more metabolically active tissue now than I did at 260 pounds. If I have more metabolically active tissue—in other words, lean muscle mass—then I am burning more fat. Muscle is metabolically the most active tissue in the body. Work that metabolism. Keep it going. My body is a fuel burner at rest and a fuel burner when working out. Fat does very little other than clog you, widen you, and destroy you. Fat is not active. Muscle tissue is. So burn fat and increase the lean muscle mass, and you'll be in much better shape than you are right now.

I've spent a small amount of time on increasing lean muscle mass. But I don't own a weight belt. Aren't they the ugliest? Whenever I can, I lift some weights. My body is a fat incinerator, and yours can be, too, if you are willing to build some lean muscle mass along with me and Jenn in the photos in this book.

Imagine what your butt is going to look like when you've burned off the fat, increased the muscle, and put on those shorts. Think about it. It's attainable and easy. Do you want it? Then strength train with us. Tired? Strength train. Want that feeling of being lifted and strong, want the aches and pains to fly out the window? Strength train.

> I didn't realize how out of shape I was until I tried to get it back.
> —Comment from a client

I had a friend who was Ms. Fitness, an aerobics queen. Beverly knew every teacher in town, went to all the classes, and had every move down. The only problem Beverly had was a genetic leg problem. The ugliest legs in town, no matter what she did. Thick, tree-trunk legs. No matter how little she ate, no matter how many classes she took, her whole body looked good except for those hideous thighs and legs. That's it—genetic. Nothing she could do about them. That's what she was born with, and that's what she learned to accept.

Her opening line when she met someone was, "Hi, I'm Beverly, I have disgusting legs and there is nothing I can do about them." So Beverly and I met, and the first thing we did was change her diet, a big thing with me. High-volume, low-fat, no questions asked. She started a weight-lifting program for her legs. She knew it all, so for me to recommend weight lifting for her legs only confirmed what she already suspected—that I was nuts. But for whatever reason—desperation, probably—she listened.

Not only did Beverly reduce her body fat to the point that she never thought possible, her legs began to take on a different shape, to look 100 percent better. Her moment of glory came one day in class after she had been working with weights for a couple of months. Another woman in class came up to her and said, "I've been staring at your legs through the whole class, and one of my dreams is to have legs that look like yours."

You want a smell-the-rose moment? That was it for her (and still is, I might add). Beverly was not born with great legs. When she puts on fat, that's where it all seems to land. Who cares why, it just does. Her legs may never be as great as those belonging to someone who was born with great gams, but they look pretty damn good. The minute they come up with that bone-extension surgery, she may be standing in line, next to me, but for now she loves her legs enough to wear nothing but skirts, shorts, and anything else that shows them off. Beverly has since quit the real world and disappointed the hell out of her family and is teaching fitness and great leg exercises to the masses. Nice ending to the story, don't you think?

Weight training is inexpensive—a couple of cheap dumbbells is all you need. It works. It will help you build lean muscle mass and change the way you look and feel. That's why I'm recommending you do it.

Follow the photos. Work with Jenn and me and get lean, strong, and healthy.

RESISTANCE TRAINING FOR MUSCLE ENDURANCE AND TONE

THINGS YOU WILL NEED TO GET STARTED

- Straight-backed chair
- Mirror (optional)
- Dumbbell weights for upper body
  Beginning: 2, 3, and 5 pounds
  Intermediate: 5, 8, and 10 pounds
  Advanced: 10, 12, and 15 pounds
- Ankle weights for lower body
  Beginning: None (use the weight of your own leg)
  Intermediate: 2–5 pounds
  Advanced: 5–8 pounds

Before you begin your resistance training program, here is some basic terminology you will need to be familiar with:

Repetition—one complete exercise movement from beginning to end. Also called a "rep."
Set—a specific number of continuous repetitions.
Rest—a short pause (about 60 seconds) taken between sets for muscle recovery. It takes 3 minutes for the muscle to replenish ATP (energy stores) completely; 80 percent of ATP can be restored in 60 seconds.
Contraction—tightening of a muscle.

These exercises can be done every other day. Make sure to take a day of rest between each day of resistance training.

GENERAL GUIDELINES:

- All upper body exercises are performed in the "postural position": chest lifted and shoulders relaxed. Shoulder blades should feel as if they are coming together. Elongate through the spine and all the way through the top of the head, as if your head is reaching toward the ceiling.
- Avoid rolling your shoulders forward or hunching (shrugging) them up toward the ears.
- Keep the natural lumbar curve. Avoid rotating your pelvis too far forward or backward (under): too far forward will hyperextend the spine and create tightness in the lower back. Too far under or tilting the pelvis posteriorly will create an over-flat back and a rounding of the upper back. Hold abdominals in tight and keep hips in a neutral, relaxed position.
- Do up to 10 repetitions of each exercise.
- Rest 60 seconds between each set of 10 reps.
- Do up to 3 sets of each exercise.
- When you can easily complete 3 sets of 10 repetitions with your lightest weight, it is time to progress to the next heaviest weight. For example, if you start with a 3-pound weight, increase to a 5-pound weight.
- Focus on the muscle you are working.
- Always remember to bend at your knees, not at your waist, when picking up your dumbbells while standing.
- By the way, it is not proper form to cross your legs while doing these exercises—I'm just striking a pose for the camera!

STOP THE INSANITY!

This is Jenn, with a face like an Irish princess and a body that's changing so fast, she stuns me every time I look at her. From 340 pounds to whatever you want to be, Jenn, here's to you . . . thanks for helping me show people how to do it right.

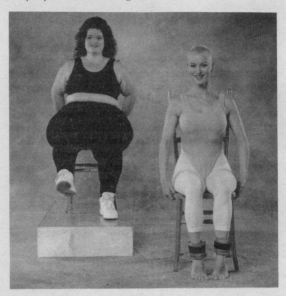

1. ALTERNATING LEG EXTENSIONS: QUADRICEPS

Starting Position:
- Add ankle weights if you want to increase your level of intensity.
- Sit on the chair with feet flat on the floor.
- Hold on to the back or bottom of the chair, placing your hands below the seat. This will help you keep your balance.

Doing the Movement:
- Extend one leg fully, straight out in front of you, contracting the quadriceps.
- Release the contraction and slowly return to the starting position.
- Complete 10 reps, then switch legs. Alternate legs for 3 sets of 10 reps per leg.

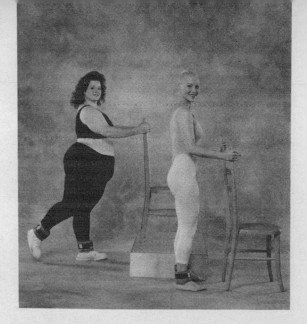

2. HIP EXTENSION: GLUTEUS MAXIMUS

Starting Position:
- Add ankle weights if you want to increase your level of intensity.
- Stand facing the back of the chair.
- For balance, place hands on the top of the chair back.
- Your feet are shoulder width apart, knees are soft.
- Remember your postural postion: abdominals tight, chest lifted, shoulders relaxed. Shoulder blades feel as if they are coming together.

Doing the Movement:
- Flex your foot and slowly extend your leg to the wall behind you, contracting the gluteal muscle.
- Release the contraction slowly and return to the starting position.
- Complete 10 reps, then switch to the other leg. Alternate legs for 3 sets of 10 reps per leg.

Things to Remember:
- Maintain proper form and keep supporting leg slightly bent. (Jennifer's leg looks hyperextended in the photo.)

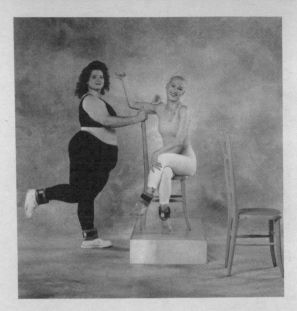

3. HAMSTRING CURL: HAMSTRING

Starting Position:
- Add ankle weights if you want to increase your level of intensity.
- Stand facing the back of the chair.
- For balance, place hands on the chair back.
- Feet are shoulder width apart, knees are soft.
- The exercising leg is bent at the knee with toes resting on the floor.

Doing the Movement:
- Flexing the foot, lift heel toward buttock and contract the hamstring.
- Release contraction and return to the starting position.
- Complete 10 reps, then switch to the other leg. Alternate legs for 3 sets of 10 reps per leg.

Things to Remember:
- The exercising leg remains parallel to the supporting leg.
- Avoid letting the knee swing forward.
- Keep the supporting leg slightly bent. (Jennifer's leg looks hyperextended.)

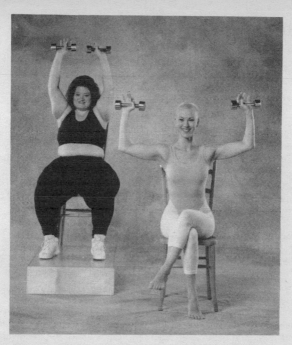

4. MILITARY DUMBBELL PRESS: DELTOIDS, TRICEPS

Starting Position:
- Sit on your chair with feet flat.
- Lift your chest, relax shoulders, and tighten your abdominals.
- Start with one dumbbell in each hand in a goalpost position.

Doing the Movement:
- Press the dumbbells to a full extension without locking your elbows. The contraction is in the deltoid, not in the elbows.
- Return to the starting position and repeat for 3 sets of 10 reps.

Things to Remember:
- Exhale on the way up and inhale on the way down.
- Maintain proper form by keeping the wrist directly over the elbow all the way up and all the way down.
- Keep the tension out of the neck by pressing the shoulders down.
- Try not to squeeze the dumbbell so tightly that your knuckles turn white—put that energy into your deltoids to lift up and press down.

STOP THE INSANITY!

5. WALL PUSH-UP: PECTORALIS MAJOR, TRICEPS

Jennifer is doing the beginner's exercise, and I am doing the advanced move on the floor. Let's start with Jennifer:

Starting Position:
- Feet are shoulder width apart and 12 inches away from the wall. (Note that the farther the feet are away from the wall, the harder the move becomes.)
- Place your hands on the wall at shoulder level, slightly wider than your shoulders.
- Turn your palms slightly inward. This will place more emphasis on your pectoral muscles. If the fingers are up and down, you will be bringing in more of the triceps.

Doing the Movement:
- Keeping feet flat, lower your chest until it almost reaches the wall.
- Keep your body in a straight line and press your entire body back to the starting position.
- Avoid locking your elbows.
- Repeat 3 sets of 10 reps.
- Increase your intensity level by moving your feet farther away from the wall. You may increase your intensity even further by standing on a box, then begin to do push-ups from your box before advancing to the floor.
- Remember to use a well-supported wall.

Advanced (that's me):
- Take the position on the floor.
- The hand position remains the same.
- If you become very advanced, move from the knees to the toes. Continue to hold your abdominals tight to help support your lower back.
- Lower your whole body to the floor, not just your chest. Pressing up slowly, repeat for 3 sets of 10 reps.

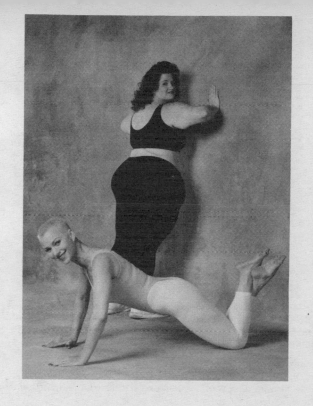

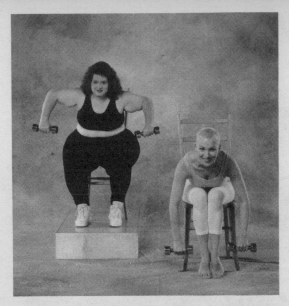

6. BENT-OVER SEATED DUMBBELL ROW: LATISSIMUS DORSI, POSTERIOR DELTOIDS AND MID-TRAPEZOIDS AND RHOMBOIDS

Starting Position:
- Sit on your chair with feet flat.
- Lean forward with your chest and keep it lifted. Avoid crunching the shoulders up to the neck.
- With one weight in each hand, extend arms toward the floor, with palms facing the back wall.

Doing the Movement:
- Lift your elbows up and toward the middle part of your back as if you were squeezing a rubber ball between your shoulder blades.
- Return to the starting position and repeat the movement for 3 sets of 10 reps. Remember to rest for 60 seconds between each set.

Things to Remember:
- If you are feeling tension in your neck, press your shoulders down and back.
- Instead of looking up, focus your eyes on a spot approximately 4 feet in front of you. This will help ease tension in your neck.

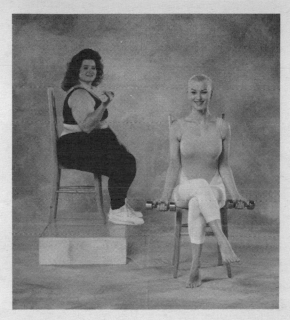

7. BICEPS CURL: BICEPS

Starting Position:
- Sit on your chair with abdominals tight and chest lifted. Elongate your spine.
- With a dumbbell in each hand, let arms hang down by your sides with the palms of your hands facing forward and elbows close to your waist.

Doing the Movement:
- Lift dumbbells up and contract the biceps at the top of the motion.
- Slowly press the dumbbells back to the starting position.
- Repeat the exercise for 3 sets of 10 reps.

Things to Remember:
- Avoid dropping or swinging the dumbbells.
- Keep your upper body in a stable position. Avoid rocking back and forth.
- Grip the dumbbell lightly instead of squeezing it. Think about contracting the biceps instead.

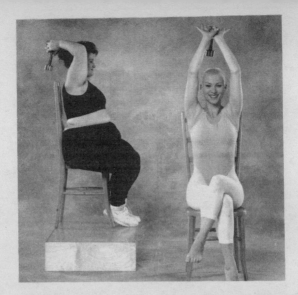

8. SEATED OVERHEAD TRICEPS EXTENSIONS: TRICEPS

Starting Position:
- Sit on your chair with feet flat.
- Hold a single dumbbell with both thumbs interlocked around the end of the weight, palms open and facing the ceiling.
- Extend arms above the head, keeping the elbows tight to the sides of the head.
- Elbows are slightly bent.

Doing the Movement:
- Bend the elbows and slowly lower the dumbbell toward the floor.
- Contract the triceps by extending the open palms toward the ceiling.
- Repeat for 3 sets of 10 reps.

Things to Remember:
- If this move is uncomfortable for you at this time, skip it. As you get leaner and stronger, you will be able to add this exercise to your program. Triceps are being used as a secondary muscle in other exercises of this routine.
- Keep the tension out of the neck by continually pressing your shoulders down and back.

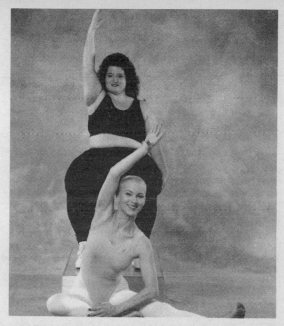

9. ONE ARM OVERHEAD STRETCH: LATISSIMUS DORSI, OBLIQUES

Beginner's Position (that's Jennifer):
- Sit on your chair, lifting up through the chest, abdominals tight, elongated through the spine, as if a string were attached to the top of your head, lifting toward the ceiling.
- Lift your right arm and reach toward the ceiling.
- Hold for 30 seconds.
- Repeat on the left side.

Advanced Position (that's me):
- Thank God we get to sit on the floor!
- Sit on floor with the left leg extended and the right leg curled in toward the knee.
- Lift through the chest, abdominals tight and elongated through the spine.
- Lift your right arm and reach toward the ceiling. Slowly bend to the left side.
- Hold 30 seconds and repeat on the other side.

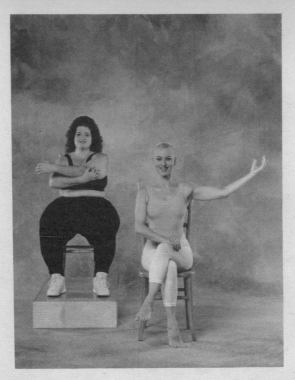

10. UPPER BACK AND SHOULDER STRETCH: UPPER TRAPS AND POSTERIOR DELTOIDS

- Sit on the chair.
- Extend right arm to the side and bring it toward the center of your body.
- Place your left hand between the elbow and shoulder of the right arm.
- With the left hand, bring the right arm toward the chest. Feel the stretch in the middle part of your back and back of the shoulder.
- Hold for 30 seconds and repeat on the other arm.

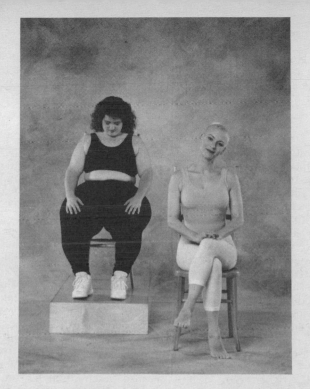

11. NECK STRETCH

- Press your ear toward the shoulder and hold it for 10 seconds.
- Rotate the head forward with chin toward the chest and hold for 10 seconds.
- Rotate the head toward the other side and hold for 10 seconds.
- Repeat as many times as you like.
- Remain in your postural position.

STOP THE INSANITY!

Now you have an option. You can stop right here and guarantee that you'll look better, or you can follow me to the next step—to something that feels wonderful.

FLEXIBILITY TRAINING

It all seems to end with training, doesn't it? Well, that's exactly what it is training you for, a better life. Training to stop the insanity in your life. It's up to you.

Flexibility training—why would you do it? Why should you? What does being able to touch your toes have to do with getting lean?

Not much of anything, is the answer to that question. For all the folks who were born being able to press their face to the ground—bully for you. Most of us are not that flexible. So who cares about it?

Here's what I think. Burning fat and increasing cardio-endurance and muscular strength are the most important things for you to do to begin, because that's what you need to do to see changes in your body. And seeing those changes is very exciting and very motivating. Flexibility training will not do much for you if looking in the mirror and seeing a leaner you is your motivation. So blow it off, right? No, don't—because even though some stretching here and there doesn't burn a ton of fat, won't increase that lean muscle mass, and in the whole picture won't do much to turn your body into the body of your dreams, it has some great side effects and absolutely helps the process.

Sure, you lengthen and stretch the muscles that contract during your aerobics activity—that's a good thing. The blood and oxygen flow through the muscles, keeping muscles flexible. That's great, and you'll be thrilled when you're eighty and the only one in your group who can bend over and pick up the puck on the shuffleboard court. But that's not why I think it's important for you to include some flexibility training in your fitness program. First of all, it feels so good. Not the bouncing, joggy motions you see people doing before they go for a run. I mean lifting, pressing through the chest, slow, controlled, resisted, extended stretching. Holding a stretch and falling into it. Shoulders relaxed, chest up—the form always applies—stretching through the muscles. . . . It's a great feeling and a wonderful balance to a cardiovascular workout.

Stretching does help prevent injuries, although flexibility isn't going to do much if you fall off a 10-foot wall. Pulling tight muscles, tendons, ligaments—all that junk is less likely to happen when you include some stretching in your workout.

But that's still not why I think you should do it. I think you should take a few moments after each fat-burning event and stretch because it helps you get back in touch with a body that you may not have thought about in years. It's a few moments of thought, connection with your body, and silence (unless you've got metaphysical music screaming at you in some aerobics class cooldown), and you have a chance to feel your body. Think about it, and maybe throw in a mental goal-defining exercise while you're sitting, standing, or lying there.

I never really put much emphasis on stretching when I first started changing my body. I mean, who cared if I ever touched my toes? I was too busy trying to figure out what all this was about and how I could get from a size 22 to a size anything other than that. Then I got fit and cool, and I threw in some stretching once in a while. I thought that was pretty good for someone who was born as stiff as a metal rod. "Relatively flexible" is how I would have classified myself until . . . I took a yoga class. I'm fit, strong, and reasonably flexible. I am a woman, so consider me capable of anything. So I take this class with a friend of mine.

News flash, guys. If you think for one second that you are flexible, go take one of these classes. The first thing the yoga teacher did was hit a big gong in the corner and start chanting. Everyone closed their eyes, except me, of course. I was still peeking through one eye. The gong gonging, the chanting loud and in some other language, and the teacher asks us to sit on our lamb's-wool rugs and begin our class. (Lamb's wool conducts energy—did

STOP THE INSANITY!

you know that? I should have hung lamb's wool over my castle in Garland. Maybe I could have gotten through the day.) Then the class starts, and within minutes I'm ready to get up and call Barnum & Bailey Circus. These people belong in the circus, no question about it. Leave out the gongs and put a brightly colored outfit on them, and crowds would gather. I couldn't believe what they were doing and what she was asking me to do.

The teacher came around to help old stiff rod—me. She was lovely, very kind and gentle—what else would you expect a yoga teacher to be, rough as a truck driver? No chance, these people have to be gentle and flowing —it's part of the job requirement. She suggested some alternative poses, modifications—I instantly loved her and thought about changing her whole disposition, putting her in a neon leotard and tights, and getting her in the aerobics industry. They certainly need anyone who understands the concept of modification, even if it's a yogi in disguise. She asked me to do a modified version of the leg-around-your-head move. "I'd need joint surgery to try that. Is there something else I could do, like sit here for the rest of the class and watch you guys flow through these unnatural moves?"

I have tried a few sun salutations and horse-fly-to-the-moon moves since then, and it's not my idea of big fun. But since my experience, I have newfound respect for flexibility, yoga people, and circus performers.

Flexibility is associated with "warming up." There are a couple of things that go on in gyms, aerobics studios, and workout centers all over this country that make me mental to be around. People doing head-and-neck sit-ups make me nuts. Those abdominal stands—that piece of equipment in gyms that people lie across, feet tucked under two pads to hold them down, and the swinging up and down they do that supposedly increases abdominal strength—the lower-back damage going on that is as obvious as anything could be is hard to watch. (There's usually a "private trainer" standing right next to the person who's ripping their lower back to pieces, counting . . . 8 more, let's go . . . HELP ME.) Another thing that's difficult to be around is the stretching that goes on all over the floor of some of these places. Sitting head bent over the knees and bouncing into a stretch or two. Standing up, arms in the air, bouncing to the left a few times, then bouncing to the right a few times. Standing up, bending over at the waist, and bouncing a few times to stretch . . . what? What are these people stretching?

We've been taught to do static stretches that must go before all workouts. Runners lunge—that's if you're able to get down to the floor. Lift here, press there, hold for a couple of seconds, and you're on. Bounce, bounce, bounce, and you're warmed up and ready to go. Ready to burn fat. And safe from injury because you've warmed up.

Hey, aerobics industry—you know better than that. You know that the best way to warm up a muscle is to get blood and oxygen to it. The best way to do that is to move. Slowly. Starting slowly, warming up the muscles and the cardio system, and getting your breathing established—then you're warm, and you can increase your level of intensity to get into the aerobics section of your workout for 30 minutes or more. Then you cool down. Slowly again. Same concept as a warm-up, but it's called a cool-down because you are coming down from your aerobic level—and THEN YOU SHOULD STATIC STRETCH THE MUSCLES. MUSCLES SHOULD BE STRETCHED WHEN THEY ARE WARM, HEATED, HOT, NOT WHEN THEY ARE COLD.

The yoga people know that—that's why they put heaters on, no matter what the temperature is outside. It's like a sauna in these classes, because they want the muscles hot, the body hot. The exercise physiologists know that. The doctors probably don't, but my questions is, Why doesn't the aerobics industry? And where do you get these dumb heel presses from?

Warm up your muscles by moving slowly.

Increase your level of intensity.

Get into that fat burning.

Cool down by moving slowly.

Then stretch, stretch, stretch, and become a yogi.

Exercise. Let's break it down.

STOP THE INSANITY!

FORM

When: Every time you move. Think form.

EXTENSION

When: Every time you move.

CONTROL

When: Every time you move.

STRENGTH TRAINING

Increase lean muscle mass so that you:
    burn more fat
    have enough strength to hold yourself up
    have a butt that looks good when all the fat burns off
    don't end up with empty sacks for arms, legs, and abs.

When: Every other day would be nice. Three times a week. One day on and one day off. Whatever works for you.

FLEXIBILITY TRAINING

Don't bounce . . . please, don't bounce.
    Stretch after your aerobics workout, when the muscles are warm.
    Fall into and think about the stretch.
    Use correct form and hold your stretches for at least 20 or 30 seconds.
    Think about your body, lengthening and stretching the muscles you just used.

When: After every workout would be nice, but if that doesn't happen, try to stretch a couple of times a week. It is important to include it, and it sure as hell feels good —so give yourself that feeling and stretch it out once in a while.

See, exercise isn't all that bad, when you understand what you are supposed to be doing. When you know how the hell you are supposed to do it, and what it is that you are going to get from it. Then you will be much more likely to do it, and you will certainly be able to live with the results.

I've been fat and I've been fit. Fit is better.

After taking the first exercise class (with lots of modification), I felt both happy and sad. Happy that I made it through the class. *Sad* and *ashamed* that I had let myself become so fat and out of shape.
—Comment from a client

ABS

The exercise chapter is over. I've explained it all, summed it up, and now we are heading into chapter 7—"Enjoying the Process."

Burn fat—very cool, we all need to do that. Increase lean muscle mass—open to that now that I understand it, fine. Increase cardio-endurance—that's a good thing. Get those pumps and filters strong and healthy, reap those rewards. But Susan, dear Susan . . . WHAT ABOUT MY STOMACH? WHAT IN THE HELL AM I SUPPOSED TO DO ABOUT THE THING THAT'S HANGING DOWN MY THIGH?

Let me give you a moment to catch your breath and tell you that I know that's one of the most hated areas on every woman's body. It's the area that your O.B., along with mine, has convinced you that you'll never get back in shape after a couple of kids. It's the area that all the sit-ups in the world don't seem to change after the age of thirty-five, and you'd pay $10,000 to have it flat, with little hipbones poking out the sides, and smooth again. Well, that's exactly why I'm devoting this whole section to explaining it.

Hang loose (pardon the pun)—we are going to solve

the problem. Never treat the symptom, always solve the problem.

That stuff hanging off your stomach is fat. The only thing that is going to burn that fat off your stomach and the rest of your body is aerobic activity. It *will* burn off—keep in mind what you learned way back in chapters 4 and 5 about not putting fat in, burning it off, and having low body fat. There is no way on earth that you will still have fat hanging from your stomach when you are 15, 16, 17, 20 percent body fat, have increased your lean muscle mass, and are lean, strong, and healthy. Think about it. Are you going to be lean everywhere but your stomach? Nope, not possible. It will burn off your stomach just the way it burns off everywhere else.

So, as you are doing aerobic exercise, dedicate a few workouts to the fat on your stomach. Focus on a picture of a flat washboard abdominal section, if that's what you want, because you can have it.

The next thing you have to do to change your stomach is to increase the strength in the muscles underneath all that fat. Sit-ups? Nope. Not in the beginning. A great way to begin to regain your abdominal strength is simply by using your abdominal wall while you are working out, sitting in your car, seated at your desk, or anywhere else you find yourself during your day. That's right. You can work on your abdominal strength wherever you are by doing one thing—thinking about it and lifting.

Sitting in your car, whether you feel it or not, lift up through your abdominal wall and hold it. Don't stop breathing—the tendency is to hold in your abs and stop breathing. But keep breathing as you lift and hold, just as you remember to press down your shoulders in your brilliant form. You may not be able to lift and hold for any length of time in the beginning. So what? That just means your abdominal area is weak, so work at a low level of intensity—building strength in the abdominal wall while you are burning fat—and change it. The stronger the muscles get, the longer you'll be able to hold them up. The less fat hanging from your abdomen, the easier it will be to hold it up—there'll be less of it, and the more you strengthen it, think about it, and get back in touch with the muscle, the easier it will be.

Everywhere you are, every time you move, during every workout, lift up and through your abdominal wall. Think about using a part of your body that may have gone to hell and back, increasing the strength in it and burning the fat off it.

When you are ready or physically able to get on the floor and do some "official" abdominal exercises, here's what you need to do.

Lie on the floor.

Knees bent.

Energy in your heels.

Pelvis slightly tucked.

Hands behind your head or by your side, depending on your fitness level. Hands behind the head makes the abdominal lift harder. Either way is fine.

Head resting in your hands, if hands are behind your head. No clasped hands, just your head resting in your hands. Your head ain't light—some of us are lugging around 10 to 15 pounds of head—so use that weight as resistance for your abdominal lift. Let it go and lift it up with the abdominal wall.

Lift your chest to the ceiling so that your shoulders are just off the ground. Immediately you'll feel your head and neck pulling up.

That's what happens when you try to compensate for the weak abdominal muscles you have. Instead of requiring the abdominal muscles to lift your chest, you are trying to get your chest up with your head and your neck. The only way to stop that from happening is to strengthen the abdominal muscles. You can't do that if you continue to use your head and neck muscles to do the lifting. (Can't get a job without experience, can't get experience without a job—same dilemma.) You lift up a couple of inches—constantly reminding yourself to relax your head and neck—using your abdominal wall to do the lifting and pressing, increasing the strength in the muscles. Think 1-inch lifts up and 1-inch presses down. Lift up, press down, lift up, press down, nothing to it. The only thing you need to do is think abdominal and make the muscles do the work.

If you want a challenge, lift your left leg, if you can.

Knee over the lower section of the abdominal wall, to protect the lower back.

Soft knee always.

Lift your chest toward your knee.

Lift an inch toward your knee.

Press your chest down an inch.

Repeat the process with the other leg up in the air.

Try both legs.

Lift both legs into the air.

Knees soft.

Chest lifting toward your feet.

Lift with the abdominal wall.

Relax the head and neck.

Breathe.

Lift and press.

What you've done by adding one leg or both legs is require more from the abdominal muscles. The movement will be harder, increasing your level of intensity immediately.

If you are a beginner, you can keep both feet on the ground, lifting your 1 inch and pressing your 1 inch. At any point when you feel you have the strength, add a leg or two. Try it for a few repetitions and go right back to your feet on the floor, lifting and pressing. You have the option. How do you know when you are ready to increase your level of intensity? The minute the old 1-inch lift is easy. Just like your strength training, challenge yourself, do the movement in correct form, with resistance, control, and extension so you avoid injury and get the most out of the movement. Don't be afraid to increase intensity. If you find that you've taken it beyond your physical limit, decrease it.

My stomach was my problem area. I remember sitting in the living room of my castle, so depressed, grabbing the rolls of fat around my stomach, hating it, pulling at it, crying because I didn't know how I was ever going to get rid of it, and I didn't know how I was going to live with it. I worked hard on reducing my body fat, and my stomach was the last to go. But it's gone. And I love the fact that it's gone. I still work hard on my abdominal strength because it's my goal to have the strongest abs on earth. I get the biggest thrill when I go to a strength-training class and make it through a really tough workout with strength to spare. No matter how my body looks, when my stomach doesn't feel strong, I don't feel strong. It is my fitness barometer, because it was my fattest and weakest part and I hated it the most.

If I told you how many times a day I just lift my abdominal wall and hold it in, feeling the strength and the control, you'd think I was a kook, because it's a little excessive—but, hey, I earned it. The only way to get a strong stomach is to build the strength—nothing can get you that strength, not lipo, not any other cosmetic surgery. Nothing can burn the fat but aerobic activity. All that crap about having C-sections and never being able to regain the strength in the muscle is just that—crap. When you cut a muscle it heals, just the way your skin does when you cut it. You can absolutely regain the strength if you work it. Having children does not automatically mean you are going to have a hanging gut for the rest of your life. Some women can birth twenty kids and have a flat stomach minutes after the birth—but who cares about them, that's not reality for 99 percent of us. You may have to work harder than those women with naturally flat stomachs, but you can develop the abdominal muscles of your dreams by burning the fat and increasing your strength. That's not genetics hanging from your stomach. It's fat. You don't have a stomach on you because you've had children, you have a stomach hanging because you have too much fat and not enough strength in the muscle.

No matter how mature you are or how well developed your self-esteem was as a child, discovering a hipbone after you've been fat for a while sends most people into a tizzy. I went mental when I started to feel a hipbone—and then when I saw it? Forget it—I could quite honestly classify that as one of the best days of my life. Now, how's that for immature? Birth, death, marriage—I've had all that, but regaining my hipbones is up there as one of the most important moments of my life. Scary. You're reading a book written by someone who is willing to admit that. That's even scarier.

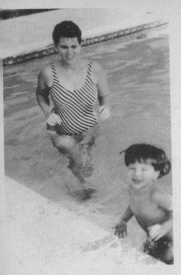

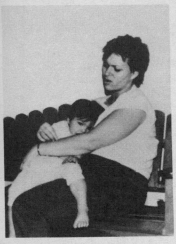

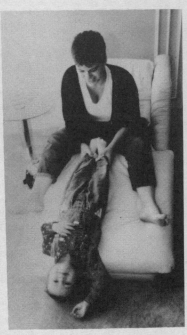

Still not a bathing beauty, but looking better. Getting into a bathing suit and swimming with my kids was a big deal. Slowly getting better—that's what these years meant to me.

SEVEN

Enjoying the Process

It is good to experience life in a woman's body.
—KAREN KATAFIASZ,
Celebrate-Your-Womanhood Therapy

Linda called me from Florida this week. She spoke with my assistant, Sally, and said she wanted to talk to me. I don't think she expected me to call her back, because when I did she almost had a heart attack.

She had called because she wanted to know what she could expect in a couple of months from eating, breathing, and moving. She really needed to get in shape for a few things that were coming up and wanted to know when the changes were going to start.

My conversation with Linda was fabulous. We went from "When is this going to happen?" to truly understanding and appreciating the process that was going to change her life. So I thought you and I could have the same conversation with me playing both parts—that dual personality comes in handy once in a while.

What can you expect from eating, breathing, and moving? A very reasonable question. You can expect, immediately, to get your life back. Resurrect from the dead, which is the way most of us are living, and gain strength, choices, and power that you've never had. You can sure as hell expect more than you could from any diet you've

241

ever been on, but that wouldn't be difficult, because you've never gotten a thing from any diet but starvation and aggravation. Stopping the insanity in your life is not painful or expensive, and it will never retard you socially.

Never again will you have to not eat when everyone else is—"No, thank you, I don't eat, I just drink liquid shakes for food, because I'm out of control, hate the way I look and feel, and am on diet number 1,000,000,000,001 in my life. Watch me, everybody, see if I fail on this one, like I have on the other 1,000,000,000,000. . . ."

Your body will get what it needs to function and will look and feel better than it has in years. And here's the big one: The internal changes you will be making by increasing your metabolic rate, building lean muscle mass, burning body fat, and pumping blood and oxygen to those 75 trillion cells and however many muscles you have in your body will make the external changes permanent.

Linda had been eating, breathing, and moving for three weeks. I asked her how she felt.

"I used to get up in the morning and my feet felt like lead. And in just a couple of weeks, they don't feel so heavy.

"The other day I went shopping with my friend, and it was six-thirty at night before I ever got tired enough to sit and take a break."

I'm loving this, Linda. Here's what I live for—discoveries like this in three weeks. What more could anyone ask? This is pretty cool and getting cooler.

"I never thought about my body before. I never thought about designing what I may or may not want to look like. The only thing I ever felt for my body was hatred. It was like living inside an enemy."

This is where I started to cry. Hearing someone say something like that—"living inside an enemy"—about the beautiful, brilliant, perfect body that they—we, all of us—have been given. All the wonders and potential of this body of ours, and we end up hating it? It's very, very sad, but something I hear all the time.

"Now I am beginning to see my body as someone I can work with." (A little schizophrenic, but understandable.)

"Hey, Linda," I asked, "how much do you weigh?"

"Four hundred pounds, and I'm five-four."

"Linda, what's the social occasion that's pressuring you to be perfect in a couple of months?" Here's reality, folks—400 pounds, and you want perfection in a couple of months.

"It's a family reunion, everybody is going to be there. I know eating, breathing, and moving are the answer, and I want to do it to show them all that I can do it."

Neon sign flashes . . . DANGER, DANGER, DANGER, WILL ROBINSON.

To all the Lindas of the world: Cancel the family reunion. Get the flu or something. Do what you do when you can't make it in to work because you know one more day is going to kill you. Lie. Don't go. Avoid it like the plague.

Enjoy the process of your feet feeling lighter than they have in years for a little while before you expose yourself to the next emotional bashing that may send you into an eating frenzy. Revel for a while in your clothes getting looser. Give yourself a chance to feel the energy coming back into your life and give this process a chance to ignite the hope that the process brings back.

Hope is not some intangible romantic notion that none of us can ever get our hands on. We are not handed hope on a silver platter by someone or something in our lives. My hope has been developed and rebuilt through lots and lots of hard work and creating something tangible and understandable to hold on to.

Changing my body and my life didn't happen by chance. God knows I never healed the emotional and mental first. I started with the physical, giving my body what it needs to function. And then I started to feel hopeful again.

Just like you, I thought the only hope I'd ever feel was in the end result. *When I get skinny, it'll be all right.* When you put that statement in print, you can really see the stupidity of it. Hope in a skinny body? What does one have to do with the other? We have been trained to believe in and attach importance to one thing—the end result—instead of learning to love and appreciate the process.

My hope grew and strengthened during the process of changing my body. Every accomplishment I made from the very beginning was fuel for the hope I was beginning to feel, the self-esteem I was rebuilding, the belief that I was capable of doing this. Getting lean, strong, and healthy.

How do you measure that? The first piece of clothing that gets looser, the first exercise class you make it through, the first person who gasps when they bump into you because you don't look like the person they remember? None of these things has anything to do with the end result—they all have everything to do with the process, and the process is glorious.

Each step of the way brought back the hope, the dreams, the excitement, and the goals I'd lost sight of. The things that blew up in the explosion, call them casualties of war. My hopes and dreams began to rebuild and got strong during the process.

What is the hope formula? Where are the how to's that guide you? It is the ultimate intangible because nobody even knows what it is. You know what it feels like, and you sure as hell know when you've lost it, but what is it, and how do you get it? As simple as this sounds, I would like to suggest that you try something to begin breaking the cycle of self-hatred, negative self-image, starvation, and deprivation. Try giving your body what it needs to get well, and enjoy the process.

Regaining hope saved my life. I changed my body, but so what? It wasn't in the end result. It was in the process.

When did I know I was capable? I didn't know when I started this process. Do you think a good-looking body makes a damn bit of difference when you are in front of three cameras doing live television for the first or two thousandth time? Or when a publisher gives you a lot of money as an advance to write a book? It is not a smaller body that gives you what you need to get up at five A.M. every morning to type before you get the kids up and ready for school and then begin your day. It's physical strength, having a body that is capable of starting and functioning at a high level of intensity for a long period of time. A strong, fit body—and then you pray. In the scope of things, changing my body—what does that mean? When people stop me in airports and ask for my advice, it's nothing but hope that gets me through—hope that I am saying what they need to hear. Hope that I'm touching the women who need the information, presenting myself properly, and making a difference in their lives.

If this book is giving you hope, I can say with everything in my being that it's worth putting your faith in. Bet on it because it works.

My hope came in the form of quality information that I could understand and apply to my life. Seeing the results as they happened, from the very first burst of energy to the black string bikini, helped me trust the fact that I could regain control in my life. Whether it's rebuilding a life or fighting menopause, it's about the same thing.

Many of the women in my studio are going through a process that every woman on earth will face. I'm so grateful to the women who have come before us and taken menopause out of the closet—where it had been hidden in shame, embarrassment, and madness—and restored the natural order and respect for a process that is a wonderful part of womanhood. My clients have shared their feelings with me, and they are dealing with some of the same issues that I dealt with when my marriage broke up and my life fell to pieces. Loss of control. The feeling that choices are being taken away and you can't do anything about it. Feeling and watching their bodies change right in front of their eyes and not being able to do anything about it.

Wait a minute. You can't do anything about it? How about getting as lean, strong, and healthy as you've ever been, during this time of your life? How about getting your body the oxygen it needs? How about doing what one of my grandma clients is doing? Yesterday she came into the studio, dressed in a yellow-and-red dress, body looking fabulous. She's been weight training in a big way and looks like a million bucks. "My granny never looked or felt like this," she said. "Even when I'm flashing hot, I look and feel better than I've ever felt in my life." Hope, hope, hope. . . .

If hope is what you need, then it's hope I'm selling. Wrap it up and take it home with you, because this works.

My friend Jill—whom I watched go from a bulimic, frightened child to the most beautiful, secure, strong, enlightened woman I've ever met—told me I needed to tell you all that you must enjoy the process, because that's the only way to rebuild the hope. And the hope is what gives you the peace and confidence that you're gonna make it, no matter what happens.

> This is the first time in my life that I can look toward the future and feel excited and hopeful about the possibilities.
>
> —Comment from a client

So, Linda. Avoid anything that is going to divert you from the process. Don't do this for your family—to hell with them. Don't do it for your husband. Forget about what people think you are capable of. Who cares? It's not about any of those things. This is about you getting well. Fit. Lean, strong, and healthy. Changing how you look and feel—not how anybody else feels about you.

If you want a system to stay on track, I've got one for you. Once you've faced how unfit you are and you've begun the process, you may find yourself doubting (of course, that is before your wall of hope is built and gets so strong that nothing could topple it). The immediate results you'll be seeing and feeling don't have much value in a society that wants instant everything. We are so far into the insanity that we expect it all to be fine right away, even if we are starting at 400 pounds and half-dead.

Here's how you can give your immediate results value.

Ask yourself these questions every day, a hundred times a day if necessary. Do it while you're breathing (two birds with one stone—what a horrible expression).

Do I feel better?

Do I have more energy?

Am I feeling stronger?

Am I shrinking?

Is this worth it?

If the answer to any or all of these is yes, keep going—keep going and don't look back. Keep moving forward.

I've got another suggestion for you. Part of the new monitoring system that's gonna make you a little nauseated.

Study your body. Wear clothes that allow you to see your body while you are working out—loving the process, remember, loving the process. Stay with me here.

I have taught hundreds of classes during the last couple of years, and my classes are filled with obese women in two-piece leotards. Exercise bras and tights, midriff bare. Not an easy thing to find until a 260-pound woman got fit and designed these clothes so that other unfit women could watch their bodies change. Fashion has nothing to do with this. These clothes are about fit, quality, and function. The function? Clothing designed to work with your body while you are getting fit. Absorbing sweat is important when you are sweating buckets. Being able to move is important. The last thing a larger woman needs is anything restricting her movement, the rolls of fat are restrictive enough. Elastic choking you, fabric binding you, and anything crawling up your butt when you are trying to move are the last things you need. You want your clothing to move with you, not against you. Have we gone from stopping the insanity to how to shop for leotards? No, right now I'm getting to why the hell you should expose your body for the world.

If you think feeling energy is a great experience—having the strength to move, great; lighter feet, no more lead in your life, fine—let me tell what Big Thrill 101 is: seeing a rib cage. The collarbone thing can't be described. It's great to watch your body go from covered in fat to leaner. But you can't watch anything when you are covered from head to toe in sweats. So uncover. Get those sweats off—you don't need any more covering, you've got enough—and look at your body. Watch it change. Get back in touch with it. You know you are fat and unfit. Look at it and change it. Enjoy the process. It may take a while to get used to it, but you will.

At 260 pounds and using the old monitoring device, jumping on and off the scale every thirty seconds, my life was controlled by the numbers shown on that piece of equipment. Talk about interrupting the process. One pound up, and my day was shot to hell. Depressed and starving all day, just to see that pound drop the next morning. Those days are gone for me and for you. You've got a new monitoring device and a new awareness of a totally different process.

I was just with Beth. Talk about enjoying the process. Beth has gone from a tight 30 to a size 14. She's standing in front of a mirror looking at herself wearing a pair of blue jeans with a white shirt tucked in.

"I love mirrors now. Every chance I get, I stare into one and look at the person looking back at me. I think I'll get my picture done by a professional. . . . Have you ever had yours done by those guys in the mall?"

She's talking and I'm not listening, because my mind is racing back to the first pair of blue jeans I could fit into. To get a pair to fit felt wonderful. Tucking something into your pants is a luxury that only an ex-fat or a fading-from-fat-to-lean person can understand.

A belt can't be described. To begin to see your waist, to know that one is under all that fat and you are going to see it one day, is beyond the shadow of a doubt the biggest and the best fun. It's similar to pregnancy. Waiting for your baby to be born so that you can meet him or her. Same questions.

What's it going to look like?
Will it be big or small?
What kind of a relationship will I have with it?
Will I love it like I think I will?
Then you get into the specific belt questions.
Will I belt it?
Hang chains from it?
Expose it to the world every chance I get?
Tattoo it?

Have my husband eat whipped cream off it?

Taken it too far? It's a question that only you can answer. I happen to like having whipped cream eaten from my midriff.

Beth has "fallen" for herself. Watching her look at herself in the mirror, admiring herself and being so proud of her accomplishment, shot me back in time to some of the greatest clothes moments during my process.

Trying on bathing suits. How's that for difficult? Every woman on earth hates the yearly process that requires you to see your body from every angle in those hideous fluorescent lighted rooms with mirrors everywhere. After the blue-and-white beached whale experience, I wasn't going anywhere near a bathing suit store for the rest of my life—until the day I pulled into the parking lot of a shopping center to buy some bread at a bakery and ended up walking into a store that sold nothing but bathing suits. Every color, shape, and size up to a reasonable number —the old 12, 14, 16, and you're-out-of-here insanity— was in this store. Bathing suits everywhere, and I was standing in the middle of them all, with no idea which end of the rack to head toward.

Positive Reinforcement 101. Dual personalities kicked in big time, and I started talking to myself like a crazy lady. "You've worked hard, you look good, you feel good, your self-esteem doesn't hang on any of these racks. No matter what happens in this store, you will be all right."

I felt like I was going into battle, volunteering for the jump right into the lion's den. I was scared, embarrassed, and worried even before I tried one suit on.

Without thinking, I headed for the size 10 and 12 rack. Sure I'd changed my body—that was obvious by the sizes I was wearing and the way I felt. But we are talking bathing suits here—very small pieces of fabric that expose it all. You couldn't have dragged me to the smaller sizes.

Everything I was doing made me feel self-conscious. My casual cruising in the size 10–12 racks made me wonder if everyone in the store knew that I had been 260 pounds and that bathing suit shopping was one of the hardest things I'd ever done. Surely they all knew just by looking at me.

Be cool, Susan.

Act like you've got dozens of these things at home and you're just looking to add to the collection.

I gathered a handful of 10's and picked up a few 8's on the way to the dressing room, just to see if there was a chance in hell they could possibly fit.

Try it, get the size 8. Go ahead, get it in a bikini.

Bikini?

Size 8 black bikini.

You'll be alone in the dressing room.

Just try it on and see how it looks.

Nobody will ever know.

Into the fluorescent I go, close the doors, and that's it —my moment of truth, trying on bathing suits.

The size 10 fell to the floor when I put it on, and I vowed from that moment on that I would always begin trying on clothes with a size guaranteed to fall to the floor. What a way to start the day.

Size 8, way too big. I had to ask the saleswoman to get the same black bikini in a 6. She looked at me, obviously wondering why in the hell I'd tried on 10's and 8's, and suggested she bring it in a size 4 or 2. Get outta here. Size 2 or 4?

She came back, and guess what? The 4 was too big. The 2 won hands down. There are no words that describe that moment. . . . It was actually a bit longer than a moment, because I stood in shock, staring from every angle. Not only did these two pieces of fabric connected with string look good on me—the lumps and clumps that had been all over my thighs and stomach were gone. I could jump up and down—and I did right there in the dressing room—and my body didn't jiggle. Sexy? Yep, it looked very sexy.

I understood exactly what Beth was saying. It's a great day when mirrors and cameras become your friends. It was a great moment standing in a room looking at my body in a bikini.

Without enough money left in the bank to pay for the mortgage that month, I bought the two tiny pieces of fabric that cost a fortune. Ms. Klein must get her fabric from the mountains of Tibet, because this bikini was unbelievably expensive. But selling the car to have this thing sounded very reasonable to me at that moment. I was not leaving the store without it. Nobody could ever accuse me of not getting my money's worth out of that suit. I've worn it ten million times—it doesn't even have to be a pool party for me to slip into that black bikini. It now holds a place of honor in my underwear drawer because it's too frayed to wear anymore. But you can bet that every time I open up my drawer, that shredded size 2 black bikini puts a smile on my face.

It's great when my sister says, "Hey, Jo, where is the other half of you?"
— Joanne, Ellington, Connecticut

Right after the birth of my second baby, a friend told me to try to enjoy the moment, the process, because it would never happen again. I would never be able to get it back.

Get it back?

Who would ever want to?

Why would I ever want to remember having babies back to back, let alone enjoy the process?

Here I was:

Heading for divorce.

Scared out of my mind.

As hormonally imbalanced as they come.

And just in case you want to add more to this list, I didn't know how I was going to get through the day, forget about the process.

Again, it took me forever to understand what she was saying, but I understand now. I missed a lot of the process, and I am sorry I did.

STOP THE INSANITY!

It was during a business meeting recently that I put one and one together and realized there was no difference in learning to enjoy the process, no matter what process we're talking about.

A very rich (and I mean the kind of rich that would blow the roof off most people's understanding of rich) businessman looked at me and said, "Susan, what you are doing is wonderful. It's well organized, has a lot of honesty and integrity, and is being done with a sharp business mind and good business sense in record time. I just hope you realize that it's more fun getting there than being there. It's getting there that you should be enjoying, because nothing's better."

At the time, in the middle of some pretty big negotiations, this advice or wisdom didn't have much of an impact on me other than to provoke a very diplomatic response. That's great, thanks for the advice, but I need your cash to get this project done so we can get this message to the millions of women who need it so they can get on with changing their lives. Thanks so much—let's get on with it.

But now I see. Changing your body, having a baby, and getting a project funded are all the same thing. The process is what will make you strong. The process rebuilds your self-esteem. The process relights your fire in a big way.

Part of it was about reaching that size 2.

But it was also about my thighs not rubbing together anymore.

About accomplishing each goal every step of the way —that felt better than anything could.

About feeling the fear leave my life and the hope creep back in.

About finding out that there was nothing wrong with me—I had not failed, the systems had failed me.

Hey, Nancy, I finally understand what you meant. Consider me a genius. Count me in as one of the most evolved people on this planet. The process is wonderful.

I've said it a million times. If you can go from a size 28

to a size 20, why can't you go from a size 28 to a size whatever you want to be? It's the same process. The power behind understanding this and going through the process is invaluable. It's glorious. Be smarter than I was. Enjoy what Beth, Penny, and all the other women who have been smarter than me have taught me. Don't let this slip by, you'll never be a size 28 again. Watch yourself change. Feel it, understand it, and enjoy the process. If I had the information you do, the support and encouragement that you have, I would have written down every feeling. Taken a full-length nude photo before and after. And remembered every moment.

Do you want to experience someone changing? Have a look at the chart of a client of mine.

Four months ago she weighed 310, could barely move, and felt horrible. She was 5 feet 4 inches and huge. Look at her before and after measurements.

	Before	After	Change
Date:	1/19/93	4/15/93	
Triceps:	18″	17″	−1″
Chest	50¼″	47″	−3¼″
Waist:	46¼	44¼″	−2¼″
Hips:	66″	64″	−2″
Thighs:	36″	33¾″	−2¼″
Pecs:	46½″	45¼″	−1¼″
		Total:	−12″

Her body has lost a total of 12 inches of fat. She's gone from 66.9 percent body fat to 58.6 percent body fat.

She's increased lean muscle mass, increased cardio-endurance, and works out at a level of intensity she never dreamed of reaching.

All she has to do now is keep doing what she's doing and watch the fat melt off and the muscle increase. She's loving the process and getting quite famous as a result. If you want to see a beautiful woman, look at the strength-training photos—that's Jenn. Watch Jenn shrink and get leaner, stronger, and healthier.

STOP THE INSANITY!

> The beginning of a habit is like an invisible thread, but
> every time we repeat the act we strengthen the thread,
> add to it another filament until it becomes a great
> cable and binds us irrevocably, thought and act.
> —Orison Swett Marden

Enjoy the process, quiet the old tapes and start playing
the new ones, increase your fitness level—all fine and
dandy things to try, but they don't always come easy. So
let's help you with it. Let's make it as easy as we can.

There are exercises for the body, and then there are
exercises for the mind. Mind modification is a whole different ball game. (My sons are baseball addicts, and although I wouldn't know a home run from a touchdown, I
threw that in for them.)

Professional athletes understand mind modification
and use it all the time. Well, aren't you in training? Training for a new body? Why shouldn't you have the advantage of mind modification so that the process is easier and
you have all the support and tools you need to make it as
easy and efficient as possible? It may be just the edge
that you need to reach the finish line—your fitness goal.

There's no reason at all why you shouldn't use all that
you can—that's how I feel about it. The Olympic runner
and you—not much difference. Both in training. Both
burning body fat, building lean muscle mass, and increasing cardio-endurance, and both with a very specific fitness goal in mind. Olympic runners may spend years
training their bodies. They also spend years training their
minds. Which, if you ask any Olympic runner, is equally
important, sometimes more important than the physical
training that goes into winning. They spend time visualizing the race. Seeing the end result. Feeling the heat.
Hearing the crowds roar, feeling the heaviness in their
legs at the end of the race, their heart pumping. Finally
they see the finish line. The ribbon shining in the sun, the
trumpets blaring . . . Well, as far as I am concerned, if
you are going to visualize, visualize big. The trumpets
blaring are my idea. Send in the trumpets—after all, I'm
running for the gold.

Mary Lou Retton (don't ask me why I picked her as an example) talked about the mental imagery she used to become the first American woman to win a gold medal in individual gymnastics. (I know why I picked her. She's a woman, and she won a gold medal, that's why.)

"I'd see myself performing in my head, and it really helped me tremendously. Since I usually had trouble on the balance beam, I'd review the beam and my routine in my mind, picturing myself landing straight, seeing the perfect landing."

If visualizing helped Mary Lou land straight, how about you? Why not use the same technique she used in her training, since it seemed to work? Mind modification involves training your brain while you are training your body.

Bambi never mentioned the technique to me. (Bambi never said a word to me, come to think about it.) If it's good enough for the athletes of the world, then it's good enough for you.

No need to sign up at your local Tibetan monastery, even if there is one in your town. It is really a very simple procedure, and it doesn't require ten years of solitude.

J. Krishnamurti said:

> A meditative mind is silent.
> It is not the silence of a still evening.
> It is the silence when thought
> With all its images, its works and its perceptions
> Has entirely ceased.

Right on, Krishnamurti. Well said. As soon as your mind is still and its perceptions and images cease, even for a second or so, you can begin to fill your brain up with new and different images.

Refilling the brain. Doing your own advertising. When you really think about it, everything we feel, think, or believe has been planted by someone or something. Whether it's family, friends, television, magazines, social rules, or regulations—whatever it is, it's been programmed into your brain and very much affects what you think and feel or how you live. Our brain is like a computer and responds to what it has been told. I am not about to touch this subject at all, other than to suggest that you consider beginning to program a different body image, end result, or physical reality that works for you.

Here's what I did. During my recovery—and that's exactly what I see my physical change as, a recovery—I worked three to five minutes a day on seeing an end result. Not the images that were being splashed at me in every direction. My end result. Exactly what I wanted from fitness.

I wanted a leaner body. So I began to see my body as lean as I wanted it to be. Let me confess right here and now, that was very, very lean. Strength was important to me. I was tired of aching and hurting, so I visualized my body as a strong body. I tried to feel the strength and see it as defined muscles. Energy was another biggie. As I pictured the body I wanted, I included enough energy to get through the day with some to spare. Certain clothes (the tiny black dress), shoes (I gotta include the spiked black heels, to be really honest with you), bathing suits (throw in the black string bikini), and social situations (visualizing people who had made me feel fat and ugly and watching the look of surprise on their faces when they saw me)—all that was definitely included.

It took a while for me to connect my body with my mind. You see, I hated the way I looked and felt so much that reconnecting wasn't easy in the beginning. It took a couple of weeks for me to see my head connected with my body, not someone else's. The models and images in every magazine that I picked up were the first to pop into my mind when I started. It was my head connected to someone else's body for so long, I began to wonder if I was capable of seeing what used to be my body. I'd forgotten what it felt like to look and feel the way I wanted so desperately to look and feel again, and within minutes I was back to the dual-personality mentality of the panic attack days. My head was connected to so many bodies within seconds of visualizing that I wondered whether this could be helpful or damaging.

It took only a couple of minutes a day—two minutes was a lot of time to devote to anything when you have children around—for a couple of weeks until my mind started to connect with my body. Susan as I was: 260 pounds. A little depressed—I was feeling better, but I didn't exactly have a Buddhist's mind—and very unfit. Finally I started seeing who I was without freeze-framing into some beautiful, tall, lean model's body, and it all started falling into place.

It was not always smooth sailing. The mental battles that went on inside my head before I ever got to anything that resembled quiet meditation were something that the *National Enquirer* would have paid good money for: TEXAS HOUSEWIFE BATTLES ALIENS INSIDE OF HEAD.

The dual personality. Susan I, who desperately wanted to look and feel better, and Susan II, who doubted every step of the way that it was ever going to happen. Susan II—who blamed the failures of the past, who stubbornly refused to believe that anything could ever be different or that this time it would turn out the way I needed it to be—was the personality that reigned most of the time. I started seeing Susan II as a monster.

Here's where I might cross a line for a lot of you. When we get into monsters and visualization, I can understand you at least putting this book down for a pause before resuming. But remember, we are talking about stopping the insanity, and although this may seem a bit insane to you right now, it's part of the process. So pause if you need to, but bear with me and consider mind modification.

My first couple of sessions with the monster of self-doubt were as far away as they could possibly be from the peace I thought was associated with sitting still, focusing, and meditating. It was constant chatter in my brain.

"No, Susan II, you don't look like that and never will."

"That's someone else's body you're seeing right now, not anything you'll ever look like."

"Get a life, Susan. If that was possible, you would have been there by now—after all, you've been on every diet there is, followed all the programs, and it ain't happened yet. So what do you think a little meditation will do? Make it happen? Ha ha, you dumb, crazy mind, it can't be that easy.''

"That looks too much like Cheryl Tiegs, put your body back. . . . OH, GOD, it's too much to take . . . stop the picture, the kids need me, gotta go.''

"Hurry, meditate, it's the last chance you'll get today. See it, feel it, hurry up, do it.''

Total craziness and confusion. So when I suggest you begin connecting your mind with your body, I'm not telling you it's going to be an instant cure-all. What I'm saying is that this technique can and should be worked on, like your fitness level, and that it is a valid technique to include in your life.

It's free, it's easy, and it works. Like oxygen, it's there and simply needs to be understood and worked so that you reach your goal faster and easier. Build it, develop it, strengthen it. Quieting the monster, learning how to turn off the constant negative self-image tapes that run through your head, is an important and valid tool.

When I started walking and was feeling so good, my brain would turn on. "This is pointless. You're so fat, you'll never feel better—why are you bothering?" I felt as if someone were inside my head turning the knobs, tuning in the negative station, and controlling the volume and frequency. There she was, Susan II at full volume. Mix Susan II with severe hormonal imbalances, add anger and hatred for the Prince, stir in a little exhaustion and Mr. Brain Control living inside my head, and you could only imagine what I had. It's a wonder I lived through it. The monster was always with me. Walking with me. Grocery shopping with me. There in the living room of my home and always with me in bed at night. It never stopped reminding me to look at my thighs, my stomach, my arms, and to get a grip on reality. Never stopped reminding me that I was the fattest person in the aerobics class. When I was tired or depressed—90 percent of the time—it had me.

"You don't need to go to class today, what's the point?"

"You'll never look like them anyway."

"Don't bother, take a break."

"It can wait until tomorrow."

Slowly I started to distinguish Susan II from Susan I. The monster from my dreams and goals. So you know what I did? I built a cage. A huge, ironclad cage with a lock and key. I had to find a way to keep the monster quiet for a while so I could begin to reprogram. Send the messages I wanted my brain to be receiving instead of the stuff playing on automatic all day and all night long. Seeing and feeling what I wanted to see and feel instead of what I was being forced to see and feel.

Some days required more of a fight than others, but I eventually learned how to put the monster in the cage, lock the door—I was in charge of the key—and keep it there long enough to think about what I wanted from fitness. Getting on with the business of locking up the monster and reprogramming my brain was one of the most powerful tools I had in the process of changing my life. Replacing the old, automatic tapes with new ones certainly contributed to my physical and mental change.

Instead of looking at the mirror and wanting to die, seeing how huge my thighs were and how far I had to go, I'd think about what I was doing to change and how far I'd come. Big difference in focus. I'd think about getting oxygen to every cell and muscle in my body and how that was helping my body get well. Strengthening my upper body, abdominals, and lower body, and what I was going to look and feel like when I was lean, strong, and healthy. I was walking and visualizing every day, and my mind and my body started working together. I began to feel it was possible. I worked daily on the physical and the mental. There was no spiritual moment or mental enlightenment that changed the way I saw myself. It was a process. Nothing guided me through the tough times, and there was no fairy godmother, voices, or newfound spiritual strength.

It was the physical (eating, breathing, and moving) and the mental (focusing for a couple of minutes a day on what I wanted from this process) that worked together to help me reach my goal. Not magical, not mystical, nothing complicated about it.

> During your cool-down/meditation to reconnect to my body, I cried! No, "sobbed" is the correct term. I could feel all the sadness I have been covering with my professionalism and my intellect.
> —Comment from a client

Visualizing the way you want your body to look and feel is not the only mind game you can play as you change your body. Learning how to focus on a muscle—whether it's to cool it down or contract it—is another fabulous mind game that increases the efficiency of the movement.

It sounds a little nutty, but when's the last time you thought about your ankles? I've taught many classes and ended with visualization. Thirty fat women lying on the floor or sitting on chairs, eyes closed, learning how to focus—and then I get to the "think about your ankle" part of the focus. Half the room opens their eyes and looks at me like I'm out of my mind. Why should they think about their ankles? Why should *you* think about your ankles?

Let's spend a minute thinking about what your ankles do for you. All day and half the night they support, in many cases, a hell of a lot of weight.

Little tiny ankles.

They bend for you.

They twist for you.

They step down for you.

Your ankles do a lot of work, are under an enormous amount of pressure, and are required to continue to function without a thought. I don't know anything that can continue to work well without a second's thought. Isn't that what women have been telling husbands for centuries? (I haven't been at it for centuries; although having to explain the same concept over and over in the middle of the second marriage makes it feel like centuries.) I need acknowledgment, attention, focus . . . and so do your ankles. Focusing on your body, spending a few minutes a day reconnecting, is the balance to the assumption that our bodies will continue functioning no matter what we do to them. They won't.

It's easy to go from thinking about your ankles to learning how to relax them. Release the tension in the joints. If you can do that, why can't you go up your leg to the calf muscle, releasing it or contracting it? Here's where the mind helps you get leaner, stronger, and healthier.

You're making a picture of what you want from fitness. Getting back in touch with parts of your body you have never thought about and focusing on the muscles and working them more efficiently through focus and control.

As I was changing my body, I thought about what I wanted. You probably thought, from the intro through chapter 7 of this book, that I have been as superficial as any one human being could get. Well, not true. My surface goals and dreams go deep.

Here's what I visualized:

Looking better than my ex-husband's girlfriend.

Feeling and looking sexy and seeing myself in tiny black dresses.

Being the leanest woman at parties or any social situation.

Having men ask me out left, right, and center, so I could turn them down if I wanted.

Having those great-looking arms that all the models have and visualizing those arms in tiny little sundresses.

Having the flattest stomach on earth, concave would have been fine.

Making love.

Hearing the gasps as I walked past people who knew me fat.

Hearing my ex-husband beg me to come back and make it work.

Don't you think Gandhi would have been proud? Consider me a disciple. Take me to the mountains in India and teach all those boys sitting on the top how it's really done. Queen of meditation comes to the mountain.

Frightening, aren't I? Notice there was never a thought, or a picture drawn, that had a damn thing to do with health. Not a healthy goal in sight, just looking better. As a studio owner, fitness representative, writer of a book about getting lean, strong, and healthy, I should lie to you. Make any reference I can to health and wellness. But the truth is, it never entered my meditation. WOW, there's an expression. It never entered my meditation. Those were my goals—I got them and more, so here's to visualization, eating, breathing, and moving.

You need to start thinking about your goals, whatever they are. Define exactly what it is you want from fitness. In the privacy of your own brain you can tell the truth. Get specific and honest and focus on it. Make it real. Develop this just like you're developing your cardio-endurance, building body strength, burning fat. There are no unrealistic goals other than being six feet tall when you are four feet nine inches tall. If you really can't visualize anything other than someone else, get some therapy along with this eating, breathing, moving, visualizing stuff—it can't hurt. We all need it.

Along with "If you can't see it, who cares?" "Use everything you've got" is what I live by. Don't expect a religious experience, although you may be surprised at what happens when you spend a couple of minutes in oxygen and silence—something we never take the time to do. Make visualization a part of your foundation of wellness. Both worlds can meet. India meets the suburbs of the United States of America. You can have the kids, the house, the bills, and the pressure and still meditate. Visualizing right after you've hung up the portable phone, turned off the TV, and set the microwave for dinner is not a sin. Who ever said you had to wear white robes and have hairy armpits if you wanted to meditate?

Hairy armpits? Where did that come from? The Prince did say something worth remembering. Something. One thing. Let me make that clear.

The Prince is very much a man's man. Great body, macho, loves to hammer and fix things, hardworking man's man. Add that to our differences. Macho man and feminist woman marry. What was I—blind, deaf, and dumb when I married him?

Anyway. One day I took him to a local health food store, because I wanted to show him some of the wonderful food hidden in the aisles of a health food store that you just couldn't find on the shelves of your local grocery store chain. I mean seaweed, burdock root, ginseng—what more could you want?

The Prince puffed up like a blowfish in this place. The walls threatened his macho pride. I'm running around showing him all of my discoveries, we get a few things, check out, and as soon as we get out the door, the Prince looks at me and says, "If those people are supposed to be so healthy, how come they look so goofy and sick?"

Now, as I look back and share this story with you, it amazes me that I married a man who used the word *goofy*, but love is blind as a bat, and the Prince had a good point. Everyone in the store looked like it was their last couple of days on earth and not one of them had seen daylight in twenty years. Drawn, pale, emaciated, and goofy—yes, goofy as hell. That's what the Prince and I —the upwardly mobile, nice, young suburban couple— thought when we considered things like meditation. Move to the mountain, give up all your worldly goods, grow the hair under your armpits and on your legs, and sit still for very long periods of time.

Not true. Here's what I did. I found a comfortable position to sit in. Sitting in pain or being uncomfortable while you are trying to focus on anything is not a good idea. Otherwise it doesn't matter where or how you sit.

Close your eyes. Take a few deep breaths. Think of these breaths as cleansing breaths. You are taking in oxygen and letting out all the tension, anxiety, worry, and negative self-images with the exhale. As you breathe, begin to make a picture of exactly what you want from eating, breathing, and moving.

If it's a leaner body you want, then see your body as lean as you want it to be. If it's strength you want, then see and feel your body as strong as you want it to be. See your muscles defined. See the cuts and lines in your thighs, butt, hips, arms, and back. Feel the strength. Connect that feeling with your body. Think about feeling lifted and strong. See yourself being able to run, jump, lift ten bags of groceries with ease. Be as detailed as you can be when you identify strength, getting lean, or feeling better.

If it's more cardio-endurance you want, see your body being able to process oxygen more efficiently. Feel the energy you'll have to spare when you are healthy. See yourself as an Olympic runner, a sprinter with air left over after the race. See your body recovering quickly after exertion. Visualize yourself running after the two-year-old—with a load of laundry in your arms, in the sweltering heat—and not being winded. It doesn't matter how you picture it, the only thing that matters is that the things that mean the most to you are included in your mental photo.

As I got used to doing this exercise, I started to create movies in my mind. I'd visualize myself walking in the tiny black dress and high heels into the party, where, of course, I was the leanest, strongest person in the room, hearing the gasps of all attending, bumping smack dab into the Prince and his girlfriend, with her having a bad hair and face day, not looking her best or anywhere near as good as I looked. The Prince falling to his knees and crying and screaming, begging me to come back and make his life complete. Apologizing for the pain and torture he put me through because of his stupidity and selfishness . . . me sweeping past both of them toward my perfect-bodied, beautiful, evolved man who adored the ground I walked on. . . . It continued from there, got more dramatic and detailed with every second of meditation, and you could only begin to imagine how it ended. Their lives end in tragedy. The Prince bloody and crying in front of the house—he's been hit by his girlfriend's car as she backs out of the driveway. She kills herself out of remorse.

So go ahead and get detailed. Include whatever you want. I needed the dramatic death ending for a long time —to give me some way to release the anger. See your body in any situation you need it to be in. If you want it all, and I hope you do because it's attainable, then you must begin to create and get in touch with a picture of your body as lean, strong, and healthy as you want it to be.

"There is only one way to change bad habits—replace them with good ones." I heard that line in some movie on drug abuse. It made a lot of sense to me as I was changing my body. I had developed some bad habits. Replacing them with good ones meant getting the foundational information I needed to change my body and applying it every day. It also meant finding as many tools, techniques, whatever you want to call them, as I could to help me keep going forward.

Getting fit has not eliminated all my bad habits. It would take an act of God to wipe out every bad habit I've spent a lifetime creating. Every day I continue to build better habits, and one of the cheapest, most effective, and easiest ways I've found to help the process is using my mind to define what I want, to see the outcome, and to spend minutes a day focusing on it.

I had a client who got the eating, breathing, and moving part of her program down within minutes. She got it right away. Mind modification was another issue. She had such trouble in the beginning creating a picture of herself as anything other than a fat, unfit person. After two weeks of working on it, she told me that it had finally worked. "I've done it. My head is off your body. It's finally my head on *my* body."

Wendy is not the same half-dead human being I met just six months ago. She's reached her fitness goal, and now she's working on a few new ones. Now when this woman wants to accomplish something, she gets the information she needs, works on it, and visualizes what it is she wants. . . . I think she's working on becoming president of the United States.

WATCH OUT, AMERICA, SHE JUST MAY DO IT. . . .

> You must do what you think you cannot do.
> —Eleanor Roosevelt,
> *You Learn by Living,* 1960

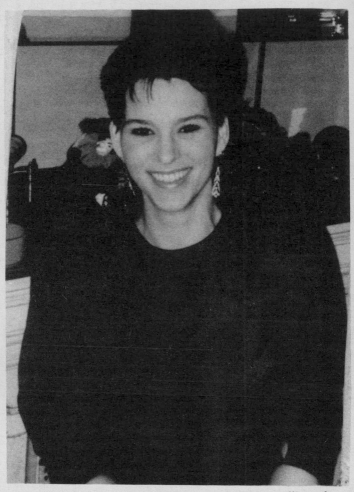

If you look closely, you'll see a couple of big rolls in the middle, but you can't say I hadn't come a long way at this point. Believe me, those rolls are gone forever.

EIGHT

Questions and Answers

> *Be patient towards all that is unresolved in your heart and try to love the questions themselves.*
> —RAINER MARIA RILKE

I've spent the last four years traveling all over this country, giving speeches and seminars about wellness to every kind of group imaginable. Large crowds, small groups, big cities, small towns, temples, churches, and hospitals. My favorite part of any seminar is the question-and-answer period at the end.

As I've said on national TV and everywhere else I've gone: I've got no pride; I'll tell you anything. I'll answer any question you've got. Combine the wonderful women who have attended my seminars, wanting as much information as they can get, with my lack of pride or shame, and you can imagine the kinds of questions that have come up.

There have been seminars where the question-and-answer section lasts longer than the whole seminar. Laughter, tears, respect, and love have all been a part of the energy and sharing that have happened hundreds of times when we get together and talk.

The question-and-answer sections in many books I've read never got to the meat (excuse the expression) of anything. My questions were rarely answered. I was always left feeling like a nosy old aunt because I wanted answers to the questions that were obviously not fit to print.

STOP THE INSANITY!

Well, I'll repeat, I've got no pride. I've answered them before and I'll answer them again—the questions that people really want the answers to.

1. How Often Should I Exercise?

Your body needs oxygen every day, and your muscles need to be worked. Thirty to 60 minutes a day is not too much to ask of your busy schedule so that you can benefit from the rewards exercise gives you—especially the extra energy! I hope exercise has a different meaning for you now than when you first started this book. Nobody should ever beat the heck out of themselves or pound themselves into the ground. But take the time to move daily within your fitness level. If you're not up to par, having a rough day, coming down with the flu or a cold, you can still move. Remember to modify your fitness level. A 15-minute walk may be more reasonable than your usual 30 minutes on the StairMaster or whatever it is that you're doing. If your fitness level is below a 15-minute walk, then try just 5 minutes.

2. I've Been Exercising for 2 Weeks and Haven't Lost Any Weight Yet. When Does the Weight Start to Come Off?

The weight will come off as soon as your body begins to use the supply of fat that you've built up as fuel. The more you burn, the more you lose.

Quick weight loss is mostly water and muscle tissue. It comes off quickly and usually goes right back on as quickly. Losing body fat is a different process. Since your scale is dead, asking yourself when the weight will come off is irrelevant. Your new monitoring system is asking yourself these questions:

- Do I have more energy?
- Am I getting stronger?
- Am I shrinking?
- Do I feel better?

The fat will come off. Give it more time than 2 weeks.

3. How Much Should I Weigh?

Every time I've ever seen a physician's chart on the average weights according to height, age, body type, whatever, I've been floored. I'd like to know where they got these numbers. When your body fat is within a healthy range, when you have the lean muscle mass that you are comfortable with, and when you look in the mirror and love the way you look and feel—that's how much you should weigh.

4. What About Special Occasions—What Do I Eat?

So often I hear, "Okay, I get this. It makes a lot of sense, but I have to go to a wedding in 2 months—what am I going to eat?" Who knows what you're going to feel like eating in 2 months? Will it be just before your period? Will you be frustrated, tired, in the mood for something salty or sugary?

Because of the deprivation and starvation that dieting causes, food in the past has been something to be afraid of, something you have to plan ahead for, and a never-ending obsession. It is no longer any of these things. You will eat what you like, what you're in the mood for, and, if fat is your concern, the lowest-fat foods at the wedding.

Food is no longer your enemy. It is your fuel. Enjoy it. Eat!

5. Will I Build Muscle Running or Walking? Are My Legs Going to Get Bigger?

Whenever you use a muscle, you build it. You will build strength and endurance. In order to build bulk, you have to lift a heck of a lot of weight— and sometimes, more often than not, have a steady diet of steroids. It is not easy to build bulk—consider how hard weightlifters work to get it. Building strength and endurance is not the same as building bulk.

6. What About the Kids? What Should They Eat?

Children should eat the same things you eat. *This is not a diet*. You stop the insanity by eating high-quality, high-volume, low-fat foods. Obesity is a national epidemic among our children. They are developing so rapidly and have so much pressure to deal with on every level in this society we live in. Who needs high-quality fuel more than our children? All the emphasis we put on education and development seems secondary to the fact that our children are living on chemicals and preservatives, instant junk. Our children are malnourished. We should be ashamed of this.

7. Does Metabolism Slow Down with Age?

Yes, your metabolic rate slows down with age. However, it's all relative. I know some 35-year-olds who do so little and are so out of shape that they are functioning at an 80-year-old level. If you eat right, move right, and breathe right, you will maintain a healthy life-style and metabolic rate. It is not a given that after age 50 you're doomed to live in a downhill spiral.

8. Is Breakfast Really the Most Important Meal?

The most important? Who knows? All meals are important. Fueling when you need fuel is important. It very much depends on the individual and his or her schedule. I don't like eating when I first wake up. But after moving for a few hours, I eat a huge breakfast.

What does breakfast mean? If it's force-feeding upon awakening, then it's not good. If it's being hungry and fueling for the first time in the day, then it's no more important than any other meal. You should eat when you are hungry.

9. How Much Water Should I Drink?

I love this water question. You should drink when you are thirsty and try to drink water.

If all it took to lose weight was water, or if drinking those 8 glasses a day that we've been taught to drink made an ounce of difference, I would be buoyant. I'd be a mermaid! All this water stuff has nothing to do with anything—like everything else we've been talking about, it's been blown way out of proportion. Don't wait until you have foam coming from the sides of your mouth to get a glass of water. Drink when you are thirsty, and eat when you are hungry. This is sane. Force-feeding water is not only insane; it has nothing to do with reducing body fat.

10. Why Did My Doctor Put Me on a Low-Calorie Diet?

Unless there is a good medical reason, you've been put on a low-calorie diet because he/she doesn't know any better. Ask your physician what you're supposed to use as fuel and if there is an alternative other than starvation.

11. How Long Does It Take to Change My Metabolism?

It takes, on the average, 6 to 8 weeks to increase your metabolic rate. That's the standard "industry" answer. But there are so many variables: Genetics. Your level of fitness or lack of fitness. The level of intensity in your training. Consistency and mental focus. Also, the foods you are eating and any medications you may be taking.

I can tell you from my own experience, and from the thousands of people I've seen changing in the last several years, that our bodies respond quickly when we consistently eat high-quality fuel and work within our fitness level. Who cares exactly how long? Just keep building and improving.

12. After I Exercise, Is It True That My Body Continues to Burn Fuel?

Yes, your body continues to burn fuel after you exercise. The jury is out on exactly how long afterward. But what's more important is that by exercising, your body functions more efficiently cardiovascularly, muscularly, and in processing oxygen.

13. Should I Ever Count Calories?

Your caloric intake is directly connected to the energy you expend. Remember, you burn fuel while doing *anything*.

The only calories you should be thinking about are the number of calories you should not go below before your body goes into starvation. If this is making you nauseated right now, go back to chapter 4 and reinforce the information.

If you do nothing—and I mean *nothing*—and eat 3,000 calories a day you will gain weight. What you don't burn off turns to fat, and you get fat. Other than that, no, don't count calories. Some days you'll eat more because you'll be expending more energy. Other days you won't want to know from food. And then there will be days when it will be something in between. Eat when you're hungry.

14. What Do I Do During the Holidays When the Temptations Are All Around?

Holidays are a time for celebration. There's enough pressure on all of us to have the time of our lives each and every special occasion. I always find them to be exhausting, never living up to the commercials on TV, and I always find myself swearing that next year it'll be different. The emotional and financial strain they put on you and your family is worth a whole other book.

But as far as food goes, you no longer have to be afraid of special occasions. You eat the low-fat foods. If you're going to someone's else's house for a meal and know they're still in the dark ages of fat education, eat before you go. Stuff yourself with your favorite low-fat foods to the point that the thought of food makes you sick. At the "occasion" have a beer or a glass of wine (unless you have a drinking problem) and forget about the junk laid out on the table.

15. Can I Lose Weight Without Exercising?

Easily. Starvation always guarantees weight loss. But in order to burn body fat you must combine reducing the amount of fat you're putting in your mouth with exercise. Exercise is not only about losing weight. So if your question is, "Can I get lean, strong, and healthy without exercise?" the answer would be, "Absolutely not!"

16. What About Cellulite?

Talk about a word that mystery and confusion have been built around. CELLULITE. There are rubs, creams, electronic devices, and even institutions built around this thing called cellulite.

Well, here it is. There is no mistake about it: cellulite is fat. There is nothing more complicated about it.

At 260 pounds I had more chunky stuff—that's my description for cellulite—on my body than you could imagine. Don't imagine it. Grab your thigh right now. Have a look at it—it's fat. The leaner you get, the less you'll have. You will get rid of it. Burn it off by eating right, breathing right, and moving right.

17. What About Liposuction?

What's the deal with liposuction? If going and having all the fat sucked out of your body worked, I would recommend it. I would have done it, and there wouldn't be a fat woman on earth, because we'd all sell everything we owned to pay for this costly procedure. I don't know all the details of liposuction, but I can tell you that getting lean, strong, and healthy is not about this.

18. What If I'm Hungry an Hour After I've Just Finished Eating?

EAT! As you are getting stronger, healthier, building muscle, asking more from your body, it will require fuel. Some days you'll eat like an animal. Who said you have to eat breakfast, lunch, and dinner at any certain time? Probably the same folks who told us "three squares a day" and all the other incorrect information. If you're hungry a couple of hours after you eat, eat!

19. What About Diet Drinks—Are They Bad?

Bad? Don't they clean the decks of naval ships with Coke? Remember the science experiment you did at school, where you put your tooth in a glass of diet soda and within a couple of days it disintegrated? If fat is your concern and your diet drink has no fat in it, drink it. If chemicals, colorings, and health are your concern, stay as far away from them as you can.

20. Is This Forever? Will I Ever Not Have to Exercise?

This is forever for me. I never want to stop exercising — because of how bad I feel when I don't and how good

STOP THE INSANITY!

I feel when I do. I hope your life-style change is forever. Making the initial changes and then maintaining them once you've reached your desired fitness level are two different things. Once you've built it, maintaining your foundation of wellness is easy and requires cardiovascular conditioning 3 to 4 times a week. I hope you'll find the challenges of a strong, lean, healthy body enjoyable.

21. How Do I Introduce This to My Husband, Who Is a Big "Meat and Potatoes" Guy?

Very, very slowly. Don't wipe out the fridge and cabinets and put a bucket of wheat grass on the table and exclaim, "No more fat in our family—it's healthy from now on!" Rebellion is what you will get.

If you're serving a meat loaf, try making a lentil loaf with low-fat gravy—they'll never know the difference. If it's chicken, leave off the skin and broil it in lemon. Add a rice salad to the plate and introduce a low-fat dessert.

Make the changes slowly. Make your low-fat food spicy and tasty. And don't make an issue out of it. Remember, you are not on a diet. You are changing the way your family eats so you will be leaner and healthier.

22. What About Eating Disorders?

I had an eating disorder. You don't get to be 260 pounds without one. It was called "eating too much fat because I was angry, hurt, and depressed." Overeaters Anonymous hates it when I say this—but while you're talking about how many times you threw up yesterday, go for a walk and get some oxygen into your mind and body. It just might help the healing process.

I'm not a therapist and don't pretend to be. I know there are emotional issues connected to getting fat. Didn't most of us grow up in some sort of dysfunctional, screwed-up family? I think we are all somewhat codependent and we all enable something or someone.

Ninety-nine percent of us are fat because we eat too much high-fat food and don't move enough. That's the problem, and it's easy to solve. The symptoms of the problem are endless. When you give your body the foundation of wellness—eating, breathing, and moving every day—you'll be surprised by how many of the symptoms disappear.

23. I Have PMS. Will This Help?

After I had my second son I was an emotional wreck. Three days before my period, shopping for groceries could bring on an anxiety attack that made me run from the store—without the food! My PMS was so bad, I was getting progesterone shots a week and a half before each period. PMS is nothing to joke about. Anybody who has had a hormonal imbalance knows how horrible it is to have to deal with every month.

Some wonderful research is being done by pioneers in this field. However, there is also an enormous amount of ignorance and denial in the medical community about this very real hormonal imbalance that affects millions of women every month.

Fitness will not cure PMS. But being lean, strong, and healthy can do nothing but help. I still have "bad PMS." But, believe me, dealing with it monthly as a fit person, feeling strong and healthy, is worlds apart from sitting in my living room at 260 pounds, hating the way I looked and felt and having to deal with it month after month.

24. Can I Ever Eat Fat Again?

Sure—if you ever want to. It's surprising what happens when you eliminate a poison from your body and then take it in, even in tiny amounts. I went to a party a couple of months into my new low-fat eating life and didn't know how much fat was in the salad dressing and some other foods being offered. I ate what I thought was a low-fat version of the buffet. Within hours I had the worst diarrhea and I felt horrible—greasy and sick. I eat low fat now because I don't want to eat fatty foods and they make me feel terrible.

Soon into your low-fat life-style your body will let you know that it will no longer tolerate a high-fat intake.

25. Do I Need to See My Doctor Before I Begin an Exercise Program?

Here I go again. NO. More important than seeing your doctor is not beginning any exercise program unless you are very aware of your fitness level and physical considerations and are being taught by your fitness professional how to modify to accommodate them.

I am not implying that if you have just had open-heart surgery, you don't need to check with your doctor before going for a run. If you are being treated for an injury, degenerative disease, or anything else and have been under the care of a doctor, then of course you should find out what your physician feels needs to be considered.

But if you are simply fat and unfit and want to begin to get well, you do not need to see your physician before taking a walk and eating low-fat foods. How could this be harmful? Your doctor should agree (unless you've been under care for a problem) that getting oxygen, eating high-quality lower-fat foods, and increasing your cardio-endurance is not harmful—it can do nothing but help.

26. Do I Have to Be a Vegetarian?

I have not eaten meat in years. Not because I care about cows (sorry, you animal lovers) but because I can't digest meat and it looks gross. I gained 133 pounds as a vegetarian. Some of the fattest clients I've had have been vegetarians. Anybody who eats dairy, nuts, tofu, and all the other high-fat "natural nonanimal foods" can get fat just as easily as the animal-eating, bacteria-filled, clogged-colon meat eaters.

There is no such thing as lean red meat—it's a contradiction. A "lean" 8-ounce steak has the equivalent of 8 teaspoons of butterfat in it. What's lean about that? The saturated fat that comes from animal products is killing us. Go back to chapter 4. It will give you the necessary information to decide whether you could or should ever eat meat again. I do not and will not eat meat. However, remember that being a vegetarian does not always keep you healthy and lean.

27. If This Is So Simple, Why Isn't Everyone Doing It?

I'm clueless. I really believe that this has been made complicated by the industries that profit when you continually fail and get sick so they can "heal" you—purposely creating their own need.

28. Do I Need to Shop in a Health Food Store?

If you can stand it. In most health food stores I've shopped in, it seems as if the employees have lost a few brain cells or are stuck in a 1960s time warp that is not to be believed. Must we wear tie-dyed shirts and have our hair in "Rastafarian" braids? Can't we live in the 1990s and be more professional about running the business?

There are more options than health food stores. The commercial grocery chain stores are beginning to pick up on the fact that American consumers are becoming educated about the quality of foods they are eating. More and more these stores are carrying lower-fat snacks, more grains, and brand names that were once known only in health food circles.

One option that I believe is very important is organic produce. If you can buy a fruit or vegetable that has not been sprayed, waxed, irradiated, dyed, or gassed to ripen —you should. They are, without a doubt, higher-quality foods.

29. Should I Exercise When I'm Tired?

Yes, you should exercise every day. The important issue is moving within your fitness level every day. If you are tired, work within your fatigue level. This means a lower level of intensity, as you focus on getting oxygen and taking time for your body and your mind.

I work within my fitness level every time I move. I may be tired from working and mad at my husband, my foot may be aching, I may be premenstrual—or whatever else may be going on. You won't always get in your six days a week. But missing a day or two is not the issue. We should move and get oxygen every day. Working within your fitness level allows you to exercise without the pressure of having to be a powerhouse every time you lace up your sneakers.

30. Each Time I Lose and Gain Weight, I Seem to Get Fatter—Am I Nuts?

No, not at all. You *are* getting fatter. Write this down, take it to your doctor or weight loss counselor, and ask them if this is true. Tell them Susan sent you and get ready to hear the truth that may make you want to lunge at whomever you're talking to.

When you lose weight through starvation (dieting) you are losing water and muscle tissue along with lots of other things—your health among them. What you lose in lean muscle mass you regain as fat. I must repeat this. . . . WHAT YOU LOSE IN LEAN MUSCLE MASS YOU REGAIN IN FAT.

Your diet, like the millions we've all been on, is making you fatter and weaker. This is not your imagination. You are getting fatter every time you lose and gain.

Please, please stop dieting forever.

31. Susan, You Look So Much Different and You Are Definitely Fit and Full of Energy. But Have You Had Cosmetic Surgery to Get That Way?

Big question that I get asked often.

Let me explain one thing about cosmetic surgery. If there was any surgical procedure on earth that could take 133 pounds off a body, increase upper body, abdominal, and lower body strength, increase cardio-endurance, and completely change the inside and outside of a body, I WOULD BE THE FIRST IN LINE TO HAVE IT DONE, and I would recommend it to every human being under the sun. Why not? We'd all be healthy, have energy, look and feel fit, and we wouldn't need anything else.

Unfortunately, there is no such surgery and never will be. It doesn't happen that way. I changed my body by eating high-volume, high-quality, low-fat foods, moving within my fitness level and increasing my level of intensity as my fitness level developed, getting oxygen to a body that was so oxygen depleted that I could barely function—giving my body what it needed to be a healthy, well-conditioned, fat-burning machine. That's how I changed my body, and that is the only way you can ever change the way you look and feel.

But have I had cosmetic surgery? ABSOLUTELY. Would I have more? By the time I'm 60, I'm probably going to look like I'm in a wind tunnel, my face will be so far back on my head. YES, YES, YES, count me in for whatever makes me feel good.

About a year after I changed my body I had a tummy tuck. My decision to have my stomach done was based on a couple of things.

First, the surgery was being paid for. There's motivation right there for most of us to have something done.

Second, my body looked really good—I liked it. The only thing that was not the way I wanted it to be was loose skin in the middle of my stomach—not from weight loss, folks, but from back-to-back birthing. You guys know what I'm talking about: that weird stuff around your belly button that looks like the skin of a 108-year-old woman.

Here's where I've gotten into trouble before. To all the groups out there trying to tell me that if I have changed anything, then I must hate myself because I'm trying to live up to an impossible image and that I'm betraying women by doing so, I say GO TO HELL.

I am not living up to any image because the male-dominated world tells me to do so. I never will and can't be forced to. I don't care what they think is pretty. Yes, I have been influenced by Barbie—I mean, who hasn't? But any woman who sleeps with a man like Ken could never be an idol of mine. Yes, I have been influenced, but that's not why I had cosmetic surgery.

I had my stomach done for me.

I had my ear done for me.

And I will have whatever else I have done for me.

The political arguments about the pros or cons of cosmetic surgery don't interest me.

What does concern me is anybody who thinks they can

have a cosmetic procedure done to solve the problem of being fat and unfit. Lipo doesn't work unless you change your life-style. Getting a tummy tuck because you are fat is insane. You will still be fat when it's over, and you will get fatter unless you change what you are eating and learn how to breathe and move.

When you are fit, do whatever you want (as I did when I was already fit). I'll probably be a different nationality by the time they lay me down, so who cares?

My stomach is a very small part of a body that is low in fat, strong, and healthy. My new ear has not changed my life, but I'm thrilled I did both.

You make up your own mind about what you want to change with the knife, but please don't have it done until you are lean, strong, and healthy. You'll come out looking even better unless they slip (which is the chance anyone going under the knife takes). I thought the risks were worth it. Thank God it worked, and now I am Susan without the skin around my belly button and with an ear that no longer looks like Dumbo's.

PART THREE

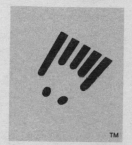

Sanity

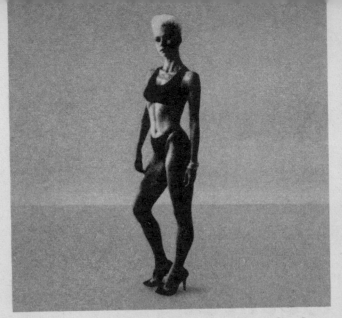

Everybody told me not to use this picture when I was talking about the aftereffects of eating, breathing, and moving. "You'll offend every woman in America." "It's too sexy." "You look too strong in it; nobody will believe it's you." "High heels with bathing suits imply sleaze, and the American woman doesn't like sleaze."

Blah, blah, blah . . .

Susan's response then and now: There isn't a woman in this country who doesn't want to be able to put on a thong bikini and jump up and down and not wiggle all over. Maybe there are some who would choose to do it in the privacy of their own homes, unlike me splashing it all over national TV. But every woman alive understands why I am thrilled to this day when I look at this photo— you don't have to have been 260 pounds to understand it. Sexy? What in the hell is wrong with sexy? Nobody will believe it's me? Who else could it be? Look at the hair. High heels and bathing suits = sleaze? Well, we better talk to the Miss America pageant, because this stuff has been going on for too long now.

NINE

Life
Changes

Regarding sharp responses and the ability to record them, it is particularly precious to me as I continue moving steadily from fog into sunlight.

—TONI MCNARON

Lose a little weight, gain some strength, and your whole life will change. You'll accomplish things you never thought possible:

Travel all over the country.

Appear on national television.

Write a book.

Sign for your own TV show . . . realistic?

Well, realistic or not, that's exactly what's happened to me.

Leslie (one of my clients) and I appeared on a national talk show together recently. If you were to search the world for two people who were as opposite as night and day, you'd find Leslie and me and end your search.

Small-town southern girl.

Devoted to her husband (not that I'm not—I mean, if it's "stand by your man" you're looking for, call on me).

An only child.

Very, very sheltered and protected.

Quiet.

Has spent her whole life learning how not to rock any boat.

STOP THE INSANITY!

Making nice.

We had nothing in common but a huge weight gain. Leslie weighed somewhere in the 300–310 range. Physically she was not functioning. She was tired all the time. Had the old fat aches and pains. Joints swollen, lower back pain, never feeling quite right. Emotionally she seemed fine on the outside, a nice, sweet, kind, non-boat-rocking type, but inside she was miserable. Leslie wanted more than anything not to be fat, but after years of trying every diet under the sun, she had resigned herself to the fact that she was never going to be anything but fat.

Leslie was in a seminar I was giving. Her face stood out in a crowd of hundreds because she was so beautiful. A couple of days later she came to my studio. In a class full of large, unfit, uncoordinated people, Leslie stood out again. But it wasn't her beautiful face. It was how painfully shy, how unbelievably unfit—she couldn't keep her arms up in the air for more than a couple of seconds —how enormously fat she was. Leslie's weight, 300 pounds, wasn't the highest in the room, but she's so short and compact that she looked huge. So big, round, and uncomfortable. I try very hard not to predict who will or who won't understand how to stop the insanity. But I gotta 'fess up. It was difficult to watch Leslie that first day and not be afraid that she'd never make it. The combination of the physical problems and the shy, scared, quiet disposition had me doubting whether she'd be able to give this process a chance.

Well, put me in my place.

Bash me over the head with my own ignorance.

Give me the emotional whiplash for the rest of my life, and get me out of the business of predicting anything.

She did learn what you are learning and has done a better job than most of us could ever do. How to eat, how to breathe, and how to move. Her body has changed tremendously. She is ten dress sizes smaller, has more muscular strength than she ever dreamed possible (a small, tight, compact cheerleader's kind of body), has cardio-endurance for days and energy for ten, is considering giving up her job, and is training to be in the fitness business. Hey, running around in cute shorts and tank tops, loving what you do and changing people's lives, has its advantages. Ask Leslie what she thinks.

Leslie's got a lot to say, and when I asked her if she wanted to say it on national TV, she said yes and agreed to meet me in New York. So she flew to New York, settled in at the hotel, and we met the next morning.

What an impact this woman had on millions of other women! That shy, polite, southern charm can bite like a snake—something I think most southern women had figured out before I came along and clued them in. The diet industry got bit that day . . . a very effective method I have yet to learn. Catching flies with honey, or whatever that old expression is. Leslie was confident, clear, and strong on camera. She acted like she'd been doing television all her life. Certainly not the same woman who had been sitting in my seminars just months before her national TV debut.

What's the point of this little story?

Who cares about Leslie and me appearing on some TV show? You should care, because this story is about you, me, Leslie, all of us. She didn't just appear on a national talk show in front of millions of people and pull it off like a pro. That's not all she did.

Leslie had never been on a plane before.

She had never been to New York before. She had spent her whole life in a small southern town hearing about the dangers that lurked around every corner in cities like New York.

Leslie had never done lots of things she did on that trip. How did she do it? Was it losing weight that gave her the courage to get on a plane, fly to New York alone, settle in the hotel, go for a walk alone that evening, meet me in the morning, and appear on national TV? Weight loss—is that all it takes? Does an increase in self-esteem give everyone the courage, professionalism, and composure to pull all that off? Was it weight loss that has created a wonderful respect and friendship between two exact opposites, Leslie and me?

No.

STOP THE INSANITY!

I'm concerned more with myself becoming fit and healthy than cosmetic reasons (of course, a benefit, too!). I'm too young to feel like an older person.
—Comment from a client

If I hear this "self-esteem" thing one more time, I'll puke. Every magazine you pick up, every weight loss brochure you read, talks about "it."

I did not increase my self-esteem.

Leslie didn't increase her self-esteem. She got well. It took a heck of a lot more than an increase in self-esteem to do what she did. If increasing self-esteem was all it took, then all that positive reinforcement junk would work. . . .

"Look in the mirror for five minutes a day and tell yourself you love yourself."

I tried that stuff, and within days I turned into Sybil:

"I love myself. . . ."

"No, you don't—you're fat and miserable!"

"I am happy being me. . . ."

"How could you? You can't function, you feel horrible, and you look like an animal!"

"I am pleased with where I am, no matter where that is. . . ."

"Stop lying to yourself! You'd sell your soul to feel and look better!"

All that positive reinforcement only added to my already complicated emotional state when I was fat and unfit. There was enough chatting going on in my brain.

We all know what it feels like when you are sick. You know, like when you have the flu. Increasing your self-esteem, positive reinforcement, or those nice little daily meditation sayings do very little to help you accomplish what you need to accomplish, whether it's cooking dinner or being the mother, wife, or businesswoman you need to be. When you are sick, you can't do it. Whatever your plans are this week—the kids, the house, your job, personal plans, goals—if you wake up tomorrow morning with the flu, your plans (even the best laid) go to hell and back.

It doesn't matter what your brain says—"I'll just get up and fix dinner." You make it to the edge of the bed and you're spent. It's over.

I was sick. Leslie was sick. Chances are, if you're reading this book, you are sick. It is physical, not emotional. IT HAS NOTHING TO DO WITH INCREASING YOUR SELF-ESTEEM!

There is only one answer to the problem. If you are sick, not well, you've got to get well. Eating, breathing, and moving will help you do that.

You don't think Leslie was nervous from appearing on national television? Being ten dress sizes smaller didn't make her any less nervous. How did she do it? She had different resources to tap into that she'd never had in her life.

She was strong. Physically strong. Nobody knows better than Leslie that anyone can get well. Nobody understands the difference being fit can make like the Leslies of the world. She had something to say, and nothing was going to stop her from saying it. That's an inner strength that only comes with going through the process and making the changes. You earn that strength. Nobody can give that to you, and nobody can take that away from you.

Before the show, Leslie had eaten a huge, high-volume, low-fat breakfast (there's that fuel thing again), gone for a walk, spent some time thinking about the show and what she wanted to say. (Meditating while walking down the streets of Manhattan—I'm not sure how safe that is.) She was physically and mentally ready when the time came to do the job. Sure, she is proud of herself. Yes, her self-esteem has improved as her body has changed, but that's not what she pulled from or tapped into to do what she did.

My increase in self-esteem is not what kept me going while I was building my studio (sounds like I took hammer to nail and actually built the joint, doesn't it?) and developing my business. The first time I did TV, I was on a live show. Never in my life had I been in front of a camera. I got to the studio early in the morning, sat around in the green room (which was actually an ugly yellow), and when someone with a headset came in, yelled my name, walked me out to a set, sat me down, and left me, it was not my weight loss that got me through until the host sat down and we began talking to each other in front of 5 million women. That 6-minute segment would never have happened—because I would have had a heart attack and died—without a lot of physical strength, without the focus (that visualization really comes in handy when you have to stop your heart from pounding through your chest from fear), without the oxygen, without the physical strength and wellness that I'd spent the time developing. It would have been almost impossible to do with the flu. Functioning while you're sick is very difficult. That's the state I functioned in for so long. That's the way Leslie lived.

If you are living in a state of illness, your body doesn't have enough oxygen to function, enough muscular strength to hold you up, a strong heart to pump the blood and oxygen through it, and if you are carrying tons of extra fat, then it's going to be harder for you to get through the day, do your job, or function. Reaching your goals, accomplishing your dreams, takes energy that you don't have.

I didn't have the energy to think about my dreams. Leslie had forgotten what her dreams were. It's ridiculous to wait around for an increase in self-esteem before you start living your life. It's too unattainable, and we are all too screwed up. There isn't a family out there that isn't dysfunctional. All of us have been abused in one way or another. Everyone has an alcoholic, drug addict, emotional abuser, co-dependent, or enabler in the family. It would take too long and cost too much for most of us to increase our self-worth.

Hating the way you look and feel is not just an emotional issue. It is also a physiological issue.

This is not about self-esteem. This is about giving your body what it must have just to function every day and having your body respond with more energy, more strength, and less fat. And you end up with more choices.

When you have more choices, you will make different

decisions. If you know how to exercise within your fitness level without feeling as if you are going to die, understanding what you are doing and how to do it, you may just go for a walk instead of heading for the fridge when you are frustrated, angry, or afraid. Whatever it is that triggers you is not the most important thing. It will all still be there when you are fit. Believe me, Leslie and I still get angry, frustrated, and afraid, but we have twenty different ways to release or work with the feelings. The only option I had at 260 pounds was to head for the fridge.

The diets weren't working. I tried them all.

The exercise classes that I went to just humiliated and hurt me.

The doctors didn't have the answers.

The dietitians and nutritionists made it too complicated for me.

The weight loss counselors spoke to me like I was a child who couldn't control herself.

What choice did I have?

Where was I supposed to put the anger, pain, frustration, and fear that I was living with every day?

> I have continuously gained weight in the last six years (mostly since my pregnancies, which I looked at as a license to eat!), and it has become *all* I think about and judge myself on. It is pretty much everything I base my "success" on ("so therefore I am a complete failure").
> —Comment from a client

Let me tell you about anger. A couple of days ago there was a reporter calling everyone I know, following my children to school, camping out in front of my house, interviewing my ex-husband, and doing everything he could to annoy me. My body is very fit. My life is wonderful. The kids are healthy. I can pay my bills, and the Prince and I are okay. But let's be honest: having some bonehead sneaking around your life trying to get some dirt on you is not exactly a low-stress situation. I have a newfound respect for Sean Penn. I understand why he punches every reporter he sees—these guys are obnoxious. The pressure and anxiety that I went through were no different from the unbelievable pressure and anxiety that I lived through as my white picket fence was exploding. The big difference in my life is that I now have many, many different ways of getting rid of or dealing with the anxiety.

Instead of yelling, screaming, or eating my way through it, I went to the studio and taught myself a class. I went nuts. Two and a half hours of pumping, sweating, focusing, and getting it all out.

I couldn't have done that when I weighed 260 pounds. The family bike ride was not an option, either. I built the tools necessary to have these choices. There may be therapists reading this book who think I am oversimplifying the issue of control and choices. Well, I disagree. While you are working on all the issues that you have to deal with, why not get some oxygen? Could it hurt? While you are talking about how many times you threw up yesterday, how compulsive you may be, or how much of an enabler you are, take a walk. Begin giving your body what it needs to live. How could it do anything but help? If this thinking is simple, then so be it, but is it wrong? Does it have any validity? Why not begin to heal the physical while you work on the emotional, the mental? I've found that it's a heck of a lot easier to heal the physical. I've got a good fifty years of therapy ahead of me before the emotional and mental are well, but in the meantime I look and feel pretty damn good, and I've got lots more choices and control in my life by getting well physically. So why not start with eating, breathing, and moving and bringing your body back from the dead? The best beginning is in your hands. It's not just your weight that's about to change.

So please, women's magazines.

Enough with the focus on weight loss.

Stop with the self-esteem argument.

Quit treating the symptoms.

Solve the problem.

I became very afraid of food. I hid it and would eat without anyone knowing. I would sneak food and would eat until I got sick. It really began to control me. I gained weight and then became obsessed with my body weight. . . . I still fear food sometimes and am still tempted to binge or fast. One extreme to the other.
—Kathy, a client

My life as a single, 260-pound, 43 percent body fat, unfit, unhealthy mother of two was very different from my life now as an independent, 14 percent body fat, strong, fit, healthy mother of two.

Two lives; same person.

I was so far into the insanity of starvation and deprivation, so physically sick, that getting out of bed in the morning was a big accomplishment. My trip to the post office overwhelmed me because it wasn't worth the effort it took to get there. I couldn't think about anything but getting through the day. If that's the way you feel, then you must go through the same process I did to get well. We all have to do the same thing to give our bodies a foundation of wellness and build from there. Build the life you want. Reach the goals you set. Fulfill the dreams you have. Weight loss has very little to do with it anymore. It's a wonderful side effect. Solving the problem will totally change your life.

My life has changed dramatically since I got well. I adore my sons—that hasn't changed. I'm the kind of mother who pulls out the family albums at the grocery store checkout and assumes the whole staff of checkers and baggers is interested in my children's photos from birth to present.

My children are old enough now that they say, after being introduced to a roomful of clients, friends, managers, and grocery store checkers, "Mom, could you leave out the brilliant and beautiful in your introduction? Just tell them our names . . . we'll say, 'Nice to meet you,' then we can leave."

Raising children is difficult. Every mother reading this knows that. Raising two who are one year apart when you are alone, depressed, fat, and unfit is almost impossible. One day, when the boys were babies—in the double stroller with the double diaper bags—we were shopping for rubber pants (no disposable diapers for me, I was too evolved; I'd rather wash ninety diapers a day—two babies, double diapers, you figure it out) and undershirts. You all know what it's like to shop with two kids—nothing relaxing or fun about it. The store was packed, the kids were trying to escape from their stroller every thirty seconds, and I was at my wits' end. All I wanted was to buy a few pairs of rubber pants and to sleep for a month and a half without being wakened. Rubber pants and T-shirts in hand, I got to the counter to pay the chirpy little 21-year-old who was scanning my purchase. Then this lady standing next to me turned, smiled at the boys, looked at me, and said: "Wow, are both of those boys yours?"

I was so frazzled at this point that I could barely speak, but I managed to answer, "Yes, they are."

Then she said, "It must be very difficult raising children that close together. Mine are two years apart, and it's hard enough for me. They look like happy, healthy children. You must be doing a very good job—I admire you."

I looked at this total stranger who had just given me what I so desperately needed—acknowledgment—and broke down in tears.

She put her arms around me and hugged me while I cried, apologizing, explaining, and sobbing.

The 21-year-old smiling girl behind the counter didn't know what to do. Two women, who three minutes before were total strangers, standing in front of her hugging and crying, talking about isolation, pain, and fear.

I left the store feeling like a babbling idiot, afraid to look at my own reflection. I really thought I was about to crack in half. That woman understood my pain—no doubt she'd been there—and took the time to comfort another cracking mother. Her acknowledgment and understanding made me feel less isolated and crazy, her arms wrapped around me offered a moment of peace and support that was a matter of survival at this point.

The boys were happy and healthy, but there were some hard times to get through. I'm not exaggerating when I tell you that getting out of bed was the most I could do many days. I wanted so badly to take them out, play in the yard, look and feel good and be the mother that I read about and saw on TV—the mother I thought I should be. You know, Doris, Harriet, Barbie's mom (does Barbie have a mom, or was she just rocketed down from heaven without the messy process of birth?). I'd try. Get everyone and everything cleaned and dressed, get in the car, go to the park, throw the ball once or twice, and feel like I was going to die.

Put the guilt, shame, and frustration of not being the best mother in the world in a pot, mix in the hatred and anger I felt for the Prince and his Princess, throw in some hormonal imbalance, and you've got yourself an explosive soup. There's at least a year's worth of late night binge eating right there.

Other mothers seemed to have it all together. You know the ones. Those special moms who fit into their size 6 blue jeans six weeks after the birth of their baby. The ones who always have their hair done, makeup on, and are wearing nice, clean, coordinated outfits. The hair and makeup I can almost understand, but those fresh, pressed coordinated outfits I could never figure out. We won't spend any time at all on my hair (there wouldn't be any point to that), and makeup didn't exist in my life for years, but I really tried to get through a day without being covered in pee, poop, or vomit. The pee and poop were accidents, rubber pants leaking, trying to change one poopy diaper on the floor of the bathroom while the other baby, who was toilet training, was about to fall into the toilet. Reaching and grabbing for the drowning child, you sometimes get a little poop on the sleeve of your shirt and don't notice it until you are falling into a coma that night. But the vomit—there wasn't a day in a three-year period that I didn't have vomit on my shirt. How do these women do it? How can anybody with a newborn wear anything but a rag? Vomit on silk, something's wrong. I was confused.

Those women seemed to have it all together, and I was falling apart. I didn't feel I was doing it right, but I knew my children were healthy, happy, and very much loved.

My most humiliating private moment with my 3-year-old daughter was when she poked my tummy and said, "Mommy, you need more exercise, you still fat."
—Lisa, Ione, Washington

Two A.M. used to scare the hell out of me. It doesn't scare me anymore. That time of the morning is so much different for me now.

Nighttime used to be very difficult for me because I was so unhappy. It was a time of silence when I couldn't face the quiet. It was a time of excruciating loneliness. I was painfully aware of the short time I had in between babies waking up and needing something from me. I didn't feel I had anything to give them. The helpless child who needs you so desperately and the mother who has nothing to give—that pain can't be explained, only understood by our mothers who have been there at 2:00 A.M.

I was fat, unhappy, lonely, and scared, and the baby would cry, needing something. Walking toward the crib, night after night, desperately wanting the other baby not to wake up, not knowing where I would find the strength to give this little person what he needed. Rock him, sing to him, be patient with him when his teeth hurt or his fever was rising, give him whatever it was that he needed from me when sometimes there was nothing there to give.

Fear does not describe what I felt during those moments. Exhaustion is not what I felt. It was beyond definition, it was like being the walking dead. Having nothing left, but still functioning.

There was nobody there to meet my needs or hold me when I cried or was afraid. The only thing I had during those times was the anger and pain of knowing that my husband—we were only separated at the time—was sleeping peacefully or making love to his new girlfriend and that he didn't have to be there for two small children who needed him now, not the next day or the next visit.

The anger and pain engulfed me so many times and took over.

I'd sing the song, rock the cradle, get the baby to sleep, make it all right, and go back to the empty bed and the pain.

That's not all that made 2:00 A.M. so intolerable. Facing myself, the way I looked and felt, my life, was the most difficult thing. It was easy to get lost thinking about the Prince, but it was impossible to get away from myself.

No matter how angry I was at the Prince or how much I believed he had hurt me, it was what I was doing to myself every morning when the sun rose that I could barely live with. The cycle started with every new day. The binge eating. The promise and belief in the next instant cure. The guilt and self-hatred when it didn't work. The constant thinking about food, dieting, getting skinny. The hope that I was going to make it out of this mess this time and the fear of failure that went with every attempt.

I've never been in a tornado, but I know what it must feel like. When I think of the *Wizard of Oz,* I think of blinding winds, pouring rain, and the swirling energy that keeps you in the same place. Never being able to get out of the grip of what is going on around you. A force so strong that you feel helplesss.

That's exactly what I felt at 2:00 A.M. every morning.

My solution or comfort at the time was eating.

I did not get myself out of the anger, pain, and self-destructive behavior by loving myself enough or forgiving the Prince and his Princess. I never got that far. Call me unevolved, simple, or immature—that's not the way it went.

I got myself well as I was living with the anger and the pain. Slowly I got lean, strong, and healthy, and amazing things started to happen. First I started to sleep better. I think anybody who knows the power of sleep deprivation —any mother out there—understands what even a couple of hours of good sleep can do for the mind, body, and soul.

Then, as I got well, my mind was busy with thoughts of what I could do for myself. Tomorrow I can go for a walk. It may sound basic to some, but it's a big deal and a hell of a choice for someone who believed there were no choices. I began to understand that if I didn't eat that pound cake, or concentrate on the Prince and Princess, I could go to sleep and wake up and get on with my life.

Things started to change as I regained the strength and cardio-endurance and reduced the body fat that was making me feel trapped without choices, caught in the tornado.

Do you know what 2:00 A.M. means now?

The boys sleep better at 9 and 10 years old. Thank God. Usually I'm dead asleep by that time of the morning because I've had such busy days that I find myself in a coma. But if I'm up, I'm up because I'm writing. Or I'm up making love with my husband, and that's the only time that we have been able to find in a week . . . late, but a pretty good reason to be up, in my opinion. I may be reading something that I've been trying to read, worrying about a business problem (and God knows I have enough of them), or getting a snack because I can't sleep.

My snacking now is not a matter of loneliness, it's a matter of eating—a big difference. My snacking now is enjoyable. Alone, for me now, is a luxury. Sometimes I just get up, get some food, go into the living room, organize my thoughts, and get ready for the next day, full of challenges and opportunities.

There are nights when I'm up sitting alone and my husband calls to see if I'm okay. Don't tell anyone this, but it has become important to me that someone who loves me for who and what I am wants to make sure I'm all right. Mind you, it does not validate me or make me feel whole—I do that for myself. It simply means that there is someone who loves me, and getting back into bed and having someone reach out and hold you is nice. (Notice as I wrote this paragraph I went from me to you. Do you think there is something wrong with me because

I use you when I'm talking about anything that resembles need, or that I say "Don't tell anyone" in a book just before telling the world that having my husband in bed making sure I am all right feels good? Call the therapist, get the padded room ready—I'm going in for a while.)

I still wake up sometimes worried about the children, concerned about the Prince—after all, he is still the father of our children and we have very different opinions —and needing some reassurance. The really big difference now is that I have so many other choices in dealing with the emotions and fears that all of us face, and so many different ways to deal with it all—simply because I am fit. I feel good about the way I look and feel. It is really, really that simple.

I am never going to lead you to believe that every morning at 2:00 A.M. you can find me making passionate love to my husband (although I'd like that), but you will find me any time at 2:00 A.M. doing things totally different from what I did when I was fat, unfit, lonely, and frightened.

It's the same time—2:00 A.M. It's the same person— Susan Powter. But it represents a totally different reality. It represents a time to be alone, a time to make love, a time to read, or just a time to organize my thoughts. It no longer means fear, loneliness, and binge eating. I am not afraid anymore because I have a foundation of wellness that nobody can take from me. I built it, and I live with the joy of it. SO CAN YOU.

> My job is very active and physical, and when your clothes are too tight to move in, it's hard to move and do a good job. I used to wear a smock to work so no one would see the weight I gained.
> —Billie, a client

If somebody had told me a couple of years ago that I would be speaking all over the country about wellness, writing a book, running the best exercise studio in the country, and doing national TV, I would have sat them down and explained that they had obviously done too many hallucinogenic drugs in their past and they should get out of the business of predicting futures.

Back then all I wanted was for the Prince to help me keep a roof over my head. The bills were minimal—diaper service, formulas, electric, and gas. I didn't need a big monthly clothing allowance, and entertainment wasn't a problem—I had no social life. I just needed the Prince to live up to his end of the bargain. Someone had to help me keep the standards we had set together, but the Prince was having trouble remembering he had two children at home who needed to eat.

It seems to happen a lot. The Princes of the world run away, get a girlfriend, and develop that special amnesia just about the same time every month—when it's time to send the check to the ex-wife and kids.

Poor things. It must be hard to remember the responsibilities they've already established when there are so many other things to think about: their broad shoulders, the new girlfriend's needs, the new families that so many of them start (there's a concept—not capable of taking care of the family you've started? Do it again, have some more kids and another wife, and if that doesn't work, go ahead and try a third time), and the most important need . . . their little willies. Yes, it's their needs and desires that must be considered before anything else. Well, the little willie, the girlfriend, and the broad shoulders came before me and the children many times. A constant fighting and groveling for money only added to the depression and anger I felt. The bills were due on the first of the month, and by the sixth or seventh the anxiety and anger were suffocating. Knowing how busy he was attending to his little willie, his girlfriend, and his broad shoulders didn't defuse the explosion when the check finally came on the tenth, eleventh, or twelfth of the month. He would drop it off, and I would blow up.

He would look at me like I was the most unreasonable, craziest woman on earth and feel justified that he had left. I could hear him thinking, No wonder I left—look at her, she's nuts. I truly didn't know what I was supposed to do. How was I going to stay home, be the kind of mom the kids deserved, and pay the bills without groveling every month?

So I thought I'd be one of those creative stay-at-home moms who seem to be able to do it all. Start a million-dollar business, look and feel great, and be the best mom in the world.

My first attempt: home baby-sitting. Just what I needed. I had

No energy.

No strength.

I was

Fat as a house.

A single mother of two.

Severely depressed.

Feeling isolated.

A little overwhelmed at the thought of getting up in the morning. . . .

Hey! Let's have twelve other kids running around and get paid a couple of bucks per kid. That'll work. Day care —just what I've always wanted to do. But, you see, I didn't have the choices; the Prince had the choices. I did whatever I could to survive. He was living—well, I might add—and I was trying to survive. Why? That's the question that made me a little nutty. Why? I still want an answer. But we'll get the answer one day. For now, it's how to make a living and raise kids without going insane in the process. Day care was not the answer for me. I hated being more isolated, having more stress, still not making enough money to get beyond the first of the month without groveling, so I tried cooking classes.

Yep, I'm a good cook. So why not teach cooking? Great thought that inspired me until I taught my first class. Four women, paying me to teach them a thing or two in the kitchen, with two children running around. That's all I've got to say. If you want to experience high stress, try getting anything done in a kitchen with two kids around. Of course the Prince never had to think about that, because everything was covered so that Daddy could work, because Daddy's work was important. Mommy trying to hang on by her fingernails didn't seem to matter as much as Daddy.

Many brilliant home-grown businesses have come from single women raising their kids and fighting for survival. But my baby-sitting or cooking classes never got off the ground. I was too much of a wreck to be the president of Susie's Baking Company. If you want to get kicked in the self-esteem pants, begging for money every month from the Princes of the world does it every time. Maybe if *they* had to do it once in a while they would understand why their "crazy ex-wives" are as crazy as they are. So until the Prince and I settled on my monthly allowance, I did whatever I could to get by. (Allowance? What was he allowing me to do—pay for the groceries? raise our children by myself?) Friends lent me money. My parents helped—now that feels good. I'm going to marry this man, have these children, and begin my own life, thank you very much, and they end up supporting me. Talk about the inner child. That turned me right back into the 10-year-old little girl begging for Daddy's approval. When someone pays for what you do or how you live, they have bought the right to be part of the decisions you make in your life. If I bought a new stroller, I felt I had to justify it, explain the model I chose, and show my parents the receipt. It wasn't really that my parents made me feel that way (although my mother had a way of making me feel like a pile of doody within minutes); that's the way I felt. Right or wrong, being in that position was poison to my psyche. It killed me. It hurt more than the aches and pains of being fat and unfit, it was darker than the cloud of depression that was hanging over my head. It made me despise the Prince.

> I'm a divorced mother of two boys. I used to get depressed about being alone. But now it just seems not to be so important. I've never felt healthier in my life.
> —Linda, Dallas, Texas

When the money issue was resolved, the monthly check gave me an ounce of independence. It didn't solve the groveling problem, because it's amazing how many times the Princes of the world forget to write the check, or say they have something more important to spend cash on, and never quite get the right amount to your doorstep or get it there on time every month. So the groveling continued, but I could live.

Going from 260 pounds—begging for child support and nuttier than a fruit cake—to running an exercise studio had its stages. But step one was getting well. I did not begin walking so that I could lose weight and start a studio. I began walking to look better than the Prince's girl-friend.

I needed to get a job. I've had so many jobs in the past, and I mean so very many, that I know what I do well and what ain't gonna happen, no matter how hard I try. The nine to five, corporate player, team thing . . . forget it. Call me a bad player if you want, but it always bothered me when I was doing Bob's secretarial work, typing all the documents, correcting all his spelling, organizing it so that it made sense, and then I'd hear, "Congratulations, Bob, brilliantly written proposal, that really helped close the account. Well done."

Well done, Bob? Without a great secretary, Bob would have been exposed for what he was: an overpaid, sexist pig who could no more write a brilliant proposal than fly. Needless to say, I didn't last long as a secretary . . . although I can type ninety words a minute, which really came in handy writing a book on wellness and regaining control. (WOW, amazing, full circle, karmic—whatever you want to call it.)

I've job hunted as a fat woman and as a lean, strong healthy woman, and let me tell you—whether you want to face it or not—it's a totally different experience. Discrimination does exist in a big way (pardon the pun). Nobody should be discriminated against. We should all be equal. It should be a perfect world, but it isn't. When I first started job hunting, I had two strikes against me. I was fat and I was a woman.

Waitressing—I've applied and applied and applied as a fat woman. Other than diners, working the midnight to

seven shift, nobody wants you. Applying as a lean
woman, no problem. Snap of a job to get if you have the
body for it.

What else was there? Librarian? Not enough pay and
booooooooooring. Modeling was out; even the big girl
modeling that was just starting to explode back then
wasn't ready for this big girl from Garland.

With the ounce of independence and the priorities I
had, it was time to decide how I was going to make a
living and not compromise what was important to me. I
got fit, then changed my body and started feeling and
looking better, and establishing some sanity in my life.
Then I made a decision that many of you may regard as
insane.

I had just lived through the inequality in women's lives.
The Prince's rules were different from mine. I looked at
the system and figured if that's the way it is, I'll not only
join them—I'll beat them at their own game.

Why waitress when you can still be at home with the
kids and make a ton more money by dancing?

Topless dancing.

I'll give you a minute to catch your breath, then I'll
explain.

Time out. . . . You ready?

I knew if I was ever going to pull myself up by those
damn bootstraps that everyone was telling me about, I'd
need money. Financial independence became very important to me after I'd been put in a position of groveling
because of someone's, the Prince's, willie. I also knew
that I wanted to be at home reading *Dumbo* to my children and taking them to the park—an activity that is a lot
easier and a lot more fun when you are feeling good and
healthy and are wearing shorts and a tank top. I wanted
a job that required no commitment and very little time,
that gave me hours that worked for me and the children
and lots of cash.

I may not have been a fat woman anymore, but I was
still a woman looking for a job with lots of things to
consider . . . strikes against you no matter how you look

at it. It's not complaining when I say there were not many options—it's a reality. Waitressing worked. Topless dancing worked better.

But before I could get on with my newfound career, there were a few things I had to take care of. One was telling someone in my family what I was doing in case something happened to me. I called my father, asked him to come over, and had a chat with him. It wasn't easy, but I explained how important it was to me that he and my mother not have to supplement my income for the rest of my life or until the kids were in college, whichever came first, and how difficult it was for me to be in the position I was in. I chose to tell him because I trusted him the most with my secret (who knew I would be writing about it in a book someday?), and I thought he could deal with it better than anyone else in the family—meaning my mother.

My father's reaction was what most fathers' reactions would be—concern for my safety and sanity. He had a few questions, and when he got the answers he knew that the decision had been well thought out and was—when you gave it a second's thought—somewhat sane.

The second part of my plan was to make sure, when I was out with the kids, that nobody ever recognized me as the topless dancer they'd seen on stage the night before. Yes, women of America, I'm here to tell you that a lot of your husbands go to these clubs. You can't imagine how many men I've seen since—in restaurants, at movie theaters, at parties—whom I'd seen hanging out and spending their money on topless dancers. I always feel so sorry for the wives or girlfriends I see with them. They have no clue what the men in their lives are doing.

So I went wig shopping. Big fun when you've never had good hair. I tried on every wig in the store until I found the perfect one. This thing looked great on me. You would have thought I'd been born with this gorgeous long blond mane.

The third and final thing was to find a baby-sitter my children loved who could become a part of our family. After weeks and weeks of interviewing, I found her. She was the most honest, truthful, and trustworthy young girl I've ever met, and she and the boys loved each other.

That's it. Time to go to work.

The boys and the baby-sitter would be settled. I'd say good-bye, get into my car, and drive to work. What no-body ever saw was the bag in the back that had the wig, some dresses, G-strings (or T-backs, as we call them in the business), and lots and lots of hair stuff—blow dryer, hairspray out the yin-yang, curlers, curling irons, bobby pins, and ribbons. (It costs a lot of money to maintain that big hair look.)

I'd pull into the parking lot of a restaurant that was close to the club, put the wig on (difficult to do in a little car), brush it out so it looked real, and go to work. No-body ever saw me without that wig on, not in that place. As far as the other girls, managers, and owners were concerned, I was Bernadette, with long blond hair.

It's not easy to write about this part of my life, because it means a lot more to me than just rebuilding my financial future and trying to fill the hole after the explosion. It was about the pain I saw. The young women I saw who were living this life, and their pain. It was about the nice, socially acceptable men who sit in their comfortable up-per-middle-class homes and go to church every Sunday and flock (pardon the pun, I think I'm going to hell for that one) to places like the one I worked in—but con-demn the women who work there. It's about the lack of choice that so many young girls feel they have and the choices they make that affect the rest of their lives. But that's a separate book.

I did dance topless, and I did make a good living, but I never lived the life-style. Other than the moral issues involved in taking your top off and getting paid for it, there are some very practical issues that I realized and faced when I started dancing.

It was the life-style that was killing—and I mean that literally—those girls. The nonstop drinking, spending the money as fast as they made it, drugs everywhere, par-tying with the men they met at these places. Believing in the men they met and not defining and planning their own lives. The same problem that housewives in the suburbs face, just different circumstances. I'd already made lots of those mistakes. Some made in my adolescence, some made in total faith in the Prince. So I was determined not to make the same mistakes twice. I danced my eight-hour shift, read, paid bills, talked to the girls until they got too drunk to talk, did whatever I wanted in the dressing room in between sets.

There were four stages in this club. Your first song was on the main stage, dancing in whatever outfit you chose. Mine were always pretty long dresses—another well-thought-out part of my plan. Everyone was wearing sleaze—tight, black, sexy, sexy, sexy things—twenty-eight girls and the same old look. Then I'd come out on stage in a long, frilly pretty pink dress—bingo. Instantly I had their attention. Then you go back stage, and the next song is the first of your topless performances. Main stage, topless, wearing only a G-string. You dance your song on the main stage. Then you go to stage number two for the next two songs. The same thing again to stages number three and four. The only set that you have control of is the first two songs on the main stage—the thought being that the main stage is the center of attention, and that's where you had to capture the attention of the money holders, the men sitting in the club.

I see topless dancing as a very honest example of what life is really like for most women. We parade our wares in front of all the men, they ogle and admire and pay cash, they pick the one they want, and we walk away thinking we have security. What's the difference between dancing topless for them and what most of us do to catch a husband? (Just a thought.) Many times during that period in my life, I remembered a line in a movie I'd seen. It was a movie about a "nice girl" consciously choosing to become a prostitute. She was responsible, clean, lived well, paid her bills, was a good citizen, but thought it was an okay way to make a living. Her parents took her to court to prove that she was obviously insane and needed to be hospitalized because no normal person would choose to do this. She was being questioned in court and said, "You think I'm nuts being paid five hundred for oral sex? I know women who roll through shit for a fur coat."

Maybe this is just a bit strong for a book on wellness, but while we are talking about stopping the insanity, it couldn't hurt to discuss some of the other insanity we face. Well, that's what I faced, and since this is about my life, I gotta say it. That "nice girl" had a great point.

You want to know how I feel about dancing? I enjoyed it. I hated it. I resented having to do it. I learned from it. It worked very well for me and my children. I was responsible with it. I am sure as hell glad I'm out of it and have other choices. And last, but certainly not least, I pray that all the girls I met while I was there have something in their lives other than dancing and men—because neither one lasts forever.

My dancing career didn't end for a while. I took a hiatus and tried something new, but right in line with the dancing. I met a man. A rich man. Yes, I met him in the club, but I wasn't naive enough to believe that this was Prince Charming. He was a very nice man who didn't go to places like that often (oh, sure) and really liked me. He came in to see me for a month and a half before I ever agreed to meet him outside the club. Now remember, there's a complication. He knew Bernadette, the long-haired dancer. Not Susan, the short-haired mother of two. (I think I have some of the funniest wig stories in history, but they can be told in the book on topless dancing.) We'll call him Half Prince, because I had stopped believing in the Prince, but he was nice and had some princely qualities. One of which was wanting to take me away from this horrible environment and save me. Typical manly thing to want—of course his wife and children didn't know what he was doing, saving topless damsels in distress.

So when it was time for our date and I showed up at the restaurant as Susan the short-haired mother of two boys, he was taken aback, to say the least. I told him the whole story, he understood, and we had a very pleasant evening. After a couple of weeks of dating he decided to tell me that he was married, was in the process of getting a divorce, had moved out of the house, and wanted me to stop dancing.

Married? How married was he, was the first issue to resolve. I heard how horrible the soon-to-be-ex-wife was, a story I'm sure the Prince had told to all of his girl-friends. The fact that it was a miserable marriage and that he'd moved out was fine with me. It had nothing to do with the relationship we were establishing, and the last thing I wanted to hear was a divorce story—I had my own. Not dancing was another story. That was my income. Whether he liked it or not was never a concern of mine. I was making a living, and there was nothing he could do about it. That was it. End of story.

We continued dating, and he met my family. Everyone liked the Half Prince, and it was fine. Making love for the first time other than with the Prince was difficult enough. I'm not pleading innocent virgin here, but I'd never been married, divorced, as fat as I'd been, and spent years without sex in my life. Call me sentimental, but it took some getting used to. After being 260 and hating my body, it was wonderful, absolutely wonderful, that someone thought I was attractive. The Half Prince loved the way I looked. He would tell me how sexy I was and how beautiful I was, and it would floor me. I'd ask him to repeat it, just to hear it again and again. He didn't know me as the fat, unfit, unhappy woman I'd been. I had told him about the Prince, the divorce, being fat—he'd seen pictures, but he never connected with the fat woman in the photos. All he ever said, in the throes of passion, was that the Prince was crazy to leave a woman like me—I had to agree with that and get on with the business of making love (something I'd missed terribly) to the new Half Prince in my life. Funny how good sex after years clouds your ability to take a stand. I never really shared anything about the whole fat issue with him—I mean, why bother? He didn't care, and I was feeling wanted and loved for the first time in years, so why harp on old news? Let's get on with the new news—someone thought I was beautiful and sexy. That's all that really mattered.

STOP THE INSANITY!

We worked out all the time, ate high-volume, low-fat food wherever we went, and my ex-life, like his soon-to-be-ex-wife, had nothing to do with what was happening. He had two sons, I had two sons, we went on trips with the kids and enjoyed spending time together. He was good-looking, intelligent, and loaded. What more could someone want? Other than the fact that his girlfriend was working in a strip club, it was just two people dating.

A couple of months after we met he mentioned that he'd like to buy me a gift, a fur coat. If anyone has the desire to buy me anything, let me tell you right now, a fur coat is not the thing to get. I would no more wear a fur coat than fly in the air, but I sure as hell needed what a fur coat would have cost him, so I told him: Instead of buying me the coat, give me the cash. He did. I got my teeth fixed—I had needed two root canals for a long time but couldn't afford them—and bought a washer and dryer with the money. That's what we did every time he wanted to buy me a gift, which was frequently. This man was used to women who needed lots of gifts on a regular basis to be happy. I never wanted the presents, but I was glad to take the cash. I redid the kitchen, new cabinets, new fridge. Paid the bills and eventually stopped going to work, because I didn't need to. One night he picked me up in a limo and handed me a small package with a black evening bag inside stuffed with cash. Well, there's the payments for the castle for a while, so why go in and dance the night away? It's not as if I quit dancing—in that business, there is no notice given for anything. Girls come and go—sometimes at the oddest times and in the most unusual ways—so I never quit. I just didn't go in for a long time.

Everyone liked the Half Prince, and the Half Prince and I enjoyed each other. That was it. Nothing more, nothing less. What we had was a socially acceptable form of prostitution. We dated and slept together, and he gave me cash. That's what it was, and never—not for a second —did I think it was anything else.

You may want to know, and I know the tabloids do, how could I possibly live with myself and do what I was doing? I think I was being honest about my situation. I was past the point of believing in fairy tales, and my reality was a mortgage and two kids I loved and wanted to spend as much time with as I could. I needed cash to do that, and if he wanted to give me cash instead of buying more rings, what's wrong with that? But prostitution it is, so if that's what you want to call it, then call it that. I've been fat, unfit, unhealthy, depressed, and a prostitute—it sounds like a segment on the "Geraldo" show, but it's not. It's the truth about my life.

Dating the Half Prince was fine, but I had a lot to say to the aerobics industry and to all the unfit people out there, even if the Half Prince wasn't interested.

> My husband told me as we were making love that he could tell "your butt's getting firmer." That felt good to hear.
>
> —Andra, a client

I suppose you could say that my aerobics career began when I was the only fat woman in a room full of fit women asking my advice. Teaching is sharing information, and that's what I was doing—sharing what I'd learned. The first real class I taught was in a club, a big, fancy health club that took itself very seriously (and still does). I had no idea what I was doing. When I tell you no idea, I mean none at all. The aerobics coordinator liked my story, and she hired me to teach. We spent some time together working on a routine for class—she thought it was two teachers sharing routines, but it was really me stealing everything she showed me and trying desperately to put a routine together before the first aerobics class I ever taught.

What it takes to lead an aerobics class is good music (something I didn't have the Monday before the Thursday class), a good "routine" (something I was stealing the week before and working on), the disposition of a frustrated performer (anything for attention, count me in), a decent body (you wouldn't believe how many unfit aerobics teachers are teaching people how to get fit), and nothing more. What it takes to be a great aerobics *teacher* is a desire to get people fit and something different to offer them. My routine may not have been the best. It was simple, straightforward, and easy to follow—something that came in handy years down the road. My music was all right—I'd copied another instructor's tape, and that's exactly what it sounded like. I had the anything-for-attention disposition, and after years of not getting much, being in front of a lot of people as the teacher was fun.

But the clients told me that what made my classes totally different from any other classes they had ever taken was the energy and passion that blasted through to everyone in the room. I poured information at people. How to move, what level of intensity, how to modify, breathe, breathe, breathe, and how to do it. Everything I wanted to know and never got the answers to in every class I'd ever been in was what I gave to every single class I taught. I still do the same thing. Call it an encyclopedia of a workout within an hour. The club called it too severe and not fun enough and asked me to change my method, but the clients loved it. Hundreds of people told me it was the only class they'd ever taken that taught them anything. For the first time during their twelve years of taking classes—these were some serious, rich, aerobic women—they were seeing their bodies change. Even though I was a bit intense, they loved it.

My life at this point was in the middle of another transition. (Another day, another transition, should be my motto.) The Half Prince and I were getting along swimmingly. I was teaching aerobics, sometimes four and five classes a day. The boys were healthy and happy, but I was feeling strangled. I wanted more. Less of the Half Prince and more of my own everything. So I made a decision, which made the Half Prince furious and turned out to be one of the biggest pivotal moments of my life. I declared my independence and told him I was going back to dancing. That was it. I'd dance a few nights a week, save the cash, teach aerobics during the day, and begin a career. I was not yet clear about what kind of career I wanted, but I didn't want one as a girlfriend, and marriage was never going to be part of my life as long as I lived.

So I danced again. One night only. And on that fateful night during my last set—main stage, second song—some guy sitting around the stage poured beer on the stage. As I was dancing for dollars, I slipped on the beer and flipped off the stage. When I say flipped, I mean I did a complete flip and landed in five-inch heels on both feet.

Girls fall off everything in strip clubs. They fall off tables, ledges, balconies, stages. So a dancer falling is not a big deal. My falling was a different story. The managers knew me, they knew that I didn't do drugs, didn't lead the life; and when they saw me fall, they were at my side within seconds. It's a good thing they were, because when I landed on my left foot, which was the first foot to hit the ground, I smashed the hell out of it. Breaking it every which way. And seconds later the right foot hit, smashing the hell out of it. The managers were under my arms carrying me to the dressing room so fast that it amazed me.

Funny wig story during all this chaos. As I was flipping off the main stage, the only thing I thought about doing was hanging on to the wig so it wouldn't fall off. Nobody knew I wore it, and I was not about to expose my secret during my foot-breaking flip. So picture it. I'm half-nude —and looking great for an ex-260-pound woman, I might add—flipping off the stage, hanging on to my head like I was wearing a hat. Nobody noticed, because nobody notices anything in that environment—it's not exactly full of alert, intelligent, caring people.

In the hospital emergency room that morning at 2:00 A.M., with smashed feet and a lot of pain, I had to make that phone call to my father. No matter how old you are, making that 2:00 A.M. phone call always makes you feel like an idiot who can't handle her own life—and enormously relieved at the same time. I was fine getting to the hospital and filling out the forms, but the minute my father walked in the door, I started to cry and fall to pieces. What is it about a parent that can turn you into a child within seconds? Well, he stayed with me while they got me ready for surgery, and I ended up with both legs in casts up to the knee and in a wheelchair for months. That's how I broke my feet, and that's why I could understand Bill's problem, or the problem facing anyone who also needs to sit while working out. Bill and I may have hurt ourselves in different ways, but both of us injured ourselves on the job, and both of us wanted to keep working out.

My broken feet helped me make up my mind about how I felt about the dancing once and for all. It was over. Not because I felt it was wrong, but that environment wasn't where I wanted to be. I had something very positive to share with people, and it was time I had some faith in myself and started pursuing what I really wanted to do. Teach people that fitness was for everyone. Reach the people the aerobics industry was not reaching. The crowd they thought was lacking the motivation to exercise. The people they believed were not interested in fitness. I wanted to get to them and explain how to do it. Big task for an aerobics teacher, ex-topless dancer with both feet in casts.

I feel sexier. My underwear looks better on me. *It's better*.

—Comment from a client.

So I had a plan. Change the face of fitness as soon as I got out of the wheelchair. I taught my wheelchair classes until I healed and went right back to the clubs—not the dancing kind—and taught my aerobics classes while trying to figure out a way to get this message out.

Part of my life transition was to begin doing some of the things I'd always wanted to do. What do I enjoy? What would I like to do? What are my interests? Questions I'd never asked myself. The early thirties were a great time in my life. I'm not sure if these are the passages that we all go through, if it was a hormonal thing, or what it was. I can just tell you that for the first time in my life I was defining my needs, goals, and dreams and had the strength to take the steps I needed to take.

My strength came from three sources, and they were bottomless. My children gave me the courage to change the patterns and cycles in my life that were handed down to me from my totally dysfunctional family. Dysfunction breeds like fungus, and unless you clean it off, give it some light and air so that the fungus can't grow, and create an environment that fungus can't grow in, it just keeps going. My love for my sons helps me make the decisions and set the boundaries within my family that need to be set so that I can grow and continue creating a healthy, functional family for us.

The second source was the physical strength I had developed, which was growing every day. I'd gone from a 260-pound housewife to a lean machine. My metabolic rate was functioning at such a high level that I was racing from the minute I got up to the second I went to bed—which also came in handy later on. And what gave me unbelievable amounts of strength was the pain and suffering that I'd gone through with the Prince during the explosion of my life.

Finally I was beginning to understand what my friend had told me in the middle of the hell—that every negative experience has a purpose and can create a positive outcome. It would be stretching the truth if I told you that I was glad at that point to have gone through what I went through, because it was still a fresh wound. Although the Prince and I were not fighting every time we saw each other, we didn't exactly love each other. What gave me strength was the vow I made to myself never, ever, ever again in my life to end up in a position of needing anyone for my financial, emotional, or physical security. I did gain strength from experience, but I'm not sure I would have volunteered to go through it again, no matter how strong I got from it. The Prince still represented the pain, so seeing him still had a sting to it.

So I'm loaded with strength and direction, out of the casts, and ready to live my life. One of the things that I'd always wanted to do was learn to play the guitar and sing.

STOP THE INSANITY!

I have a good voice and played around with singing in my past. I knew that if I could accompany myself on the guitar, I could take my protest to the masses in song. My fitness protest songs. All I needed was guitar lessons. I'd always fancied myself as a Joan Baez type. We both have short hair, we both stood up for causes, dispositionally we were probably pretty similar, and really the only thing missing besides the angelic voice was the guitar lessons. So I signed up at the local guitar shop.

With my newfound independence, health, and direction, I guess you could say that I went kind of mad. Newly recovered anything is always somewhat extreme; then add the focus and determination I had to have to rebuild my—and only my own, nobody else's—life. And you've got it: mad with strength. That's what I was.

I barreled into this music store and told the guy behind the counter that I was an independent, strong woman who was here for her first guitar lesson. This guy had been up for days or was just brain dead and could not have cared less about my speech. He just stared at me. I was standing in front of the brain-dead counterman and looking right past him to a man sitting at the back of the store playing the most beautiful jazz guitar I'd ever heard. It would not have been so bad if the music was the only beautiful thing going on in the corner. But the man playing the beautiful music had a face that had been chiseled from stone. He had a drop-dead, perfect face—sexy as hell. I pretended not to notice or care—just what I needed in my life, a good-looking, guitar-playing man—and went in for my first realize-my-dream guitar lesson.

The problem was that when I came out, after coming to my senses, he was still there, standing right next to the exit. I'm telling you, my knees went weak. (Wouldn't you think after what I'd been through that weak knees were beyond me? I did.) If I thought my knees were weak just looking at him, I never expected what was coming next. He was next to the front door of the shop, looking at a guitar. The manager said something to me about guitars—after all, that had been my motivation only an hour before—and something to him, and we began talking. If looking at him was orgasmic, you wouldn't believe what talking to him was like. He was intelligent. Funny (very important to me). Had the greatest eyes and teeth you've ever seen. A smile for days and interesting enough to stand and talk to for hours. Between his face and his conversation, he had me standing there for about three hours before I thought about my life. The kids, the house, the newfound direction—to hell with all of it, I was as starry-eyed and stupid-looking as they come. Madly in love seems to be the only way I fall.

I tore myself away from our conversation, but before I drove off he invited me to a gig he was playing the following Sunday night. I got into my car and drove off feeling like someone had hit me in the head with a baseball bat. Scientists studying the phenomenon called love have connected the starry-eyed and stupid feeling with some hormonal explosion theory. But when I met the guitar-playing gorgeous man in the store, articles weren't being written in every newsmagazine you picked up with answers for what I was feeling. At the time, I was a woman who had just pulled her life out of the gutter and was making it on my own, had my sons to think about and take care of, and there I was walking around like an idiot thinking about this man. Standing in parking lots in the cold, talking to a beautiful, younger man (oh, that's recurring theme number 103—younger men. We probably need to get out the old psychology book from college and search for the explanations for these obviously screwed-up things in my life), losing keys, paying the bill and walking out of the store without the groceries, and dying for Sunday to get here—these were not things I needed or wanted to be happening in my life.

By the time Sunday came, I'd talked enough sense into myself to bring along a friend. I fully intended to fix the beautiful guitar-playing man up with her and walk away from this whole thing. We went to the gig, my friend and the guitar player talked—of course, he couldn't help talking to her because I kept shoving her in his face. I made up some excuse and left them there together and went home. Forget him. It's over. He may be beautiful, but no more falling head over heels with any more Princes. That's it. On with my life. Back to the business of forging ahead with my plan.

Fine and dandy until the next guitar lesson. I barrel in again, and there he is. DANGER! WILL ROBINSON. He was standing in the store. I thought I was going to have a heart attack.

They say I learned well, picked up the guitar quickly. Who's to know? I only took four lessons, because I soon had my own private guitar teacher, if you know what I mean. Under the pretense of needing a musical question answered, I asked him to come over one day. Let's fill in the details with the snowstorm that was going on (a rare occurrence in Dallas), the children being with the Prince (a rare occurrence in my life), the house perfectly cleaned, and me looking like a million bucks. Sure, it was music we both had on our minds. He drove through a blizzard to answer this musical question . . . devoted, wasn't he? And it was over. Fallen, that's what I'd done. Head over heels fallen in love.

> When you have a better self-image, you seem to enjoy it more. In fact, sometimes I feel more attractive because I know that my body is changing. The only bad aspect is sometimes I can outlast my boyfriend!
> —Comment from a client

Six weeks after we met, he asked me to marry him.

"Can you make vegetarian pizza?" he asked.

"Yes, the best in town," I answered.

"Can you make vegetarian lasagna?" he asked.

"Yes, better than the Leone family," I answered.

"Will you marry me?" he asked.

"Yes," I answered.

"Tomorrow?"

"Absolutely," I answered.

We were married the next day by the justice of the peace with two nonspeaking witnesses we grabbed from the hallway. Nobody was told, nobody was invited.

You can imagine how his conservative Dallas family

felt when he called and said, "Mom, Dad—guess what? Remember the woman you met a couple of weeks ago— you know the one, no hair, two sons, older than me? We just got married."

Now love is love, but we all know that marriage is marriage. Another thing the scientists have concluded in their love research is that the hormonal explosion and the wonderful feelings of fuzziness that go with it only last a couple of months. No joke, boys. Give me the million bucks you spent on that research—I could have told you that. There was no white picket fence around this marriage. This Princess was requiring more from this Prince. I had crawled through dirt to get to where I was.

The rules had changed.

My most rewarding private moment was when my husband and I were in bed becoming intimate, and he said, "Oh, you feel different, what happened to you? I can feel your waist again." That really made me feel like I have finally done it. Lost the fat! And I'll never go back!

—Joanne, Ellington, Connecticut

There were only a couple of things I wanted from this relationship: support, love, and intimacy. Real, evolved, deep intimacy.

Intimacy requires trust, self-confidence, and peace of mind to achieve. I'm not touching the trust or peace of mind issues with a ten-foot pole. I'd have a leather couch and would be paid $100 an hour if that's what I was discussing here.

What I do know a little bit about and have spoken to thousands of women about is the self-confidence connected to the intimacy—connected to making love—that is very much grounded in the way we feel about our bodies.

Fat women don't get many dates.

Before all the fat rights groups burn this book at their next meeting, let me just say that I didn't get asked out on many dates when I was 260 pounds. My sex life didn't exist. It had nothing to do with no men wanting to date me—although they weren't exactly lining up at my front door. It had everything to do with how I was feeling.

I was in a walking coma 98 percent of the time. When you are sick, the last thing you usually think about is sex. When you are fat, unfit, and tired as hell all the time, sex becomes quite unimportant in your life. Having two kids around doesn't help your sex life much. Say "I have two children" to most men, and "see Jack run."

I despised the way I looked, I felt awful, and I looked like a balloon-a-gram in most of the clothes I wore—the odds were against a good, strong, healthy sex life. If you need a couple more strikes against sex ever happening in a lot of fat, unfit women's lives, think about the very few men in our society who prefer to date heavy ladies and the millions of women who are unfit and fat in this country, and you've got some sad stats on your chances for an active sex life. This is the truth. It is reality for millions of fat, unfit women in this country.

Despising the way I looked and felt was the problem. The room could have been black as a cave, and men could have been begging to have sex with me, but I wasn't taking my clothes off in front of anyone.

If you are fat, proud, and walking around naked every chance you get, then you are a more evolved, mature person than I am or ever will be. My hat is off to you. That's wonderful. However, that's not the way I felt, and it isn't what I hear women saying everywhere I go. Never once have I said that we had to live up to the *Playboy*, Barbie image in order to feel comfortable taking our clothes off in front of someone who loves us. Yes, love is love, and what you look like should be less important than how you feel about each other. Yes, making love involves much, much more than what shape your body is in—it should be deeper than the physical and should cross over into the spiritual and emotional. This is all true and real, but let me tell you something else that's true and real, and I'll use myself as an example.

A 260-pound, unfit, unhealthy, severely depressed woman (or man) is not a pretty sight naked. Take it from me, it doesn't exactly get you started, whether your sense of sexuality has been warped by *Playboy* magazine or not—it ain't pretty, no matter how you look at it.

I'd be a dog-faced liar—I may be lots of things, an ex-stripper, twice married, ex-fat woman, but I think you know by now that I'm about as honest as they come—if I told you that I don't enjoy slithering around in those pretty panties and bras that I can now order from the catalogs and actually fit into and look fabulous in. If putting on the black thigh-high stockings, push-up bra, and black spiked heels—just before the dress goes on, before going out on the town with the husband—and looking over and seeing his jaw drop to the ground and loving every moment of it are rooted in some warped sexual representation . . . then, so be it. Fine with me. Consider me sexually screwed up. Because it feels great and I enjoy every minute of it. It's big fun parading around in those sexy things, and for all the feminists of the world reading this book, I am not doing it for him. I'm doing it for me. I enjoy it. It's big, big fun for me, and that's why I do it.

Yes, my sex life is better now because

1. It exists.
2. I feel strong, sexy, and good about myself.
3. I love making love.
4. I love my husband.
5. We are working on the deep intimate stuff while we are having great sex, and it's a whole lot of fun getting there.

I know women who put on 10 pounds and won't take their clothes off. Maybe that's based on some sick social definition of perfection—Barbie-or-nothing thinking—but that's real different from being 260 and not feeling sexy or comfortable enough to walk around the room naked. My issue was about the way I felt—not just the way I looked on the outside, but the way I was feeling on the inside. I felt horrible.

I showed my new husband my "before" picture and

asked him if he would have dated me. He was being very honest when he told me that he would have really liked me and been my friend because he thinks I'm funny and intelligent and enjoys spending time with me, but he would never have slept with me because he wouldn't have been physically attracted to me. If that's wrong, then consider us both sexual deviants. I would rather be his friend and sleep with him than just be his friend. With that face, every time I see him I want to have sex with him—even when I'm angry at him. It's the face.

> For years we have given scientific attention to the care and rearing of plants and animals, but we have allowed babies to be raised chiefly by tradition.
> —Edith Belle Lowry,
> *False Modesty,* 1912

Intensity? I've had plenty of that. But one of the most intense experiences has been having children. It was only by the grace of God that pregnancy was never an issue during my less-than-perfect adolescence. Until I was madly in love and married and unexpectedly pregnant, I never thought about it. Kind of fairy-tale of me, don't you think?

Birthing back to back is not the easiest thing on a marriage. But that's not what blew my white picket fence to pieces. The Prince and I were not equipped to have a healthy, functional relationship, but I had to learn fast to be a good mother. First the white picket fence exploded, and then the kids and I began our journey together. We have been through a lot. We have all suffered, and we have all grown. They had a basket case of a mother some days, and I lived with the guilt of not "bonding" with my babies and enjoying every second of their lives.

My sons have watched me change my life and have been the center of it all for me. Without them there is no point. My children have taught me discipline, honesty, and commitment and have given me what I've been screaming for all of my life—unconditional love. They love me. As I am. Me. My sons have put the innocence and purity back into my life that I'd lost a long time ago. They have made me angrier, happier, and more frightened than I've ever been in my life. To think of life without them isn't possible for me. I have never loved anyone that much.

Both boys are beautiful, brilliant, and the best kids in the world. They have a mother now who is healthy and happy. We don't sit around and talk about the change in my body and my life during the last couple of years. It is just a part of their lives, and they accept it. A reporter asked me recently what my sons thought of their mom being on TV. Absolutely nothing, other than what a drag it is that I have to fly to Los Angeles every week. They don't think about it.

Of course, I still spend a lot of energy trying to figure out the species. Men, that is. With an ex-husband, a husband, and two sons, I'm surrounded by a species I don't understand.

Why, when there is a sink full of dishes, can't these guys take sponge in hand, add the soap, and wash? You know, that circular motion that cleans those dishes. Socks and underwear on the floor? How about bending over, picking them up, and putting them in the laundry basket? Explaining that walking over the underwear, socks, towels, and stuff lying on the floor is not the solution to the problem is where a lot of my energy goes.

I came home one night, very, very tired, and premenstrual as hell. The Prince, the kids, and the husband (have no fear, I'll be explaining why the Prince was there later) were upstairs getting ready to go play baseball. I walked in to a sink full of dishes, clothes on the floor, the bathroom looking like they had washed circus animals in the tub, and I exploded. I'd spent the whole day working hard and eating salt, so when I say exploded, you know what I'm talking about. Seeing colors.

"Why am I the only one in this house who can clean anything?

"I've been working hard all day.

"The bills are paid.

"The business is successful.

"The book is almost finished.

"I am woman; I am strong; I am anything I want to be. . . .

"Why, why"—tears streaming down my face—"why do I have to come home to a house that looks like this?

"Is it because I have a . . ."

All of the men/boys were standing staring at me like I had finally, once and for all, lost it and there was no chance of my ever coming back from the edge; slowly they started backing up to the back door with a look of shock and fear on their faces. All four, the husband, the ex-husband, and the two sons, creeping step by step away from this lunatic woman.

Ages 8 through 30, all staring at me with a wide-eyed-fear-of-God kind of look, while I screamed out the questions.

"Why am I the only one who can do the dishes?

"The only one who understands how to use a washing machine?

"Is it because I have a—"

Before I could finish the sentence, my beautiful, brilliant, older son says, "Mom, are you going to tell us the uterus story again?"

"Uterus? Is that why I know how to do these things and you don't? Let me tell you, this is not innate, I've learned how to do all these things, and so can all of you. . . ."

They left the house, I had my fit and got on with the evening. Later that evening, my husband and sons came into the bedroom, slowly, and told me that although they didn't have a uterus, they would make an effort to pick things up, wipe things down, sweep anything in sight, and help with the house so that I wouldn't be the only one keeping the house clean, and they would never have to hear the history of the uterus ever again. Talk about expending energy. . . .

I came home after a really good segment a couple of months ago and premenstrual again, called the whole family into the living room. Another family meeting. Crying, I said:

"Every week I do a part of my job on national TV in front of millions of people. The country watches what I do, and I get responses from thousands of strangers.

"My family, on the other hand, never watches, has no idea what the segments are about, and gives me no feedback at all.

"What's the deal here? I would appreciate to be appreciated, thank you very much. . . ."

All the boys were sitting across from me, with that she's-a-crazy-woman stare, and agreed to watch the segments and appreciate the hell out of me; then they asked if being appreciated was all I needed, because they all had something they needed to do outside the house for at least the couple of hours it would take me to calm down.

Now my sons watch the segments; we tape them so that they can watch them after school, because I told them it was important to me. Not because they care that their mother is on national TV. That means nothing to them. One of the things I love most about the children is how unimpressed they are. My kids love me and I love them, no matter what I look and feel like. I know that, but it's pretty cool to have your mom have energy, feel good, and participate in your life. It's pretty cool to go on vacation and your mom can ride the banana boat. (Warning to all the mothers of the world—there is nothing cool about the banana boat for us. I hung on for dear life, afraid for the safety of the banana crew and its passengers—it was the kids who labeled it a really cool experience.) It was also really cool to ride dirt bikes and scuba. (Again, as wonderful as this sounds, Old Man Sea and me don't get along. Who wants to be swimming in the same large body of water as those giant sea turtles, long pointy things that look like they can sting you, crabs, and all the other brightly colored strangers? Not me, but anything to be with my kids.)

I'll tell you what's cool. When I think about the depressed, tired, sick, 260-pound mom that my children were living with and I compare that with the energy, love, involvement, and potential that our new future holds . . . that's cool.

STOP THE INSANITY!

But the problems, decisions, fears, and anxieties of life are still there. Fit or fat. When I screw up now I don't have the added burden (pardon the pun) of 133 pounds, no strength, and not being able to move without gasping for air. I still feel like the worst mother in the world, ready to call the child abuse hot line when I lose patience with my children. When I make the dumbest business decision in the world, and calling myself president of anything feels like a joke, I still want to lie down and die. Marriage number two, and I still haven't learned how to do this wife thing properly. How do you think that makes me feel? The growing and the changing never stop. Without the labor there is no birth, and the labor goes on forever sometimes.

The pressure is still on from all angles. The only thing different is that I have a lean, strong, healthy body that can help me cope with all the junk that we've all got to live with, whether we like it or not. That's life. The truth is that going from one crisis or problem to the next is a whole lot different when you are fit, well, and healthy enough to have what you need to get through it and on to the next one. That's what changing my body has meant to me and my family. Yeah, it's cool that I do national TV, write books, do seminars, and own and operate a very successful business, but it's even cooler that I'm in control and have choices now. Here's my motto: Pretty cool and getting cooler. That means pretty strong and getting stronger, pretty together but growing more, pretty smart but constantly learning, very happy and getting happier.

My children, mother, and husband are my best allies. My mom and husband are always patting me on the back for my good efforts.
—Andra, a client

It's time to get back to the Prince. After all, he ruined my life. Dumped me with two small children in Garland, Texas. I fell to pieces because of him. But something happened to the new husband and me that started to clear up this whole Prince issue.

The new husband and I went to the place we all end up going when new marriages meet reality—the marriage counselor. Things were not going well. I felt he should be communicating with me more—supporting and understanding me and sharing his deepest, darkest feelings and needs with me—and he had no clue what I was talking about and thought I'd gone crazy.

Sound familiar? We love each other and are committed to this marriage. It's the nineties. So off we go to therapy to figure it all out.

After pleading, crying, and discussing why I was so angry at the husband for not understanding what I needed in this marriage—remember, I'd been through this before and had less patience this time around—the therapist looked at me and said, "Susan, you are not angry with your husband. You're furious with yourself. You've compromised your standards. You're not living the way you want to live, and you are angry with yourself."

I left thinking she was out of her mind and obviously missed the point. My husband was acting like Fred Flintstone. That's why we were here. My being angry with myself had nothing to do with the problem.

Then it hit me.

In the parking lot.

She was right.

But I wasn't thinking about my current relationship, it was the Prince I was thinking about. I immediately began babbling—or sharing, as we say in therapy—explaining everything I was thinking with my husband. This wonderful, enlightened information about the Prince and me.

The Prince had not ruined my life. I had ruined my own life. He was not responsible for my getting fat. He didn't force feed me in the middle of the night—he was too busy having sex with his girlfriend.

Oh—excuse me. So I wasn't, and never will be, fully evolved.

I had made the choices. I had made the decisions, and only I was responsible for lowering my standards and suffering the consequences. I needed to forgive him.

Before you get teary-eyed and write the Prince a sympathy note, don't forget that he didn't handle himself too well. Showing up for his twice-a-month visitation with his girlfriend in the car was not a smart move, no matter how you look at it. Let's not be too grown-up about all of this and forgive him totally.

So, there I am in the parking lot of the therapist's office, where the husband and I had gone to solve the problems of our new marriage, sharing, babbling, explaining all of this about the Prince to him. He missed the connection totally and was convinced that I needed hospitalization and that this situation could only get worse.

I had choices.

So do you.

You have more than I had, because when I was trying to figure it all out, there was no bald woman screaming "Stop the insanity!"

You have lots of choices.

The answer to your problems is not in the diets. It doesn't come in the form of pills, shakes, drinks, or formulas. It's not in the health clubs, aerobics classes, and neon-clad world of the fitness industry. The answers are here. In the book you have in your hands. It's about getting the correct information, learning how to apply it to your life-style, your fitness level, and your physical considerations, and getting physically lean, strong, and healthy.

Remember, when you have the strength to get up in the morning, life is a hell of a lot easier to muddle through. We all have different circumstances and situations that make us feel trapped and lead to destructive behavior. That never changes. You and I will spend the rest of our lives working through the pain and the dysfunction of our childhoods. But every day is about making decisions. Decisions about the children, the marriage, the business . . . the list goes on and hopefully always will.

Stopping the insanity in your life is about making it easier to live your life. If I'd gone for a walk knowing that jogging wasn't the only way to get fit, if I'd increased my calories rather than starving myself to death, if I'd decreased the fat in my life and begun to build basic muscular strength, I could have avoided a hell of a lot of pain. I would have been able to get out of the mess I was in quicker instead of digging a deeper hole and falling in.

During the past couple of years I've heard it all from my clients and the women I've met. Lives very different from mine. Backgrounds and emotional issues that are as different as night and day. I walk down the streets of New York City with Leslie. Peggy tells me that she's found the strength to leave the abusive marriage she's been in for the last twenty years of her life. She questions why as a southern lady she was never allowed to sweat and why it took a mastectomy before she thought about her health. And dear, sweet Jill is starting to see how beautiful, sexy, and intelligent she is and how she can be anything she chooses to be without throwing up and living in fear every day.

I see and hear these things, and all they tell me is that we are all the same. We are all screwed up, afraid, have millions of issues that need sorting out, and there is not a person out there who doesn't want to look and feel good.

Stopping the insanity physically is the first step in the healing that will continue for the rest of your life. Eating, breathing, and moving your way toward a foundation of wellness is the most important step. It's easy, cheap, and attainable. What more do you want? It makes the process of solving the problems you have from your past, the problems of the present, and the problems of the future so much easier to deal with.

It is about a lot more than losing weight. Stopping the insanity is about regaining your physical strength and your sanity . . . as Sally said, it's about going sane.

I've arrived at this outermost edge of my life by my own actions. Where I am is thoroughly unacceptable. Therefore, I must stop doing what I've been doing.
—Alice Koller,
An Unknown Woman, 1982

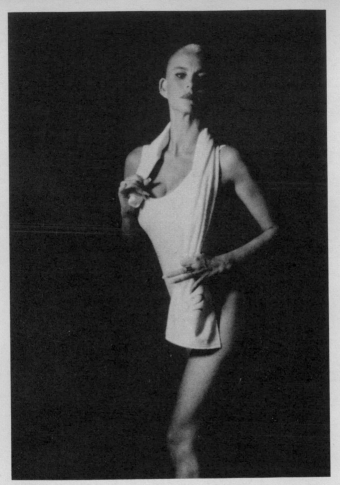

Here is the official Susan Powter portrait. The leotard is from my line of clothing, the towel has Susan Powter *embossed on it, and I just scream fitness, don't I? This is not one of my favorite shots. It just isn't me—the bikini-and-high-heels photo is much closer to the truth. This one is . . . I don't know, too stuffy, too merchandisy, too queer. That's it, it's a queer picture.*

TEN

Life on the Other Side

> *Men, their rights and nothing more.*
> *Women, their rights and nothing less.*
> —SUSAN B. ANTHONY

Dear Friends:

My life now, by Susan Powter.

Until very recently, I felt that it was my moral obligation to spend the rest of my life torturing the Prince for what he did to me.

I have grown—matured, if you will—since then, and although I may slip once in a while, all in all, the Prince has been forgiven.

Being healthy, having the body I want, running a successful business, and, of course, writing this book (every writer I've ever seen interviewed says that writing their masterpiece was a purge of sorts—well, consider me purged, pardon the pun)—things are going well, the kids are healthy, brilliant, and beautiful, and I know that I can and will create my own life. So it's safe to tell all of you that it never was, and never will be, a matter of mind over matter or loving myself enough that has solved the problems the Prince and I had. Stopping my insanity was about increasing my cardio-endurance, rebuilding muscular strength, reducing body fat, increasing flexibility, and regaining my health. If your body's not healthy, how could your head be? The same blood and junk that flow through your body flow through your mind, so the healthier it is, the better off you are. Being mentally clear enough to make better decisions has helped me much more than any affirmation ever could. If the Prince makes me mad now, I defuse the anger and solve the problem. Back in the castle, I had no choices. The anger just engulfed me.

As I've watched other women get well, I've seen the same sense of calm, peace, and inner strength—whatever you want to call it—emerge as they get well. You don't even have to conjure it up, it's just there. It's a mental/emotional strength that develops right alongside the physical strength.

> Don't forget that compared to a grownup every baby is a genius. Think of the capacity to learn. The freshness, the temperament, the will of a baby a few months old.
>
> —May Sarton,
> *Mrs. Stevens Hears the Mermaids Singing,* 1965

Since I've aired my dirty laundry to the world, I'd like to finish this book—this sweeping saga, this romance novel gone mad—by letting you know how it's all turned out. We'll start with the children because that's always the best place to begin.

My children are perfect.

They deserve whatever they want in life, and they also deserve a father. Both parents are important, and although the Prince didn't do too well in the princely department, he is a very good father. The good Catholic boy from a large family was raised seeing a baby at his mother's breast nonstop, has 20 million cousins, aunts, and uncles, and does the family thing much better than I ever did.

One night the Prince and I had a talk. We sat outside on the sidewalk in front of my father's house until 4:00 A.M. We did not discuss the past (we all know who screwed that up), we discussed the future. I told him that we were going to have a relationship for the next twenty years whether we liked it or not. We had our children together, and it was completely up to us—the parents, the adults in this situation—what kind of relationship it would be and how that relationship would affect our two kids for the rest of their lives.

I don't think there is a person alive who doesn't understand the deep connection between parents and children. Our parents' love means more than anything. No matter how crappy, mean, or useless our parents were, we spend the rest of our lives searching for their approval. I wasn't going to do that to my children. If my kids were ever going to have a chance at a healthy, responsible, evolved life, they'd have to learn it somewhere. You can talk till you're blue in the face, but it's what you do and how you live that teach the children.

Well, the Prince and I had a lot of work to do before we could teach maturity. There was a lot of anger to work through before we could teach love. There were and still are parenting issues that need to be worked through. PTA meetings for the next seven, eight years. High school graduations, college graduations—the Prince thinks a degree is the most important thing in the world; I think it's a load of crap. (Get out there and work, apprentice with someone, learn how to sell—there's my 1800s version of how it should be done.) But say college to the Prince and he thinks you are assured a successful future. See the conflict? Even in print, it screams, "You guys have a lot of work to do!" There are life's events—celebrations, births, deaths, successes—that we'll be facing together for a long time, and it makes no sense to me that we pretend we are not a family and do it all separately and dysfunctionally.

The Prince agreed on the sidewalk at 4:00 A.M. that we would co-parent our children. We agreed that I would go to work and he would take over the making of the school lunches and picking the kids up from school. He wanted to go to school—medical school. His dream is to become a doctor. This schedule works well with the children's—same hours, same vacations, same everything, everyone doing homework every afternoon. In agreement, great—now how do we make this all happen?

If ever my argument for the connection of physical health and mental stability could be proven as fact, the best case study would be during the last couple of years with the Prince and our rather unusual living situation. The fact that we've been able to pull this off would prove the point. Shuttling the children from one house to another was not fair to our children and impossible for me. It gets old fast, as I'm sure a lot of you understand that. So do what I did—move in with your ex-husband. There's the solution, America. Live together.

This is not another Texas cult (we've all had our fill of them)—it is a practical solution to a complicated problem.

I rented a duplex—three-bedroom apartment upstairs, three-bedroom apartment downstairs—right down the street from the boys' school, with a public swimming pool and park across the street, shopping down the block, and work ten minutes away, and I moved everybody in. The Prince lives downstairs. The husband and I live upstairs. The kids live in both houses. The fire escape stairway leads to both houses, and the kids go back and forth.

I pay for it all. I'd rather, thank you. Another thing I've learned is that taking money from a man is a very expensive thing to do. It has always ended up costing me a lot more than I took. It's easier and feels better for me to pay. As I type this chapter, my sons are asleep in their bedroom. It's 5:00 A.M. (diligent, aren't I?). I'll wake them at 7:00, they'll go downstairs. I go to work. The Prince gets the boys ready for school, makes the lunches, and drops them off. Each morning we check the schedule board that he has updated for the week—who's got a dentist appointment, where and when the basketball games are, what book report is due. If there's a question or a change, I'll call downstairs or he'll call up to discuss it, and it's onward with our days.

The Prince picks the boys up every day at 3:30, unless I can get a break from a meeting, photo shoot—puff, puff

—interview, seminar, or whatever I'm doing. I try to be home for snacks and homework a couple of times a week. Otherwise, I'm home every night by 5:00, 6:00, or, at the latest, 7:00 P.M. One week a month I'm gone for a week. The rest of the month I try not to leave for more than forty-eight hours. My week away is coming up this Monday, and you should see what's been packed into the week. My schedule is literally hour to hour, with plane rides late at night so I can get into the next city by early morning, and go, go, go all day.

These are jam-packed weeks, but it's by design—if I am going to run a business, do a TV show, write books, and have a family, then it's got to be organized so that it can all get done without the kids suffering. The boys have never—except when their mother was a topless dancer—spent much time with a baby-sitter. They have always had a parent with them. The Prince and I talk at least once a day about the kids, their schedule, or anything that's going on in their lives. We go to all the school functions and meetings together. It's the two boys and the Prince, who looks like he stepped out of a Ralph Lauren ad—crisp, clean, very conservative khaki pants, sky blue shirt (you know, the whole Polo thing). Then there's the husband, who—although he's getting better—looks like he pulled something out of the bottom of his closet, threw it on, and showed up at the meeting, which is exactly what he does. As for Mom, you all know what I look like—very little hair and wearing sweats. This is the family at the school function, birthday party, relative's wedding, or backyard barbecue.

The operative word here is "family." I've learned—and God knows my family should have taught me this one—that it's not what you look like, act like, or seem to be, it's what's going on in the family as a unit that counts. "You are only as sick as your secrets"—someone said that. The one thing I can say about my family—the kids, the Prince, and the husband—is that there are not many secrets (and none after the publication of this book).

The Prince and I went to a meeting last week with both

...' teachers and the principal of the school. We talked about a lot of things, and at the end of the meeting the principal said, "Whatever you and Nic"—whoops, I told you the Prince's name; there it is, the final secret out of the bag: his name is Nic, and he is and always will be the father of the two most important people in my life— "whatever you and Nic are doing and however you are living, you are doing something right. Your sons are two of the most polite, well-adjusted boys in this school." Nic looked at me and I looked at him, and both of us puffed up like blowfish—we were so proud of our boys and each other. We have done a good job. We've worked hard to be a healthy family, and we are one. I'm real proud of that.

So now you know why the Prince was upstairs when I had my pre-menstrual fit. He was borrowing some soy sauce and getting the boys' uniforms from the upstairs laundry room.

> Mama exhorted her children at every opportunity to "jump at de sun." We might not land on the sun, but at least we would be off the ground.
> —Zora Neale Hurston,
> Dust Tracks on a Road, 1942

While I'm taking care and working on that relationship with the father of the children, there's another one upstairs. The husband.

That's what I, and everyone else I know, call him. The husband. He calls me wife. I call him husband. Don't ask me why, we just always have.

This men issue confuses me no end. I say that as an adult woman with more men in her life now than some women have in a lifetime. Living with an ex-husband, a current husband, and two sons has done nothing to help me clear up the confusion.

I like men. I seem to collect them. It's me and Liz. Miz Taylor may be more beautiful than I am, but I'm right behind her in the marriage department—only six to go. The first person in a room full of people who would have to admit to not being very good at this wife thing would be me.

It's not the same the second time around. The rules are very different. I couldn't imagine what the rules would be the seventh time around. Wow, think about it . . . it just may be perfect by then. Who's to know, except Liz.

As I ask my husband every day of his life with me, if we don't have support for each other, love, intimacy, and a very strong connection, why, oh why would I ever want to be married? I married the husband because he is the brightest human being I've ever met. His mind challenges me constantly. I'm not trying to imply that we sit around and play challenging board games all day long—it's simply the way he sees things that I love. What has been considered by some who knew him long before I ever met him as a warped way of seeing and interpreting the world is in my opinion brilliance and works very well with the way I see things. He is extremely funny. We laugh a lot together.

Then there is that face. It's a good thing when looking at your husband's face makes you want to jump into bed with him . . . in this high-stress life, sometimes you only have a two-minute face look to warm up, if you know what I mean, so it has come in handy many times. I like the concept of building a life with someone and sitting on the porch swing eighty years from now reflecting together (makes us sound like sheets of metal facing the sun on that porch, but you understand—reflecting on all the wonderful moments and so on). All this is fine. The insanity comes up when you talk to Liz, me, and the scientists about how long the love stuff lasts—a couple of months —and then when you consider all the work that has to be done before you can even think about making it to the reflections on the porch.

I don't think we are very honest about marriage. "It's a lot of hard work" hardly tells you the truth about what you are getting into when you say "I do." The bills, the kids, the jobs, the lack of time spent, the old baggage that we all lug around. Throw all this at any marriage and it's going to have a hard time. We all work hard on the same stuff to try to build a life with someone we feel it is possible to build it with. The magic and mystery fade fast, and reality hits all too quickly. Our reality is that an ex-husband lives downstairs—we co-parent our children. The father is the father, and the stepfather is the stepfather, very different roles. The husband and I both have full-time careers, lots of bills, and very little time. I also have a few stipulations this time around. I want and will accept nothing less than the deepest connection, the most evolved working relationship, and the best sex life on earth. That's it. Nothing less. Otherwise I see no reason to be married.

I don't need your money, don't want your last name (I have one of my own, thank you), don't want presents, houses, cars (I can buy my own). The only thing I want from you and with you is something I don't have with anyone else. "Grow up or get out" is my motto. If I want another child, I'll birth one. I will not raise another man. I want one who's already raised or is willing to put a lot of effort into raising himself really fast so that we can get on with the equality, love, and intimacy that marriage should be about.

My husband and I have had the best of times and the worst of times. There is no one I'd rather grow old with, or at least have sex with, than the husband. If I'm willing to continue working with Nic, can you imagine how hard I am willing to work on my current marriage?

I've got to say it again. There is no way I could continue to work on the marriage, the ex-marriage, the job, the kids, and myself without the physical strength to do it. If I were still walking around physically sick, it would be impossible. I wouldn't even have the option.

The kids, Nic, the husband and I work hard. Every day making choices that can make our situation better or worse. Easier or harder. Developing, growing, and designing our life. That's what we are all doing—then there's my life. I am a part of all of the parts, and I am also separate.

At work, you think of the children you have left at home. At home, you think of the work you've left unfinished. Such a struggle is unleashed within yourself. Your heart is rent.

—Golda Meir, 1973

"So tell us, Susan, what does all this success feel like? How has it changed your life?" The reporter who asked that question didn't know what to do with the answer I gave her. Other than making it possible to pay my bills, the only thing success has done for me is enable me to do it the way I want to do it.

Freedom. That's what it's given me. The freedom to express an opinion and have people read about it. Very cool. The freedom to teach—whether it's an aerobics class, talking about food and fat on national television, writing a book, or whatever. Who could ask for more than that? The freedom to design a life that works for me and share information. It's all very, very exciting. I can't believe I get paid for doing what I do. I know you hear that in every interview you see on television with someone who's just completed a blockbuster movie, but I *really* can't believe I get paid to do what I do. Being given the opportunity to share what I've learned with so many other women and having it make a difference in their lives. The cash payment isn't all there is—it's the validation I get when someone tells me they love my tapes, watched the "Home" show and learned something, saw the infomercial and couldn't stop watching, came to a seminar and walked away knowing how to begin changing their life. Maybe I'm just the lost child looking for love, the wounded inner child needing affection—well, I got it, didn't I, and it sure feels good when I get the acknowledgment, respect, and love from all the women I meet. That's one of the things success can bring, if what you're selling, producing, or talking about is quality. I did "Good Morning America" recently. The show was on infomercials and I was so proud of the product I sell. I love my tapes. That feels good. If I were walking around in airports being recognized as a schlocky seller of junk who had made a fortune doing it, I'd hate it. It's important to me to be proud of what I'm doing. Success, measured by cash only, ain't it. The cash is nice, no doubt about it, but that's not how I measure success in my life.

There is more than one "before" and "after" in my life. Going from sitting on the bed at 260 pounds to the black string bikini is not the only transition I've gone through. Going from the topless dancer to the owner of a corporation is a big transition. Healing the anger and pain from the white picket fence explosion and learning how to face the reality of marriage without lowering my standards—now that was hard. Just defining my standards was new to me. No social rules or regulations, no past baggage or fear, not considering the husband, just me. What did I want? Then accepting the answers. Accepting who I am and what I wanted was one of the first and biggest shackles I've ever unhinged. It all works together. The end result, and I know it's not over and never will be, is that where I am at this point in my life is the best stage, the sweetest, for me.

I'm telling the truth about my life without shame, fear, guilt, or embarrassment. The first thing that happens when a woman gets successful is her morality is attacked in the hope that other women will turn away from her in disgust, and she will be knocked down. The tabloids already tried that. It didn't work.

I never knew that I was going to end up on TV. Writing a book never entered my mind. I changed my body and started teaching aerobics classes. That's all. Never in my wildest dreams did I think that the world would know that I danced topless. I wasn't prepared for the hatred, jealousy, and greed that some people reacted with as my career started taking off. Some "old friends," a relative, and some "new friends" attacked like piranhas when the press offered cash for some dirt. That hurt, and to go through it I had to grab on to my grown-up side that I'd spent years developing.

My genius, brilliant, dear friend, agent, and manager, Rusty Robertson, said to me the other day, "Suse"—she cuts everyone's name in half—"you've been through hell and back, and everything you've been through has value because you are willing to share it honestly with other women and turn it into something positive. This is going to be the best time of your life."

That's exactly what this is. I've spent years wading through the mud. I didn't always make the right choices and still don't. Some of the other before-and-afters in my life are the confused teenager getting unconfused. The girl who thought she had no choice but sex, drugs, and rock and roll, creating other choices. The woman who has gone from afraid, confused, and always feeling out of place to living without fear—what freedom that is—feeling very focused and clear, and waking up every day with such peace in my soul. That peace is what I've been looking for all my life. There isn't anything I've done as I was climbing out of the mud that I would lie about or not discuss. The more people I meet, the farther out of my own little world I go, the more I see that we are all alike. And there isn't one of us who can afford to pick up the rock in the glass house.

It is scary to be a woman out there talking, working, trying to make a difference. We are absolutely judged differently from men, and we are judged harshly. If this all blows up tomorrow, you'll still find me in my studio in Dallas, teaching my classes and loving it.

The last couple of years have taught me that nothing is free. Along with the success comes the busy schedule and less time for anything else. No matter how good I am at managing time, when the husband puts together a romantic weekend (a feat worth acknowledging in itself) and I fall asleep in the middle of the candlelit dinner, it creates some problems. If you think you felt pressure when you had a book report (as far as I ever got in school) or a thesis (whatever that is) due in school, try having a deadline for a publishing house that has paid you a whole lot of money for that special book report on your life. Sweating bullets every morning at 5:00 A.M., making sure that I've said everything I needed to say, and that at least some of it makes any sense or difference to you, ain't easy.

And if you ever worry about your children getting enough attention, nurturing, and guidance, mix together worrying about all that with traveling all over the country every week, having to be in every meeting and not being able to tell the big boys that you have to go because your son has a plantar's wart that needs to be removed.

The other day I called my father, and I explained something to him. I explained that I am raising a family, paying the bills (all of them), running a business, doing exactly what he did. But I'm getting one-third the credit.

Whenever Daddy came home from a business trip, we all knew that he worked hard and needed some time to get settled before we bombarded him with family matters. But when Mommy comes home from a business trip, she's been away and needs to make up for the time she's been gone. The house is a mess—she needs to clean up. The kids haven't eaten real food for three or four days—she needs to cook some meals. And God knows the husband needs a little attention. Nobody picks up my dry cleaning. Nobody packs my business bag. Nobody makes sure that everything is covered so that I can do my job. I am financially responsible for a family of five. I have lived up to that responsibility and kept the priorities in the right order—kids, me, job, husband—and I'm proud of that.

There are lots of benefits in my life now that I never dreamed possible. There's a lot more responsibility, work, and challenges than I ever thought I could handle. Walking into a store and being able to fit into anything that strikes my fancy is loads of fun. Eating like a cow at a restaurant and being not judged but admired for the metabolic rate that I have is great. Traveling all over the country and meeting the most wonderful women in the world is better than anything I could imagine. TV is amazing—the power of the medium and the response you get never cease to amaze me. Recognition is wonderful.

But the two things that run head to head as the most important consequences of the last couple of years are my freedom from fear and my health. I know I tell everyone I run into that it's not about health, and it wasn't. But as I get older and wiser and create the life I want to live, I realize how precious life is. How lucky I am for each day I'm given. I want to live until I am 150. I want to baby-sit for my grandchildren and then my great-grandchildren, and in order to do that I've got to be healthy. That 85 percent control—consider me learning how to regain more of that every day. When you think you've got a lot to lose—and I'm not talking cash here, I'm talking self—you begin giving yourself and your brilliant body what it needs to live. You do have a lot to lose —your health and your self-esteem. But they are easy to regain, and *Stop the Insanity!* will help you regain what you never thought you could. You cannot fail. This is not a diet, this is eating. It's learning how to do it correctly that changes your life. It's about that oxygen you are going to begin pouring back into a body that has lived for a long time without it. It's about the strength you've lost and the aches and pains that are a result of losing your strength, which you will regain.

Yep, we all have different wounded children living inside of us—we are all wounded, addicted, living in fear, and not 100 percent. The more wounded you are, the less you are functioning. The less you are functioning, the more you need the foundations of wellness.

It all started for me by getting well. It has turned out nicely, and I'm grateful for that; however, either way I would have had to expend energy, whether it was going around and around in the cycle I was born into or breaking the cycle and creating my own straight line forward. Either way, you are going to be expending energy for the rest of your life. It's nice to have it to burn. It is real nice to have the choices to make, and if the end result goes beyond your wildest dreams, give me a call. We'll chat.

We have too many high-sounding words and too few
actions that correspond with them.
—Abigail Adams,
Letter to John Adams, 1774

STOP THE INSANITY!

My friend Ruth just called. Ruth and I met years ago. Me, the fat, newly divorced, somewhat angry, very passionate single mother of two, and Ruth, perfect, no children, happy, loving wife of the studying-to-be-a-minister and big-time born-again Christian.

I had left the castle and moved into an apartment that was one of five in a fabulous old home. Always preferring the old and original to the new and practical, I moved into one of the apartments upstairs—very practical with two little babies. The drop to the backyard could have killed any adult, forget the toddlers. Paying rent I couldn't afford, anything for independence, and having to keep the kids quiet for the downstairs neighbors, Ruth and her soon-to-be-minister husband, Jeff.

The house was leased by a wonderful man who was also born again, and his policy was to lease to born agains only. Maybe he was hoping in my case, but I was the only tenant who didn't attend the daily Bible meetings in the Garden of Eden backyard this guy had created.

The day I moved in, Ruth was cooking a southern feast, complete with cornbread and gravy for the husband. I'm moving alone with two kids to the upstairs apartment, cussing and dragging things up and down all day. Ruth came up to see what was going on, who was moving in, and to offer a coffee break. We sat for a few moments, drank some coffee, and talked. The only thing we had in common was the children I had and the family she and her husband were planning. So birth was the topic of conversation. During our talk I suggested some books, tapes, and classes that had helped me make my birthing decisions, lent her the books that I'd unpacked on the subject, and off my new neighbor went.

Within minutes Mr. Ruth—which is what I called him when he came to my door with smoke coming out of his ears—was at my door. "I don't want this stuff in my home or my wife reading it," Mr. Ruth said.

My newly divorced comments went something like this: "Since when do you decide what another adult reads? You are a self-righteous pig and a danger to women and society. Women are in the position they are in today because of men like you." And I think I ended up with, "I hate you, and so should your wife."

It was, to say the least, a rocky beginning, but years later we are all very good friends and have a mutual respect and love for each other that has lasted through time and children. (They have since had three.)

Ruth had no idea what had been going on with me in the last couple of years. When you are at home raising three children, it is perfectly reasonable and understandable that you don't know anything that's going on for at least a couple of years. She called to find out how the kids and I were. During our conversation—as is the case with so many conversations with fabulous women—we began talking about how we were both feeling and what was going on in our lives. Apart from the husbands, kids, jobs, and responsibilities—how we were feeling.

She made a comment that fascinated me. She said, "Susan, you've always known what you wanted. The first day I met you, and we were talking about babies, I walked away feeling so powerful and energized. You motivated me and made it clear to me what it was that I needed to do next. You've always been a teacher and a communicator."

She was right. I am doing now the same thing I'd been doing for years—I just didn't know what I was doing or that what I was doing had any value. The real difference is how I feel about myself.

My belief in myself is stronger. Going from 260 pounds to where I am today certainly helped me believe that I could do anything.

My health has improved . . . hand in glove, I'd say.

I broke it to Ruth during our conversation that she had been motivated and made decisions based on the advice of someone who at the time was physically, emotionally, and spiritually depleted. Dead. Gone.

There are millions of books on the market that have been written to help us all find ourselves. Self-help books up the wazoo, every one with an answer. *Stop the Insanity!* is not a self-help book. *Stop the Insanity!* is the truth about what your body needs to function. It's been written to help you understand how to apply this basic information to your life and work within your fitness level and physical considerations, so that you get well. Our school systems are full of tests designed to teach us what we are good at and what we should or should not pursue. Thank God I didn't make it to the test and never listened. In the teacher's comment column of my report cards, in that perfect nun handwriting, it always read, "Susan could do so much better in her schooling if she would only apply herself and stop talking so much." One of my best friend's mothers, during one of my turbulent adolescent periods, said to me, "Susan, if you could make a living talking, you'd make a million dollars." So there, Sister Mary, what do you think of that? Why I didn't drop out of school right then and there, take my friend's mom's advice, and hit the speaking circuit is beyond me.

I've been talking all my life. I was born talking. When I was shooting the infomercial—standing on a stage in front of 1,500 people, five cameras, big production day, doing a live seminar—I was at total peace. I was exactly where I belonged. I told Rusty later that night that I came out of the womb to be standing right where I was that night. It felt right.

Talking to Ruth about birth or sharing my experiences with you about going from a fat person to a fit person is all the same thing. I'm talking and sharing my last thirty-five years and gazillions of mistakes with you. The fact that the best publishing house in the country paid me to write about it all is one of the big differences in my life. Otherwise, I'm doing the same thing now that I've been doing my whole life.

Ruth and I had a wonderful conversation about some of the things she'd like to do. Her dreams, her goals. The children are growing up and becoming wonderful human beings, thanks to the energy, love, and devotion that their parents have put in. Her husband is doing what he wants to do, thanks to Ruth's support, encouragement, and love. Now she's seeing herself as more than a mother and wife. She's thinking about Ruth, the person separate from the other roles. What she wants, the other things in her life that are important to her.

I asked myself the same questions as I was getting well, and I came up with the answers. What do I do well? Talking is the obvious answer. What do I enjoy? Teaching is what fills me up. It feeds me. Breaking down the information and explaining it. There is no magic or genius involved. I read something, understand it, and explain it —what's so difficult? Getting well was the key for me to begin questioning, focusing on, and pursuing what I enjoyed doing. Believe me when I tell you none of what's happened in the past couple of years has been easy, and I've worked my butt off for anything I've got. But my dreams have come true, and who could have asked for more than that?

Ruth sings. She sings beautifully. She's good at it and loves doing it. Hey, Ruth, get well and take your singing from the shower to the stage. Remember, there are no unrealistic goals.

The body is shaped, disciplined, honored, and in time, trusted.

—Martha Graham,
Blood Memory, 1991

When all this started, it was about fitness. Teaching aerobics classes in my studio and talking to anyone who would listen about moving within your fitness level, about building some cardio-endurance, upper body, abdominal, and lower body strength, and about fitness being for everyone. Everywhere I went, I saw so many people who needed to know how to change the way they looked and felt. My goal was always to get this information to as many people as possible.

The Betties, Cynthias, Carols, Sheryls, Janes, Jennys, Thelmas, Louanns, Jills, Debbies, and all the women who have been resurrected from the dead simply by learning how to eat, how to breathe, and how to move have taught me more than I could ever have taught them.

STOP THE INSANITY!

These women, their experiences and courage, have renewed my faith in the human spirit.

All ages.

All weights.

All kinds of physical considerations.

Defining and reaching their fitness goals. Getting well and feeling better about themselves. Making different choices and changing their lives. It has been a privilege to be a part of this process. The energy and passion that the last couple of years have required would have been impossible if I didn't have the you-know-what to get through the day. If I'd known what was involved a couple of years ago, I'm not sure I would have done it. The reality of it would have scared the hell out of me. The months and months of sitting in my studio, frozen in fear because I hadn't made the $25,000 that it took to keep the place open. Payrolls that I couldn't afford. Classes that weren't filling up but that I wouldn't cancel because of what it meant to the two or three people who were coming. When I taught my first new-to-fit class, there were three people in it. For months the three of us worked out. I taught my heart out, and they worked their fat off. We sweated bullets together, and it was worth it.

I taught a class yesterday—forty people who had never taken an aerobics class. They classified themselves as the fat, unfit, and uncoordinated. You should have seen that room. Perfect form, resistance, extension, everyone modifying for one reason or another. We were rocking. Not much has really changed. What it took to get here is blood, sweat, tears, and a whole lot of work, but when I was in that room yesterday, every second of the work was worth it. The staff of women I work with are the most devoted I've ever met. Rusty Robertson, my manager and friend. You couldn't find anyone more determined to get out to the world what she believes to be the most important information women can get for their health and wellness. Anything I've done, she's done equally. Women wouldn't be getting this information and changing their lives if it weren't for Rusty, her brilliance and her phone. So when we meet in airports, hotels, grocery stores, and parking lots, the redhead on the phone is whom you should ask for the autograph; she's the star.

Rusty and her family have sacrificed to get this message out. My family has paid a price. The time and energy I've spent building the business, doing the traveling, writing, and working the projects, have been time and energy taken from them.

The other day after weeks of running at 150 miles an hour, I took the boys out of school and went to the mall to "spend some cash." You understand, the feeling of spending just for the sake of spending—whether it's five bucks or a hundred, buying nothing that's necessary, just stuff you want—is fun, no matter how you look at it. Sometimes, when that dress calls your name, there's nothing you can do.

We go to the mall, not as a bribe for time not spent, but for pure fun. First we hit the underwear store—I just had to have an outfit I saw in the catalog. Real useful in my life. If you think there hasn't been enough time spent with the kids, can you imagine how much time the husband, our sex life, and I have together? Sex, it's the first to go when I have fifty gazillion things to do . . . but maybe that little outfit will help. Anyway, I had to have this thing.

Then we hit the toy store. The boys filled their bags with the latest noisemakers and video gadgets, and I threw in some of those educational toys that end up sitting on the shelves and never get touched.

Walking out of the mall with our bags of unnecessary stuff, I thought about all the times that I couldn't afford the health insurance—let alone the $60 video game. We've all paid a price, but the rewards, the growth, the fulfillment, the joy, the knowledge have gone beyond my wildest dreams.

My goal was to get this message out to as many women as possible. There are lots of women out there who still need to get it. A lady in my class yesterday asked me —after she had taken a 1½-hour class and understood everything I said (I saw the light bulb going on in her head halfway through)—why she hadn't been told any of this information after her open-heart surgery. During her breast cancer surgery, and as they were "watching" the lumps that were filling her other (or should we say only) breast. She said, with tears in her eyes, that she felt better after just 1½ hours. "I could do this easily and regain some of the control I've lost in my life. Taking some action to try to get well would make me feel like a human being again."

She is forty-eight years old, beautiful, and dying. Inside and out. What she said speaks for millions of women. You don't need to have gone through open-heart surgery or breast cancer. I felt like I was dying, and stopping the insanity in my life gave me the control to feel like a human being again. It gave me something to hold on to and work with so I could get out of what I was living in daily. Feeling out of control. Scared. Physically and mentally sick. I do not and will not continue to do what I'm doing to be known as a fitness expert.

I'm not.

I don't ever want to be known as a diet expert.

I'm not.

You know what? The doctors, the dietitians, and the nutritionists wouldn't have me.

I am a housewife who figured it out. Call Nic and ask him one question: "Nic, what's the most dangerous animal on earth?"

Nic will tell you that the most dangerous animal on earth is an intelligent, angry/passionate woman. The woman who started MADD, Mothers Against Drunk Driving, got angry/passionate when her child was killed and nobody did a thing. She changed the laws of our land. Well, diet and fitness industries, watch out—the women of America are right on your butt, we know how to figure it out, we know you've been lying and stealing our money, we are angry/passionate, and we are making better choices, so pack up your bags and get the hell out of here.

I still get mad when I see how simple and effective learning to eat, breathe, and move is, and then some moron from the industry says that it's oversimplified or that women don't want the responsibility. They're not smart enough to follow a formula. Don't require them to do math, they won't do it. Give them a gadget instead, they love that stuff. Don't waste your time on fat women, they don't have what it takes. . . .

Yeah, I get mad when the higher-ups in the industry flat out say these things. I know this after spending time in the meetings and cutting the deals where some of this thinking comes from. It starts with the men in positions of power making the decisions about what you and I need, and then it trickles down to us. After it's packaged and made pretty, it still screams, "You aren't smart enough to make your own decisions—so here, eat our instant food that we've made nice and pretty for you. You can't make your own decisions, so we'll do it for you. Don't think, darlin', just do what I say."

Well, we've taken the train out of Petticoat Junction, boys. I say to the women of America, if you are spending your hard-earned money on a diet, ask the counselor a few questions. Take this book with you, and if you don't get the answers you need to make your decision, walk out.

If one liquid shake didn't work, don't try another one. Try something new—eating. It works.

Use your fat formula and let the manager of your store and the manufacturers know what you think of the lies they thought you were too stupid to figure out. Stop feeling out of control. You have more control than you know, and you are a hell of a lot more powerful than you know. Use this information, get well, and help me get on with what I'm really trying to do.

Here's why I do what I do.

I believe women are the most evolved species on earth. We are the healers and the nurturers.

In our world right now, we have air we can't breathe. Water we can't drink. And in every community in the country, children are dying in the streets.

Our world needs help.

Healing and nurturing.

Organization and reconstruction.

STOP THE INSANITY!

If you wake up every day without enough oxygen to function, how can you contribute everything you have to contribute? If your body is loaded down with fat, it's too hard to keep going. As you lose strength, you can't hold yourself up—forget about healing and nurturing the world.

When I was 260 pounds, depressed and miserable, I didn't give a damn about the ozone layer. Who cared about some hole in the sky when I was trying to make it through until bedtime? Pollute the rivers and oceans, who cares? The inner cities are crumbling, let 'em crumble. Whales, schmales.

Here's why I do what I do. So that the women of this country can get well and take over the world.

Get healthy, make the changes in your life that you need to make simply by giving your body what it needs to live. You'll be surprised by how many other people you will affect just by doing it yourself. Count me in as the most surprised person on earth. You may be surprised at how many things you are concerned with outside your immediate circle as your mind and body get well. I know you won't be surprised at how effective you can be when you put your mind to something, because as women we already know how cool we can be when it comes to getting something done. Nothing will bring you more happiness, peace of mind, and pride in yourself than getting lean, strong, and healthy. There is nothing, in my opinion, that is more important or worth investing in than getting well. You can buy all the cars, makeup, homes, jewelry, whatever you want. But if you wake up every day hating the way you look and feel, it means nothing. It is all for naught. You lose your health, you've got nothing.

Don't believe anyone (that includes me)—believe the energy you feel the minute you get oxygen into your body. The strength you regain as soon as you start using those muscles that have turned to jelly, softened, the fabulous feeling of shrinking as you reduce the fat you've built up and stored all over your body, the clarity and peace of mind as you apply this information to your life and know that you have the control and can make the choices that will change your life forever. Enjoy the process, it's big, big fun.

Health and happiness to all of you.

Susan Powter

P.S. So a couple of weeks ago I'm in New York for a lot of very fast-paced meetings, going from early morning to late at night, nonstop. The third and final day of the meeting blitz had me flying from New York to Oklahoma late in the afternoon. I was giving a speech at the very large (very impressive) and well-run medical center. Flying from New York to Oklahoma in one day is enough of a culture shock for most people, but for a woman with very little hair and strong opinions about the medical community's responsibility for the health of overweight women, it's a bigger shock.

If I ever decided to stop what I'm doing, or if the diet and fitness industries end up trying to have me killed, tying a cement slab around my ankles and dropping me off the nearest bridge, I'd like to work for the tourism department of Oklahoma. I'm not sure they would like me to work for them, but I could do a hell of a good job. I'd sell the state alone, based just on the friendly people I met at the medical center.

My welcome could easily have been that southern "Hi, nice to meet you, glad you're here for a very short time —hope you're not planning to stay, because then we wouldn't like you" kind of welcome. But it wasn't. The OK Oklahomans were wonderful, and we had a great time.

I got in late, went to bed, and began my day at seven the next morning with an aerobics class. I taught at a fitness facility associated with the hospital—lots of clinicians, dietitians, and aerobics instructors on staff. This facility was basically a cardio rehab, so there were heart patients of all ages mixed with people who were just trying to burn the fat.

I was getting ready to teach the class with a room full

of people who had never laid eyes on me before. They were filtering in as I was setting up, and I was checking out the mixture of fitness levels walking into the class that I was about to teach. Some of the fittest aerobics people had come to see what I thought was so different and so special about what I do—you can always see that attitude (lots of sighs) on the faces of people in the industry, it's a smug, intolerant face that you get every time. Then there were the totally unfit, very large people, who were coming for the right reasons, and some intermediate fitness levels. They all got ready to take this early morning, who-is-this-woman class.

I begin my classes with slower music than anybody has ever heard in an aerobics class. The old increase your level of intensity by increasing your range of motion, not by picking up the pace of the music. You guys know what I mean—it's the aerobics industry that hasn't realized it yet. Anyway, the music started slow, and the "superfit" looked bored stiff and began rolling their eyes within minutes. There was no fancy choreography, another reason to be totally bored by this stupid class. No flipping from one move to another, no attitude—and the class was actually being taught. The clients in the class were being instructed. Hard for these aerobics people to understand.

I may have lost the superfit for a moment, but they figured it out real quick when I suggested they go a couple of inches lower into the move, reach a little higher, complete their range of motion, and press a bit harder. But the intermediate and beginners who didn't know me from a hole in the wall lit up like Christmas trees, and the focus, work, and energy in that room full of strangers in OK Oklahoma was fabulous.

Great class.

Big fun.

Beginning of a great day. Back to the hotel. Huge breakfast. Two bowls of oatmeal, four dry bagels, lots of strawberry jam, a pitcher of OJ, and that all-important pot of coffee. The guy who delivered the food was ready to call the *National Enquirer:* EX-FAT WOMAN BINGEING AND PURGING IN HOTEL ROOM IN OKLAHOMA.

After the Jed Clampett breakfast, going over my speech that I was giving in a couple of hours was next on the agenda. A nice hot bath, get dressed, and load on the makeup—three days on the road, lots of fake airplane air, not enough sleep, missing the kids desperately, and I'm looking about eighty-five years old before makeup. Loads of non-animal-tested, very expensive, well-packaged makeup, and I'm looking like a million bucks. It's time to go to the medical center and speak about health, wellness, fitness, and the Prince.

If I ever get sick enough to need a hospital, I'm crawling to the Baptist Medical Center in Oklahoma and checking into their women's wing. What a great facility. Dr. Woman took me on a tour of the women's wing, explaining the care and planning that have gone into meeting the needs of women in health care today. Very impressive. Consider me there when and if I ever need you guys. After the tour I'm taken downstairs to the luncheon room, which has been beautifully decorated and was packed with women for our lunchtime speech.

An unusual crowd. White lab coats everywhere, taking notes—you mean you guys don't know this stuff? A little scary. Professionals everywhere, ready to rip me to pieces—similar look that's on the faces of people in the aerobics industry, that bored, who-do-you-think-you-are look—and a room full of women eating their low-fat (out of respect for me, thank you very much) lunches.

There was one woman right in front of me who didn't look happy to see me at all. She had Christian fishes hanging from her earlobes. Now there is nothing wrong with fishes—I'd be on the express train to you-know-where if I were to say one bad word about them, and I wouldn't. But call me sacrilegious or a fashion nut, I'm just not sure they were ever meant to hang from earlobes. A pair of earrings? I'm just not sure. The fish earrings, combined with the body language, arms folded tightly across the chest, and the look on her face, tight-lipped and hateful. I felt like she'd be the first in line to throw me into the lion's pit and watch me get eaten alive.

When you're giving a speech and you have someone

right in front of you who looks like they despise you, it's hard enough. But when you also look out into a sea of white lab coats frantically scribbling notes, it can be nerve-racking.

But when the lab coats start nodding their heads in agreement, when the women in the audience connect with the pain and frustration of feeling out of control and unhealthy, when you hear the laughter from everyone about the insanity of the diet and fitness industries, when we all are in agreement that we've got to make some changes, then you realize it's okay.

We are no different.

We all struggle with the same issues.

Oklahoma, New York, Dallas, Los Angeles, and everywhere in between.

We are all sisters in wellness.

We are all sisters in health.

We are all sisters in wanting to look and feel better.

We are all sisters in wanting to change.

Sounds like a revival. Well, it pretty much was, except for the fire coming out of the eyes of my sister-in-religious-jewelry at the front table. No matter how many people in the room responded, she wasn't about to crack. Not budging an inch. I was not going to get a smile, any acknowledgment, or any feeling that anything I was saying made an ounce of sense to her.

The speech ended and it was great. We were all so connected, hundreds of women ready to commit to wellness, understanding how to apply eating, breathing, and moving to their lives and be strong and healthy forever—except, of course, for our friend in the front. I'm winding up, spewing my guts out, finishing my seminar, and the fish lady's eyes glazed over—dulling the glare for a minute. Then she did something that amazed me.

She raised her hand, and the woman I thought had hated me passionately, the one I thought I hadn't reached at all, made the most sensitive, evolved, helpful comment.

She told us that she finally understood if she gave her body daily what it needed to function, she could begin to regain the self-esteem and self-respect that she'd lost long ago. Regaining her self-respect meant rebuilding her body. And with it would come the rebuilding of her pride. Her pride was something she desperately needed to rebuild, and the possibility of eliminating the fear that had been controlling her life for the last ten years was overwhelming to her. In front of the whole room full of women, the fish lady thanked me for coming, stood up, and hugged me.

Wow. Fish lady. Send me running back to the convents and confessional booths of my childhood.

Bless me, Father, for I have sinned.

It has been twenty years since my last confession—that puts you in front of the line, into hell right there, and these are my sins.

The list is really, really long, but the biggest and most recent is the judging of the fish woman.

I judged her big time, and she came back and taught me more than I could ever have taught her in any wellness seminar.

Talk about feeling as if you've just been hit by lightning.

We have so many words for states of mind, and so few for the states of the body.
—Jeanne Moreau, 1976

AFTERWORD
Tabloid 101

Out of the strain of the Doing.
Into the peace of the Done.
—*Julia Louise Woodruff,*
"Harvest Home," 1910

It ain't easy, guys. I mean it. Riding in a limo to Linda
Bloodworth-Thomason's office—you know, Hillary's
friend—and the driver is clueless. I'm forty-five minutes
late. Now there's a meeting you want to be late for, the
biggest producers in Hollywood. Yeah, let's show up late
and blame it on a limo driver.

I'm not telling you this so you can sit back and ooh and
ahh over how well I'm doing. I'm telling you because this
experience was the last straw at the end of a week from
beyond hell.

I was initiated into Tabloid 101 this week. Yep, they
got me.

It wasn't the snooping around my home, business, or
children's school that was too much to handle, although
that was pretty difficult. The thing that really tilted it over
the edge was when a family member sold out to the rags.
We've all got some dysfunctional elements in our families, the inner child screaming from within, and the pain
and suffering that goes with it all. But what most of you
will never have to deal with is being forced to display all
of your family junk on national television and in the pages
of those brilliant magazines that let the world know that

"Flipper has tried to kill himself," that aliens have landed in New Jersey, or that everyone is having an affair with everything. Imagine if someone in your family went to these programs and print rags that soak up this crap like a sponge and talked about everything that you've ever done, said, or thought, taking it totally out of context. Can you imagine how you'd feel? How do you defend yourself against allegations based on nothing?

How does the rest of the family deal with the pain of having to talk about all that stuff because of one member's problems?

We haven't worked it all out yet. There's the real issue. Defending and explaining what we don't understand or haven't talked about was very, very difficult.

Let me tell you, if you think your family dynamics have caused your eating disorder, I've got a real disorder for you.

All this did happen to me. And I am here to tell you that as a fit, successful, pulled-myself-up-by-the-boot-straps kind of woman, I did not handle it well. What should have been a ten-minute interruption in my schedule—a television interview that I didn't want to do, a tabloid article that I didn't want to respond to, answering accusations that I should not have had to justify with an answer—turned into a very painful, badly handled, four-day ordeal. The worry, stress, anger, and pain that I felt the minute I found out what my brother had done threw me off.

My family coming into town to answer his allegations that I never really was fat also threw me off. Family visits tend to do that anyway. Going through my closets, looking through every picture that had ever been taken of me fat took me for a walk down Memory Lane that I'd rather not have taken. Picture (pardon the pun) this—my kids and I sitting on the living room floor with every family album out, photos spread out all over the floor, trying to find ones that were dated so that I could prove I was fat, with the kids asking: "Mommy, why are we going through all of these?"

I had to explain, without anger, because I don't want

anger in my life anymore: "Because Uncle Mark has gone on television and said that Mommy was never fat, and I have to prove that I was."

My oldest son looked at me and said with the beauty of a child, "Mommy, I'll go on television and tell them how fat you were. I remember sitting on your lap. You were really, really fat because my head would sink into your body, and I'd feel safe and secure."

Then comes, "Mommy, why are you crying?"

"Because I love you. I've been hurt badly by Uncle Mark. I don't want to be sitting here going through this, and my heart is breaking."

That's how my family spent the next couple of days. I knew I was facing a six-minute interview or witch-hunt, which is what it was, and had to explain why this happened—something I was not looking forward to at all.

The first thing I did after looking at the pictures was smoke a cigarette. A habit I thought was long gone. It is amazing how easy it is to run right back to the old comforting habits. I spent the night crying and smoking. Great night. The unanswered questions, unexpressed feelings, and unsorted anger—put that all together and you might find yourself as off track as I was for the next couple of days.

I stopped working out. Cigarettes and not working out for a couple of days—there's a feeling I'd forgotten about, the filthy-chimney, sloppy, unable to breathe feeling, I missed that like the plague. Throw in the loads of food I stuffed into my mouth—low-fat, but loads—and you'll understand that at the end of a couple of days I was a wounded child having a temper tantrum trying desperately to pacify it all. Shove into your mouth food, cigarettes, drugs (don't worry, I didn't go that far)—whatever was available—that was and has always been my way.

Amazing how little has changed. It didn't matter when this was happening that I was lean. Having a successful business was the last thing on my mind. The people who love and support me were in the background, and the emotional sledgehammer that was bashing me in the head was all I could feel or hear. What I had to do, when I decided it had to stop, was rebuild. Start from the beginning and rebuild. Now, granted, I didn't have as much to rebuild last week as I had when I was a 260-pound, depressed, unfit housewife and unfit mother of two. But it's hard to balance the emotional impact of thirty-five years of dysfunction coming to a head on national television against the weight and circumstances of the past. Which is harder? Don't ask me, because they both felt like death.

I got up after days of feeling like hell and worked out. It was the last thing I wanted to do—just like that walk years ago—but I did it. It was easy after that class to remember why I'd given up smoking. Do me a favor, smoke for a couple of days, then go do some high cardio —God, it feels awful. Then I made a conscious effort to give myself the things that nurture and heal me. Time with my children. Good music, a good book, a massage, time alone, and the best food. High-quality, high-volume food. I rebuilt. Got back on track. I was the only one who could do it, and it was up to me to fuel myself and keep moving forward. That's all you and I can ask of ourselves. Screw perfection. Just continue moving forward and learning. If you think you are never going to slip, just ask me, you can hang it up. As long as you continue to move forward, grow and learn, then you are doing better than most.

Now, I would like to say something to my brother, Mark. The only pain left after all is said and done is the worst pain of all.

Whatever it is that has brought you to this point of anger, hatred, and revenge has taken away a brother who was the funniest, brightest, best-looking, most talented person I knew. I love my brother and will not justify his craziness by fighting back. I had to answer the questions and defend myself against the allegations because you forced me to, Mark, but you know the truth and you know what you did was wrong. That's yours to live with, not mine or my children's.

* * *

The limo ride was the final straw.

I was frazzled getting out of the limo at MTM Studios in Hollywood, just like I was when the Prince didn't send the check in time and I was sitting at home with two small babies waiting.

The fear that I felt getting out of the car forty-five minutes late for the most important meeting I've ever been asked to attend was similar to the fear of not having enough money to pay the electric bill at the castle or having to meet the payroll in the early days of the studio. That cold fear you feel running through your veins. I wasn't afraid of the people who had been waiting for forty-five minutes for me to show up (although any sane person would have considered that)—I was afraid that I would break down and act like a blithering idiot because I was so stressed out. After the week I'd had and the limo ride from hell, that's exactly what I felt like walking into that meeting—ask me a question and I'll start to cry.

Not much has changed in the last couple of years. Nervous? Don't ask. Frustrated? The most. Angry, stressed to the nines, the whole bit. I was choking on anxiety. The only difference between my meeting and years ago is that my recovery rate was quicker. Like a strong, well-conditioned heart, I didn't have to work quite as hard to come back—to recover from the anxiety brought on by a driver who had no clue where he was, a phone that didn't work (so calling and saying I was going to be late was out of the question), the guilt of wanting to choke a ninety-year-old driver who was doing his best, the attack by my brother, the family reunion, the tears, fears, and pain of it all. This time it didn't take me as long to regain my composure, walk into the meeting, pull myself out of the tabloid tragedy, and do my job.

When you have a lean, strong, healthy body, there is something to draw on. You have more to rely on during times of stress, anxiety, fear, or confusion. The strength and balance that come with a well-tuned body help center and focus you. The oxygen pumping through a healthy body gives you the energy and fuel you need to pull everything back together in a shorter period of time. Different things threw me off track in the past, because my circumstances were different. A limo ride was as far away from my reality then as cash falling from the sky. But fear is fear. Anger is anger, and getting thrown off track is getting thrown off track—no matter what throws you. You're off, but getting back on is faster and faster when you are lean, strong, and healthy. Faster and faster, not easier and easier. It just takes me much less time to pull it all together.

I'll tell you what felt great. Knowing that I have the ability to be okay, that I can make it, no matter what's around the next corner. Winning the fight and dancing around the ring with the boxing gloves held high—that's what it feels like now. Years ago it would have gone on forever. The pain, the anger, and the confusion never seemed to end. Now it gives me a couple of black eyes, and I come back.

The really big difference now is what I come back to. My life, after years of hard work, is a good life. I am strong, healthy, and fair and capable of learning and growing.

I am not a fraud. I was a 260-pound woman, and now I am fit and healthy. I adore what I do. My children, husband, ex-husband, and I have a very healthy, functional, happy life, and nobody can take that away from me, not even the family that used to throw me for a loop within seconds. It's over. My life has begun, and I love it.

My recovery is faster and faster, not easier and easier, and yours will be also. Maybe someday it won't hurt? Naw . . . it will always hurt, because I love my brother. My life now is healthy and happy, and I've broken the cycle of anger, pain, and insanity that I was raised in. Mark, I hope you find the peace that goes with the recovery and healing that must take place before the cycle is broken. It's such a gift.

APPENDIX

Fat Content
of Foods

Breads and Flours	Serving	Total Fat (g)	Calories
bagel, plain	1 medium	1.4	163
honey wheatberry bread	1 slice	1.1	70
pita, plain	1 large	0.8	240
raisin	1 slice	1.0	70
sourdough	1 slice	0.5	68
whole wheat, commercial	1 slice	1.1	61
whole wheat, homemade	1 slice	1.6	67
croissant	1 medium	11.5	167
French toast			
frozen variety	1 slice	6.0	139
homemade	1 slice	10.7	172
pancakes			
blueberry, from mix	3 medium	15.0	320
buckwheat, from mix	3 medium	12.3	270
buttermilk, from mix	3 medium	10.0	270
homemade	3 medium	9.6	312
"lite," from mix	3 medium	2.0	130

APPENDIX

	Serving	Total Fat (g)	Calories
Cereals			
Fruit Loops	1 cup	0	111
Frosted Mini-Wheats	4 biscuits	0.3	102
granola			
commercial brands	⅓ cup	6.9	186
homemade	⅓ cup	10.0	184
Nutri-Grain			
barley	¾ cup	0.2	106
corn	⅔ cup	0.7	108
wheat	¾ cup	0.3	102
Wheat Chex	1 cup	1.2	169
Wheaties	1 cup	0.5	99
Cheeses			
American, processed	1 oz.	8.9	106
CheezWhiz	1 oz.	6.0	80
Kraft American Singles	1 oz.	7.0	90
Monterey Jack	1 oz.	8.6	106
mozzarella			
part skim	1 oz.	4.5	72
part skim, low moisture	1 oz.	4.9	79
whole milk	1 oz.	6.1	80
whole milk, low moisture	1 oz.	7.0	90
Parmesan			
grated	1 T.	1.5	23
hard	1 oz.	7.3	111
Combination Foods			
pizza			
cheese	1 slice	10.1	183

	Serving	Total Fat (g)	Calories
cheese, French bread, frozen	5⅛ oz.	13.0	330
tuna salad			
oil pack, w/mayo	½ cup	16.3	226
water pack, w/mayo	½ cup	10.5	170

Fast Foods/Restaurants (all listings are for standard servings for the given establishment unless otherwise noted)

	Serving	Total Fat (g)	Calories
Arby's			
curly fries	1 order	17.7	337
regular roast beef sandwich	1	18.2	383
Burger King			
biscuit with bacon	1	20.0	378
biscuit w/bacon, egg	1	27.0	467
biscuit w/sausage	1	29.0	478
cheeseburger	1	15.0	318
cheeseburger, deluxe	1	23.0	390
chicken sandwich	1	40.0	685
Chicken Tenders	1 order	13.0	236
hamburger	1	11.0	272
hamburger, deluxe	1	19.0	344
Kentucky Fried Chicken			
breast	1	18.0	286
breast, extra crisy	1	21.0	353
breast fillet sandwich	1	22.5	436
chicken nuggets	6 nuggets	17.4	276
Long John Silver's catfish fillet dinner	1	58.0	980

APPENDIX

	Serving	Total Fat (g)	Calories
Fast Foods/Restaurants (cont)			
McDonald's biscuit			
w/sausage and egg	1	34.5	520
cheeseburger	1	13.8	310
McChicken	1	28.6	490
McDLT	1	36.8	580
McLean	1	10.0	320
McLean w/cheese	1	14.0	370
Quarter Pounder	1	20.7	410
Quarter Pounder w/ cheese	1	29.2	520
Wendy's			
baked potato, plain	1	2.0	270
baked potato w/cheese	1	15.0	420
Big Classic	1	33.0	570
cheeseburger, single	1	34.0	580
cheeseburger, double	1	48.0	800
chicken sandwich	1	19.0	430
hamburger, double	1	40.0	670
Meats (all cooked without fat unless otherwise noted)			
beef, regular			
chuck, ground	3½ oz.	23.9	327
hamburger, regular	3 oz.	19.6	286
beef, highest fat			
brisket, lean & marbled	3½ oz.	30.0	367
rib roast	3½ oz.	30.0	367
ribeye steak, marbled	3½ oz.	38.8	440
steak, chicken fried	3½ oz.	30.0	389
processed meats			
bologna, beef/ beef & pork	1 oz.	8.0	85

	Serving	Total Fat (g)	Calories
hot dog			
beef	1	13.2	145
chicken	1	8.8	116
turkey	1	8.1	102

Milk and Yogurt
low fat milk

	Serving	Total Fat (g)	Calories
1% fat	1 cup	2.6	102
2% fat	1 cup	4.7	121
skim milk			
liquid	1 cup	0.4	86
nonfat dry powder	¼ cup	0.2	109
whole milk			
3.5% fat	1 cup	8.0	150
dry powder	¼ cup	8.6	159
yogurt			
coffee/vanilla, low fat	1 cup	2.8	194
frozen, low fat	½ cup	3.0	115
frozen, nonfat	½ cup	0.2	81
fruit flavored, low fat	1 cup	2.6	225
plain			
low fat	1 cup	3.5	144
skim (nonfat)	1 cup	0.4	127
whole milk	1 cup	7.4	139

Pasta, Noodles and Rice (all measurements after cooking unless otherwise noted)
macaroni

	Serving	Total Fat (g)	Calories
semolina	1 cup	0.7	159
whole wheat	1 cup	0.6	183

APPENDIX

	Serving	Total Fat (g)	Calories
Pasta, Noodles and Rice (cont)			
noodles			
Alfredo	1 cup	29.7	462
egg	1 cup	2.4	200
rice	1 cup	0	140
rice			
brown	½ cup	0.6	116
fried	½ cup	7.2	181
long grain & wild	½ cup	2.1	120
white	½ cup	1.2	111
spaghetti, enriched	1 cup	1.0	159
Poultry			
chicken			
breast			
w/skin, fried	½ breast	10.7	236
w/o skin, fried	½ breast	6.1	179
w/skin, roasted	½ breast	7.6	193
w/o skin, roasted	½ breast	3.1	142
fryers			
w/skin, batter dipped, fried	3½ oz.	17.4	289
w/o skin, fried	3½ oz.	11.1	237
w/skin, roasted	3½ oz.	13.6	239
w/o skin, roasted	3½ oz.	7.4	190
turkey			
breast			
barbebcued, Louis Rich	3½ oz.	5.0	135
oven roasted, Louis Rich	3½ oz.	3.0	115

	Serving	Total Fat (g)	Calories
dark meat			
w/skin, roasted	3½ oz.	11.5	221
w/o skin, roasted	3½ oz.	7.2	187
Vegetables			
artichoke, boiled	1 medium	0.2	53
avocado			
California	1 (6 oz.)	30.0	306
Florida	1 (11 oz.)	27.0	339
blackeyed peas			
(cowpeas), cooked	½ cup	0.5	99
corn			
cream style, canned	½ cup	0.4	93
frozen, cooked	½ cup	0.2	67
frozen, w/butter sauce	½ cup	2.6	105
whole kernel, cooked	½ cup	1.1	89
corn on the cob	1 medium	0.9	83
potato			
baked w/skin	1 medium	0.2	220
french fries			
frozen	10 pieces	4.4	111
homemade	10 pieces	8.3	158
hash browns	½ cup	10.9	163
potato pancakes	1 cake	12.6	495
twice-baked potato			
w/cheese	1 medium	9.9	180
soybeans, mature, cooked	½ cup	7.7	149
sweet potato, baked	1 medium	0.1	118
tofu (soybean curd), raw,			
firm	4 oz.	5.4	86

APPENDIX

	Serving	Total Fat (g)	Calories
Vegetable Salads			
Caesar salad w/o anchovies	1 cup	7.2	80
coleslaw			
w/mayo-type dressing	½ cup	14.2	147
w/vinaigrette	½ cup	5.5	77
potato salad			
German style	½ cup	3.5	140
w/mayo dressing	½ cup	11.5	189

IT'S LIKE NO OTHER VIDEO ON THE MARKET!

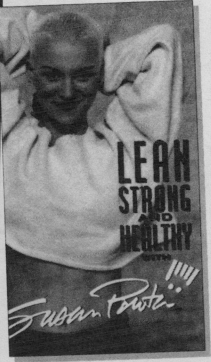

DON'T MISS OUT...
GET LEAN, STRONG,
AND HEALTHY WITH
SUSAN POWTER.

Susan's sensible approach to getting fit combines motivation and modification. This cardiovascular workout is perfect for all fitness levels. Susan's program is designed to help you get as **LEAN, STRONG, AND HEALTHY** as you want to be.

 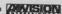